500 Paleo

Anti Inflammatory

Instant Pot,

Bone Broth and Dessert Recipes

By

Mercedes Del Rey

500 Paleo Anti Inflammatory Instant Pot, Bone Broth and Dessert Recipes By Mercedes Del Rey

500 Paleo Anti Inflammatory Instant Pot, Bone Broth and Dessert Recipes By Mercedes Del Rey

Dear Reader

Thank you and congratulations on getting this book today, which contains a selection my favourite recipes. I hope that you will enjoy all of them.

My hope is that you enjoy the best possible health every single day.

Please do leave a book review if you can as this will help me in writing more of the books that you want to read

Merche

FOR MORE BY

MERCEDES DEL REY

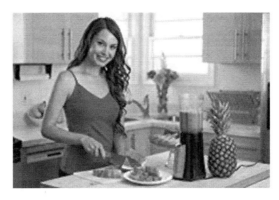

Please search this page over the www.amazon.com

amzn.to/2kSzZnU

500 Paleo Anti Inflammatory Instant Pot, Bone Broth and Dessert Recipes By
Mercedes Del Rey

FREE FROM THE PUBLISHER

DOWNLOAD YOUR FREE PALEO EPIGENETIC DIET EBOOK

AND START LOSING WEIGHT TODAY

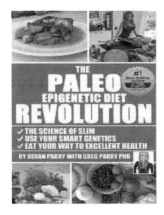

Please search this page over the internet

www.skinnydeliciouslife.com/free-epigenetic-diet-ebook

500 Paleo Anti Inflammatory Instant Pot, Bone Broth and Dessert Recipes By
Mercedes Del Rey

Table of contents

500 Paleo Anti Inflammatory Instant Pot, Bone Broth and Dessert Recipes By Mercedes Del Rey

365 Days of Paleo Keto Diet Recipes

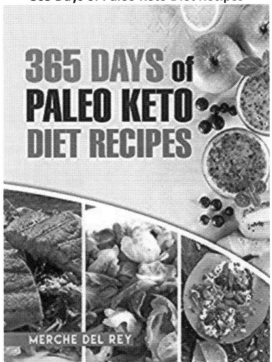

Please search this page over the www.amazon.com

amzn.to/2sXsvSz

365 Days of Anti-Inflammatory Recipes

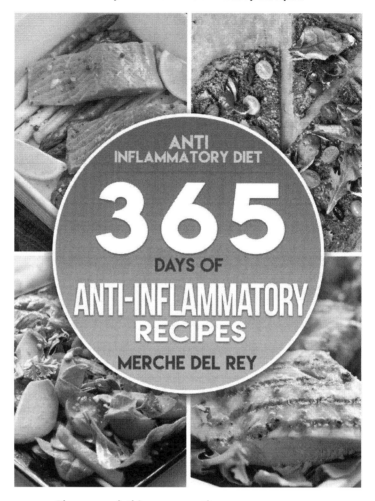

Please search this page over the www.amazon.com

amzn.to/2tgANEF

365 Days of Perfect Paleo Air Fryer Recipes

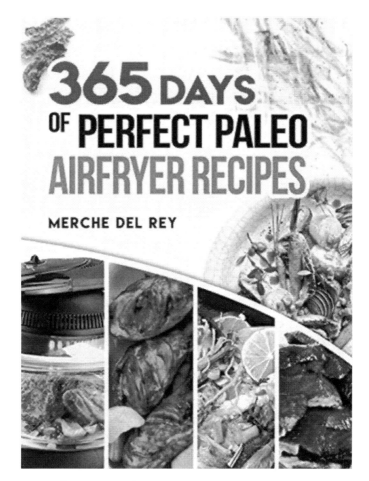

Please search this page over the www.amazon.com

amzn.to/2sv7Dm2

1.   Spiced-Smoky Brisket

Servings: 5 max

Time: 1 hour 10 mins

Ingredients

- 1.5 lb. beef brisket
- 10 drops stevia
- 2 tsp. smoked sea salt
- 1 tsp. black pepper
- 1 tsp. mustard powder
- 1 tsp. onion powder
- ½ tsp. smoked paprika
- 2 cube bone broth
- 3 fresh thyme sprigs

Directions:

1.   Firstly, blend all the spices by combining the stevia, smoked sea salt, pepper, mustard powder, onion powder, and smoked paprika.

2.   Coat the meat generously on all sides.

3.   Set your Instant Pot to "Sauté" and allow it to heat up for 2-3 minutes. Grease the bottom with a bit of high heat cooking oil and add the brisket.

4.   Brown on all sides until deeply golden but not burnt.

5.   Turn the brisket to fatty side up and add the broth and thyme to the Instant Pot.

6.   Scrape the browned bits off the bottom and cover with the lid. Then, cook for 50 minutes.

7.   Once finished, allow the Instant Pot to release steam. Remove the brisket from the pot and cover it with foil to rest.

8.   Sauté again to reduce and thicken the sauce with the lid off for about 10 minutes.

9.   Slice the brisket and serve it hot.

2. **Hearty Beef**

Serves : 4 max
Time:1 hour 10 minutes
Ingredients:
- 1 lb stewing steak
- 1/2 lb bacon tips
- 5 medium carrots (cut into sticks)
- 1 large red onion (sliced)
- 2 cloves garlic minced
- 2 tsp rock salt
- 2 tbsp fresh tyme(chopped)
- 2 tbsp fresh parsley(chopped)
- 2 tsp ground black pepper
- 1/2 cup beef broth
- 1 tbsp olive oil
- 2 large sweet potato (cubed)
- 7 drops stevia

Directions:
1. Switch Instant Pot to Browning Setting. Add 1 tbsp of olive oil and warm
2. Cot the meat with spices and then saute in batches to give them room in the Instant Pot to brown. Set aside.
3. Slice Bacon into thin strips and brown with onions
4. Add Back Beef and then add all remaining ingredients
5. Switch Instant Pot to High Pressure Setting and Set to 30 Minutes.
6. Pour the braising liquid into a blender and blend until smooth, then transfer back to the pressure cooker. Bring to a simmer over medium heat about five minutes.
7. Then add pepper to taste and sprinkle with parsley. Serve hot.

3.   Sweeto Chunky Beef

Serves: 6 max

Time: 55 minutes

Ingredients:

- 3 lb boneless chuck grass-feed beef
- 1 1/2 tsp salt
- 1 tsp ground ginger
- 2 tbsp olive oil
- 1 cup bone broth
- 1/2 cup coconut aminos
- 8 drops stevia
- 1 tsp garlic (finely chopped)

Directions:

1.   Mix salt, ground ginger into a bowl, then use to season meat

2.   Switch Instant Pot to Browning Setting. Add olive oil and when that is warm, place the beef brown on all sides about 20 minutes. When the meat is well browned transfer it to a plate and set aside

3.   Select the sauté setting and add the finely chopped garlic for 1 minute, then add broth, coconut aminos and stevia. Stir until contents are mixed well.

4.   Return the beef to the Instant Pot. Secure the lid and set to High Pressure Setting. Cook the meat for 25 minutes and rise, so set the timer of the pressure cooker to 35 minutes.

5.   After the pressure cooker has completed 35 minutes, allow the pressure to release by using the quick release method.

6.   Then, use 4 tbsp arrowroot powder with 4 tbsp of water, mix until smooth, then add it to the pressure cooker, and stir well. Then, cook over medium-high heat for about 5 minutes.

7.   Serve hot

4. Porto Deli Beef Short Ribs

Serves: 4-6 max

Time: 1 hour 15 minutes

Ingredients:

- 5 pounds grass fed beef short ribs, (cut into 3inch chunks)
- 1 tsp Kosher salt
- Freshly ground pepper
- ½ ounce porcini mushrooms
- 1 cup boiling water
- 1 tablespoon coconut oil
- 1 large onion, chopped medium
- 3 carrots, chopped medium
- 2 celery stalks, chopped medium
- 6 cloves garlic, peeled and smashed
- 1 cup coconut amino
- ½ cup bone broth
- 2 tablespoons apple cider vinegar, divided
- 4 drops stevia
- ¼ cup chopped Italian parsley

Directions:

1. Firstly, season the short ribs liberally with salt and pepper.
2. Place the porcini mushrooms in a bowl and cover with boiling water until softened for 15-30 minutes.
3. In a pressure cooker add coconut oil on high heat. Sear the ribs in batches until well-browned and transfer them to a platter.
4. Chop up the veggie and toss the onions, carrots and celery into the empty pot while the ribs are browning. Lower the heat to medium, season with salt and pepper.
5. Sauté the vegetables until softened.
6. Fish out the softened mushrooms and squeeze out the liquid and chop up the mushrooms and toss them in the pot along with the garlic. Stir the pot for another minute and add in the coconut amino, stevia, apple cider vinegar and broth
7. Add the ribs back into the pot, mixing well
8. Then, increase the heat to high and bring the stew to a boil. Cover the pressure cooker with the lid and let the contents come to high pressure. Once the pot reaches high pressure, decrease the heat to low and maintain on high pressure for 30 minutes
9. Take the pot off the heat and let the pressure come down naturally for 15 minutes.
10. Simmer the stew for at least 20 minutes and top with minced parsley.

5.   Shaky Beef Vege Mania

Serves: 4 max

Time:1 hour 20 minutes

Ingredients:

- 4 pound corned beef brisket
- 4 cups water
- 1 small yellow onion, (sliced)
- 3 garlic cloves, (smashed)
- 2 bay leaves
- 3 whole black peppercorns
- 1 tsp all-spices powder
- 1 tsp dried thyme
- 1 head cabbage (cut into wedges)
- 3 medium carrots (peeled and cut into chunks)
- 1 pound broccoli (cut head)

Directions:

1.   Place corned beef, water, onion, garlic, black peppercorns, allspice, and thyme in InstantPot. Lock lid in place and press "manual" and set time for 90 minutes.

2.   When cooking is complete, switch pressure cooker off and allow pressure to release naturally for 10 minutes, then quick release any remaining pressure.

3.   Remove the meat from the liquid and transfer to a plate. Cover with tin foil and allow to rest for 15 minutes while you prepare the vegetables.

4.   Add cabbage, carrots, and broccoli to liquid in InstantPot and lock lid in place. Press "manual" and set time for 10 minutes.

5.   When cooking is complete, quick release pressure. Use a slotted spoon to remove vegetables and serve with slices of corned beef, using some of the cooking liquid to moisten the meat and vegetables if necessary.

6.   Chew- E-Beef Vege Mania

Serves: 4 max
Time: 1 hour 25 minutes
Ingredients:
- 4 pound corned beef brisket
- 4 cups water
- 1 small yellow onion, (sliced)
- 3 garlic cloves, (smashed)
- 2 bay leaves
- 3 whole black peppercorns
- 1 teaspoon all-spices
- 1 teaspoon dried thyme
- 1 head cabbage (cut into wedges)
- 3 medium carrots (peeled and cut into chunks)
- 2 stalk celery (cut into 2 inch)
- ¼ cup corn kernel(frozen)

Directions:
1.   Place corned beef, water, onion, garlic, black peppercorns, allspice, and thyme in InstantPot. Lock lid in place and press "manual" and set time for 90 minutes.
2.   When cooking is complete, switch pressure cooker off and allow pressure to release naturally for 10 minutes, then quick release any remaining pressure.
3.   Remove the meat from the liquid and transfer to a plate. Cover with tin foil and allow to rest for 15 minutes while you prepare the vegetables.
4.   Add cabbage, corn, carrots, and celery to liquid in InstantPot and lock lid in place. Press "manual" and set time for 10 minutes.
5.   When cooking is complete, quick release pressure. Use a slotted spoon to remove vegetables and serve with slices of corned beef, using some of the cooking liquid to moisten the meat and vegetables if necessary.

7.   **Cracky Nyum Corned Beef**

Time: 2 hours 20 minutes
Serves: 6 max
Ingredients:

- 4 pound corned beef brisket
- 4 cups bone broth
- 1 small yellow onion, (sliced)
- 3 garlic cloves, (smashed)
- 2 bay leaves
- 3 whole black peppercorns
- 1 teaspoon all-spices
- 1 teaspoon dried thyme
- 2 medium sweet potatoes(cubed)
- 2 medium carrots, cut into bite-sized chunks
- 2 turnips, cut into bite-sized chunks
- 2medium rutabagas, (wedges)
- 1 medium parsnips, cut into bite-sized chunks

Directions:

1.   Place corned beef, water, onion, garlic, black peppercorns, allspice, and thyme in InstantPot. Lock lid in place and press "Manual" and set time for 90 minutes.

2.   When cooking is complete, switch pressure cooker off and allow pressure to release naturally for 10 minutes, then quick release any remaining pressure.

3.   Remove the meat from the liquid and transfer to a plate. Cover with tin foil and allow to rest for 15 minutes while you prepare the vegetables.

4.   Add sweet potatoes, carrots, and beets to liquid in Instant Pot and lock lid in place. Press "manual" and set time for 15 minutes.

5.   When cooking is complete, quick release pressure. Use a slotted spoon to remove vegetables and serve with slices of corned beef, using some of the cooking liquid to moisten the meat and vegetables if necessary.

8. **Tender Succulent Stewed Beef**

Servings: 8
Time: 1 hour 10 mins
Ingredients:
- 3 lbs stew beef (chuck roast or short ribs) cut into chunks
- 1/2 tsp salt
- 1/2 tsp black pepper
- 2 tbsp almond flour (optional)
- 2 tbsp grass-feed butter
- 1/2 onion, (diced)
- 2 cloves garlic, (minced)
- 2 tbsp tomato paste
- 3 cups beef broth
- 3 carrots (cut into chunks)
- 3 parsnips (cut into chunks)
- 3 celery stalks, (cut into chunks)
- 1.5 lbs sweet potato (cut into chunks)
- 3 sprigs fresh thyme (chopped)
- Salt and pepper to taste
- 2 tbsp lemon juice
- 1 small handful parsley, (chopped)

Directions:
1. Combine the beef, salt, pepper, and almond flour; toss to dust the beef evenly.
2. Add the grass-feed butter and warm until melted and shimmering, about 3 minutes.
3. Add beef and sauté until browned about 20 minutes.
4. Then, add the onion and sauté until softened, about 4 minutes, then add the garlic and tomato paste. Sauté until aromatic, about 30 seconds, then add the broth.
5. Bring to a simmer, scraping up any browned bits from the bottom of the pot. Add the beef, lemon juice, carrots, parsnips, celery, sweet potatoes, and thyme. Wait until it depressurizes, about 20 minutes
6. After depressurizing, remove the lid and carefully remove the short and place on a plate, loosely cover with tin foil.
7. Pour the braising liquid into a blender and blend until smooth, then transfer back to the pressure cooker. Bring to a simmer over medium heat about five minutes.
8. Then add salt and pepper to taste
9. Plate your dish by pouring the liquid into a shallow bowl and placing the ribs on top.
10. Serve hot.

9.   Terigarlic Deli Beef

Serves: 6 max
Time: 55 minutes
Ingredients:
Steak
- 2lb flank steak
- 2 cloves finely chopped garlic
- 1 tablespoon ginger

Teriyaki Sauce
- ½ cup coconut amino
- ¼ cup pineapple juice
- 1 ½ tsp ground ginger
- 1 clove garlic(minced)

Directions:
1.   In a bowl, mix together marinade ingredients, add sliced beef and allow marinating for at least 10 minutes.
2.   Select Sauté or Browning on Pressure Cooker and allow to fully heat.
3.   Cut steak into strips
4.   Mix up all teriyaki sauce ingredients (coconut aminos, pineapple juice, ground ginger and garlic)
5.   Place everything in the Instant Pot. Lock lid in place, choose the High Pressure setting and cook for 40 minutes
6.   Serve hot.

10.   Teriyaki Deli Beef With Bell Pepper And Broccoli

Serving: 6 max
Time: 1 hour 10 minutes
Ingredients:
Steak
- 2lb Flank Steak
- 2 Cloves Finely chopped garlic
- 1 tablespoon ginger
- ½ red bell pepper
- ½ green bell pepper
- 2-3 heads fresh broccoli

Teriyaki Sauce
- ½ cup coconut amino
- 1 cup arrowroot flour
- ¼ cup lemon juice
- 4 drops stevia
- 1 clove garlic(minced)
- 1 ½ tsp ground ginger
- 1 tsp olive oil

Directions:
1.   In a bowl, mix together marinade ingredients, add sliced beef and allow marinating for at least 10 minutes.
2.   Select Sauté on Pressure Cooker and allow to fully heat.
3.   Cut steak into strips
4.   Mix up all teriyaki sauce ingredients coconut aminos, olive oil, arrowroot flour, stevia, ground ginger, lemon juice and garlic
5.   Place everything in the Instant Pot. Lock lid in place, choose the High Pressure setting and cook for 40 minutes
6.   Remove the meat from the liquid and transfer to a plate. Cover with tin foil and allow to rest for 15 minutes while you prepare the vegetables.
7.   Add bell peppers and broccoli to liquid in InstantPot and lock lid in place. Press "manual" and set time for 10 minutes.
8.   Serve the vegetables with meat

11. Teriyaki Zucchini Delicious Beef

Serves: 6 max
Time: 55 minutes
Ingredients:
Steak
- 2lb Flank Steak
- 2 Cloves Finely chopped garlic
- 1 tablespoon ginger

Vegetables
- 4 large zucchinis, spirallized
- 1 large red bell peppers, (deseeded and cut into strips)
- 1 large green bell peppers, (deseeded and cut into strips)
- 1 large yellow bell peppers, (deseeded and cut into strips)
- 2 cups broccoli florets (chopped head into small)
- 2 tablespoons olive oil

Teriyaki Sauce
- ½ cup coconut amino
- 1 cup arrowroot flour
- ¼ cup lemon juice
- 4 drops stevia
- 1 clove garlic(minced)
- 1 ½ tsp ground ginger
- 1 tsp olive oil

Directions:
1. In a bowl, mix together marinade ingredients, add sliced beef and allow marinating for at least 10 minutes.
2. Select Sauté on Pressure Cooker and allow to fully heat.
3. Cut steak into strips
4. Mix up all teriyaki sauce ingredients (coconut aminos, olive oil, arrowroot flour, stevia, ground ginger, lemon juice and garlic)
5. Place everything in the Instant Pot. Lock lid in place, choose the High Pressure setting and cook for 40 minutes
6. Remove the meat from the liquid and transfer to a plate. Cover with tin foil and allow to rest for 15 minutes while you prepare the vegetables.
7. In the skillet add olive oil and heat it over high heat. Add the red pepper strips and broccoli florets and fry for 2-3 minutes. Add the garlic and ginger and cook, stirring, until fragrant, about 30

seconds. Add the zucchini noodles and fry for 1 minute. Add the remaining teriyaki sauce and cook, stirring occasionally, until mostly evaporated, about 1 minute.

8.   Top on the meat and serve

12. Teriyaki Mushroom Beef Delight

Serves: 6 max

Time: 1 hour 10 minutes

Ingredients:

Steak

- 2lb flank steak
- 2 cloves finely chopped garlic
- 1 tablespoon ginger
- 16 ounces mushrooms(sliced)
- 1 carrot(shredded)
- 2-3 heads water chestnut

Teriyaki Sauce

- ½ cup coconut amino
- 1 cup arrowroot flour
- ¼ cup lemon juice
- 4 drops stevia
- 1 ½ tsp ground ginger
- 1 clove garlic(minced)
- 1 tsp olive oil

Directions:

1. In a bowl, mix together marinade ingredients, add sliced beef and allow marinating for at least 10 minutes.
2. Select Sauté or Browning on Pressure Cooker and allow to fully heat.
3. Cut steak into strips
4. Mix up all Teriyaki Sauce ingredients (Coconut aminos, olive oil, arrowroot flour, stevia, ground ginger, lemon juice and garlic)
5. Place everything in the Instant Pot. Lock lid in place, choose the High Pressure setting and cook for 40 minutes
6. Remove the meat from the liquid and transfer to a plate. Cover with tin foil and allow to rest for 15 minutes while you prepare the vegetables.
7. Add vegetables to liquid in InstantPot and lock lid in place. Press "manual" and set time for 10 minutes.
8. Serve the vegetables with meat

13. Tasty Delight Ribs

Serves: 2-4 max

Time: 2 hours

Ingredients:

- 2 tablespoon grass-feed butter
- 1-2 lbs short ribs, (cut)
- 1 onion, (chopped)
- 1 carrot, (coarsely chopped)
- 1 sweet potato (cut)
- 2 cloves garlic, (minced)
- 1 tsp dried thyme
- 1 tsp salt
- 1/2 teaspoon black pepper
- 5 drops stevia
- 2 cups bone broth

Directions:

1. Heat the grass feed butter in your pressure cooker over medium heat
2. Add the short ribs and brown, in batches if needed, about 3 minutes per side, then set aside.
3. Add the chopped onion, carrot and sweet potato. Sauté until softened, about 5 minutes.
4. Add the garlic and sauté for 1 minute.
5. Then add the thyme, salt, pepper and stevia. Allow to sauté about a minute and add the bone broth. Cook for 50 minutes.
6. After depressurizing, remove the lid and carefully remove the short and place on a plate; loosely cover with tin foil.
7. Pour the braising liquid into a blender and blend until smooth, then transfer back to the pressure cooker. Bring to a simmer over medium heat about five minutes.
8. Then add salt and pepper to taste
9. Plate your dish by pouring the liquid into a shallow bowl and placing the ribs on top.
10. Serve hot.

14.   Short Ribs With Spring Vegetables

Serves: 2-4 max

Time: 4 hours

Ingredients:

* 2 tablespoon grass-feed butter
* 1-2 lbs short ribs, (cut)
* 1 medium leek, white and pale green parts only, coarsely chopped
* 1 onion, (chopped)
* 1 carrot, (coarsely chopped)
* 1/2-pound shiitake mushrooms, stems discarded and caps sliced 1/4 inch thick2 cloves garlic, (minced)
* 1 teaspoon dried thyme
* 1 teaspoon salt
* 1/2 teaspoon black pepper
* 5 drops stevia
* 2 cups bone broth

Directions:

1.   Heat the grass feed butter in your pressure cooker over medium heat

2.   Add the short ribs and brown, in batches if needed, about 3 minutes per side, then set aside.

3.   Add the chopped onion, carrot, mushroom and leek. Sauté until softened, about 5 minutes.

4.   Add the garlic and sauté for 1 minute.

5.   Then add the thyme, salt, pepper and stevia. Allow to sauté about a minute and add the bone broth. Cook for 50 minutes.

6.   After depressurizing, remove the lid and carefully remove the short and place on a plate; loosely cover with tin foil.

7.   Pour the braising liquid into a blender and blend until smooth, then transfer back to the pressure cooker. Bring to a simmer over medium heat about five minutes.

8.   Then add salt and pepper to taste

9.   Plate your dish by pouring the liquid into a shallow bowl and placing the ribs on top.

10.   Serve hot.

15. Sweetheart Tender Beef Stew

Serves: 6 max
Time: 1 hour 35 minutes
Ingredients:
- 1 - 2 tbsp grass-feed butter
- 2 lb (1kg) grass-feed beef (cubed)
- 1 tbsp coconut aminos
- ½ tsp sea salt
- ¼ cup arrowroot flour (optional)
- ½ tsp ground cloves
- ½ tsp ginger powder
- ½ tsp turmeric powder
- 1 large onion, sliced into wedges
- 2 large cloves garlic, chopped
- 1 tsp ground cinnamon (or a 3 inch cinnamon stick)
- 1 cup bite-sized pineapple chunks
- 1 bay leaf
- 2 tbsp dates (pitted and chopped)
- 1 cup bone broth
- 1 bunch Swiss chard, stems separated from leaves (stems finely chopped, leaves halved lengthwise and cut into 1 inch thick strips)

Directions:
1. Marinate the beef cubes with the coconut aminos, sea salt, arrowroot flour, ground cloves, ginger powder and turmeric powder for approximately 1 hour (you can also marinate just before cooking but the flavor will be less apparent in the meat)
2. Press 'saute' and heat up the Instant Pot until the display reads 'Hot'
3. Add the grass-feed butter to melt, then add the onions and saute for a minute or so, followed by the garlic, until the onions are translucent and the garlic is fragrant
4. Remove onions and garlic and set aside
5. Add another tablespoon of grass-feed butter if necessary, and brown the marinated beef cubes in batches
6. Set the grass-feed beef cubes aside and deglaze the pot with the bone broth
7. Return the beef, onions and garlic to the pot
8. Stir in the cinnamon, pineapple chunks, finely chopped Swiss chard stems, bay leaf and kumquat jam
9. Seal the Instant Pot and set the valve to 'sealing'
10. Select " Stew setting for 35 minutes

11.   Once the Instant Pot beeps and the cooking time is up, do a quick release by turning the sealing valve to 'vent' .

12.   Select 'sauté' setting and add in the Swiss chard leaves

13.   Simmer until the leaves are cooked and the gravy is slightly thickened. Add 1 tsp arrowroot starch mixed in 2 tsp water

14.   Remove bay leaf, season to taste and enjoy!

16.   Sweetheart Tender Beef Stew With Cabbage And Bell Peppers

Serves: 6 servings

Time: 1 hour 40 minutes

Ingredients:

- 1 - 2 tbsp grass-feed butter
- 2 lb (1kg) grass-feed beef (cubed)
- 1 tbsp coconut aminos
- ½ tsp sea salt
- ¼ cup arrowroot flour (optional)
- ½ tsp ground cloves
- 1 ginger(chopped)
- ½ tsp turmeric powder
- 1 large onion, sliced into wedges
- 2 large cloves garlic, chopped
- 1 tsp ground cinnamon (or a 3 inch cinnamon stick)
- 1 cup bite-sized pineapple chunks
- 1 green bell peppers (sliced)
- 200gm cabbage(chopped)
- 1 bay leaf
- 2 tbsp dates (pitted and chopped)
- 1 cup bone broth
- 1 bunch Swiss chard, stems separated from leaves (stems finely chopped, leaves halved lengthwise and cut into 1 inch thick strips)

Directions:

1.   Marinate the beef cubes with the coconut aminos, sea salt, arrowroot flour, ground cloves, and turmeric powder for approximately 1 hour (you can also marinate just before cooking but the flavour will be less apparent in the meat)

2.   Press 'saute' and heat up the Instant Pot until the display reads 'Hot'

3.   Add the grass-feed butter to melt, then add the ginger, onions and saute for a minute or so, followed by the garlic, until the onions are translucent and the garlic is fragrant

4.   Remove onions, ginger and garlic and set aside

5.   Add another tablespoon of grass-feed butter if necessary, and brown the marinated beef cubes in batches

6.   Set the grass-feed beef cubes aside and deglaze the pot with the bone broth

7.   Return the beef, onions and garlic to the pot

8.   Stir in the cinnamon, pineapple chunks, finely chopped vegetables, bay leaf and dates

9.   Seal the Instant Pot and set the valve to 'sealing'

10.   Select "Stew" setting for 35 minutes

11.   Once the Instant Pot beeps and the cooking time is up, do a quick release by turning the sealing valve to 'vent' (watch out for the steam!)

12.   Select 'saute' setting and add in the Swiss chard leaves

13.   Simmer until the leaves are cooked and the gravy is slightly thickened. Add 1 tsp arrowroot starch mixed in 2 tsp water

14.   Remove bay leaf, season to taste and enjoy!

17. Luxurycious White Creamy Beef Stew

Ingredients:
Time:50 minutes
Serves 4-6
- 6 cups water
- 450g grass-feed beef, (cubed)
- 2 cups veal bone broth
- 1 cup white onion, (diced)
- 2 cups white turnips (chopped)
- 1 cup or 2 carrots, (chopped)
- 2 cups or 1 medium-ripe plantain, (peeled and halved)
- 2 garlic cloves, (peeled and chopped)
- 1 tsp sea salt, divided
- 1 bay leaf
- 1/2 tsp dried basil
- 1/2 tsp cinnamon (or a stick of cinnamon)
- 500mL coconut milk
- 1/4 cup coconut flour
- 8-10 drops stevia
- 2 cups broccoli, (cut into large florets)

Directions:
1. Select 'Sauté' function and adjust to 'more'
2. Add 6 cups water and bring to boil
3. Add meat and allow to boil for 3 minutes before draining and setting aside
4. Rinse inner pot and return meat to pot
5. Add veal bone broth, vegetables (except broccoli), 1/2 tsp sea salt, herbs and cinnamon
6. Stir to combine, cover, set valve to 'sealing' and select 'Manual' function for 15-20 minutes
7. Once cooking time is up, unseal lid by quick release and remove meat and vegetables from the pot and set aside, leaving broth in the pot
8. Select 'Sauté' function and add coconut milk, coconut flour, and stevia stirring to mix
9. Add broccoli florets and allow to simmer until cooked and gravy is thickened
10. Discard bay leaf and cinnamon stick (if using)
11. Return meat and vegetables to gravy and stir gently to mix
12. Season with remaining 1/2 tsp sea salt or to taste and serve hot

18. Pistacapolicious Roasted Beef

Servings: 4-6 max

Time: 2 hours 15 minutes

Ingredients:
- 2 lbs Grass feed beef
- 1 cup Chicken stock
- 4 tbsp Coconut oil
- 2 lbs sweet potatoes (diced)
- 1 lb carrots, (sliced)
- 1 bunch of parsley, (chopped)

For the crust
- 120gm Pistachio Nuts (smashed and salted)
- 1 tbsp of Black Pepper
- 2 tbsp of Fresh Thyme(chopped)

Directions:
1. Combine the beef with pistachios, black pepper and thyme toss to dust the beef evenly.
2. Preheat the pressure cooker. Add coconut oil and when that is warm, place the beef roast in and sear it the in pan well on all sides about 20 minutes while spoon out pistachios that have fallen off.
3. Meanwhile, add a cup of chicken stock. Close and lock the pressure cooker lid and cook under high pressure for 30 minutes.
4. Then, add the carrots and cubed sweet potatoes and sauté until softened, about 5 minutes. Close and lock the pressure cooker lid, again. Cook under high pressure.
5. Open the pressure cooker and take out the carrots, slice them and put them on the serving platter. Remove the potatoes Take out the roast, and place on a plate tented with aluminum foil to rest.

19. Succulent Roasted Beef With Beets

Servings: 4-6 max
Time: 2 hours 35 minutes
Ingredients:

- 2 lbs Grass feed beef
- 1 cup Chicken stock
- 4 tbsp olive oil
- 2 tbsp tarragon(minced)
- 1 lb carrots(chopped)
- 1 gold beet (peeled and cut into wedges)
- 1 red beet (peeled and cut into wedges)
- 1 chioggia beet (peeled and cut into wedges)
- 2 tbsp chives(minced)
- 2 tbsp of parsley, (minced)
- 2 tbsp Lemon juice
- 3-5 drops stevia

For the crust

- 120gm Pistachio Nuts (smashed and salted)
- 1 tbsp of Black Pepper
- 2 tbsp of Fresh Thyme(chopped)

Directions:

1. Combine the beef with pistachios, black pepper and thyme toss to dust the beef evenly.
2. Preheat the pressure cooker. Add coconut oil and when that is warm, place the beef roast in and sear it the in pan well on all sides about 20 minutes while spoon out pistachios that have fallen off.
3. Meanwhile, add a cup of chicken stock. Close and lock the pressure cooker lid and cook under high pressure for 30 minutes.
4. Then, add the carrots and beets and sauté until softened, about 5 minutes. Close and lock the pressure cooker lid, again. Cook under high pressure.
5. Open the pressure cooker and take out the carrots, slice them and put them on the serving platter. Remove the beets Take out the roast, and place on a plate tented with aluminium foil to rest.
6. Add lemon juice, minced herbs, and stevia to bowl with pistachios and whisk to combine. Drizzle in remaining 3 tablespoons (45ml) olive oil while whisking constantly.
7. Season to taste with salt and pepper.

20. Pistavege Classic Roasted Beef

Servings: 4-6 max
Time: 1 hour 30 minutes
Ingredients:
- 2 lbs Grass feed beef
- 1 cup Chicken stock
- 4 tbsp Coconut oil
- 1 medium turnip(quartered)
- 2 carrots(quartered)
- 2 stalk celery
- 1 ½ cup cherry tomatoes(sliced)
- carrots, (sliced)
- 1 bunch of parsley, (chopped)

For the crust
- 120gm Pistachio Nuts (smashed and salted)
- 1 tbsp of Black Pepper
- 2 tbsp of Fresh Thyme(chopped)
- 1 tbsp rosemary(minced)

Directions:
1. Combine the beef with pistachios; black pepper, rosemary and thyme toss to dust the beef evenly.
2. Preheat the pressure cooker. Add coconut oil and when that is warm, place the beef roast in and sear it the in pan well on all sides about 20 minutes while spoon out pistachios that have fallen off.
3. Meanwhile, add a cup of chicken stock. Close and lock the pressure cooker lid and cook under high pressure for 30 minutes.
4. Then, add the carrots, celery, turnip and cherry tomatoes and sauté until softened, about 5 minutes. Close and lock the pressure cooker lid, again. Cook under high pressure.
5. Open the pressure cooker and take out and put them on the serving platter. Take out the roast, and place on a plate tented with aluminium foil to rest.

21. Tasty Lamb Rack Rosemary Curry

Time:50 minutes
Servings:2-4 max
Ingredients:
- 1-2 lbs lamb rack
- 1 tsp Himalayan pink salt
- 1 tsp turmeric
- 1 cup chopped carrots
- 1 cup chopped celery
- 6-8 cups roughly chopped cabbage
- 3 fresh rosemary sprigs

For the Sauce:
- 2 cups cooked pumpkin
- 1 cup bone broth
- 2 garlic cloves
- Inch of fresh ginger
- Juice of 1 lime
- 1/2 tsp Himalayan pink salt
- 1 tsp turmeric
- 5 mint leaves

Directions:
1. Rub the lamb with pink salt and turmeric.
2. Add lamb, carrots, celery, cabbage, and rosemary to instant pot.
3. Blend all sauce ingredients in blender until smooth.
4. Pour sauce over lamb and veggies.
5. Cook on meat/stew option for 35 minutes. Enjoy!

22. Brown Rice Rainbow Congee

Serves: 7 cups
Time: 1 hour 15 minutes
Ingredients:
- 1 rice measuring cup brown rice(180ml)
- 7 cup water
- 100gm frozen peas
- 200gm crab meat
- 1 egg
- 7 conpoy (dried scallop)
- 1 tablespoon ginger (chopped)
- Salt to taste

Directions:
1. Firstly, rinse rice under cold water
2. Add 7 cups of water and crab meat, egg, frozen peas, ginger and conpoy into the pot.
3. Close lid and cook at high pressure for 30 minutes in an Electric Pressure Cooker.
4. Turn off the heat and Natural Release for 15 minutes. Manually release the remaining pressure by carefully turning the venting knob to the venting position. Open the lid carefully.
5. Add salt to taste.
6. Turn on the heat (Instant Pot: press sauté button) and stir the congee until the desire thickness.
7. Serve warm.

23. Brown Rice Seafood Congee

Serves: 7 cups
Time: 1 hour 15 minutes

Ingredients:
- 1 rice measuring cup brown rice(180ml)
- 7 cup water
- 150gm shrimp
- 50gm squid (cut and cleaned)
- 1 egg
- 7 dried scallop
- ¼ carrot(shredded)
- 1 celery stalk
- 1 tablespoon ginger (chopped)
- Salt to taste

Directions:
1. Firstly, rinse rice under cold water
2. Add 7 cups of water and shrimp, squid, egg, celery, carrot, ginger and dried scallop into the pot.
3. Close lid and cook at high pressure for 30 minutes in an Electric Pressure Cooker.
4. Turn off the heat and Natural Release for 15 minutes. Manually release the remaining pressure by carefully turning the venting knob to the venting position. Open the lid carefully.
5. Add salt to taste.
6. Press the "sauté" button in Instant Pot and stir the congee until the desire thickness.
7. Serve warm.

24.   King Protein Banana Pancakes Recipe

Time: 20 minutes

Serves: 2

Ingredients:

- 1/4 cup almond flour
- 2 tablespoons coconut flour
- 3 tablespoons vanilla whey protein powder
- 1 cup banana(cubed)
- 1/2 teaspoon baking powder
- pinch of sea salt
- 1 tablespoon chia seeds
- 1 tablespoon coconut flakes
- 1 egg
- 4 tablespoons almond milk

Directions:

1. Combine all the dry ingredients in a bowl. Then add wet ingredients and stir together.
2. Heat a pan and coat with coconut oil. Pour 2 tbsp of batter to form each pancake.
3. Cook a few minutes. Once it starts to bubble on top, flip and cook an additional 1-2 minutes

25. Magic Strawchia Pudding

Serves 4-6

Ingredients:
- 1kg fresh strawberries, hulled
- 2 cups coconut milk
- 1/8 tsp stevia
- 1 tsp vanilla scraped
- 3/4 teaspoon finely grated lime zest
- 1/2 cup chia seeds

Directions:
1. Place the strawberries, coconut milk, stevia, vanilla, and lime zest in a blender and blend until smooth. Taste and add more stevia if desired.
2. Place the chia seeds in a large bowl, pour the strawberry mixture on top, and whisk thoroughly. Let stand for 10 minutes and
3. Garnish with sliced strawberry whisk again.
4. Cover and refrigerate for at least 4 hours and up to 3 days. Stir the pudding before serving. The longer it sits, the thicker the pudding will become.
5. Add some coconut water for a thicker pudding
6. Serve

26. Cutie Darling Cup

Time: 40 minutes
Serves: 1 max
Ingredients:
For Muffin
- 1 tablespoon grass fed butter
- 50gm unsweetened applesauce
- 1 egg
- 1/4 teaspoon vanilla
- 2 drops stevia
- 3 tablespoons almond flour
- 1/2 teaspoon cinnamon
- 1/8 teaspoon baking powder
- Pinch of salt

For Streusel Topping
- 1 tablespoon apple, finely chopped
- pinch of crumbled walnuts
- pinch of grass-feed butter

Directions:
For Muffin
1. Preheat oven to 350°F
2. Melt the grass-feed butter and grease in mound
3. Whisk in the applesauce, egg, vanilla and stevia until well combined
4. Add almond flour, cinnamon, baking powder, and salt and stir for about 30 seconds.
5. Bake for 25 minutes

For the topping: Combine the ingredients and then sprinkle on top before microwaving

27.   Yummy Strawberry Chia Toasted Oatmeal

Serves: 2-4 max

Time: 45 minutes

Ingredients:

For Jam

- 17oz strawberries

- 2 drops stevia

- 1 tablespoon chia seeds

Toasted oatmeal

- 2 tablespoons coconut oil

- 2 cups rolled oats

- 1½ cups coconut water

- ½ cup coconut milk

- Pinch kosher salt

- Pinch of ground cinnamon (optional)

- Pinch of ground ginger (optional)

- 1 tbsp shredded coconut

- 50gm toasted cashew nuts and almond nuts

Coconut whipped cream

- 1 can coconut milk

- 2-3 drops stevia

- ½ teaspoon vanilla extract

Directions:

For Jam

2. In a medium saucepan, combine strawberries and stevia.

3. Cover and bring to a simmer over medium heat, stirring frequently.

4. Once the berries are warmed mash the berries with fork.

5. Reduce the heat to medium low. Stir in the chia seeds and cook for 20 minutes, stirring frequently, until the jam is reduced and jammy

6. The jam will further thicken up as it cools. Remove the pan from heat and add more stevia to increase sweetness.

Make the oatmeal

1. In a large skillet heat the coconut oil over medium heat.

2. Add the oats and toast over medium heat, stirring occasionally, until it well toasty, around 6 to 8 minutes.

3. In a large, heavy bottomed pot, combine the milk, water, salt, cinnamon and ginger. Bring the mixture to a slow boil over medium heat.

4. Add the toasted oats and gently stir once or twice to incorporate the oats into the liquid. Cover the pot and turn off the heat. Let the oats sit on the burner, untouched, for 7 minutes. After 7 minutes, uncover and check the oats

5. If the oats in wetter in a covered pot continue to absorb water for a few more minutes.

Make the coconut whipped cream

1. Refrigerate can of coconut milk, 8 hours or overnight.

2. Place metal mixing bowl and beaters in the refrigerator or freezer 1 hour before making whipped cream.

3.   Open can of coconut milk, do not to shake it. Scoop coconut cream solids into cold mixing bowl.

4.   Beat coconut cream using electric mixer with chilled beaters on medium speed; turn to high speed. Beat until stiff peaks form, 7 to 8 minutes. Add stevia and vanilla extract to coconut cream; beat 1 minute more. Taste and add more stevia if desired.

28. Classic Peach Bisquick Recipe

Time: 50 minutes

Serves: 8-10 max

Ingredients:

- 3 cups peaches, peeled and chopped
- 2 cups almond flour
- ¼ teaspoon coconut flour
- ½ teaspoon baking soda
- ¼ teaspoon sea salt
- ½ teaspoon stevia
- ½ cup grass-fed butter (softened)
- 2-3 drops almond extract
- 3 tablespoons chia seeds
- 9 tablespoons warm water
- 1 tablespoons apple cider vinegar

Directions:

1. Preheat oven to 350 degrees F.
2. Grease pan with coconut oil.
3. Pour peaches into the pan.
4. Mix the almond flour, salt and baking soda in a bowl.
5. In a separate bowl, mix the grass-feed butter, stevia and extract.
6. Combine both mixtures.

7.   In a separate small bowl, combine the chia and hot water and allow sitting and thickening for 5 minutes. After 5 minutes, add to other mixture.

8.   Once well combined, add vinegar and stir.

9.   Pour batter onto peaches and bake for 30-45 minutes

29. Fruit Jungle Salad

Time: 20 minutes

Serves: 4 max

Ingredients:

- 3 drops stevia

- 2 tablespoons coconut yogurt

- 2 tablespoon muesli

- 2 tablespoons chia seeds

- 1 cup mangoes, (diced)

- 1 cup watermelon(diced)

- 1 cup strawberries, (sliced)

- 1 cup kiwifruit, (diced)

- 1 cup honey dew(diced)

- ½ cup blackberries

Directions:

1. In a large bowl, combine the mangoes, honeydew, watermelon, strawberries, kiwifruit, and the blackberries.

2. Add chia seed, coconut yogurt, stevia and muesli on the fruits

3. Mix and Enjoy

30 Indulgence Bar

Time: 1 hour

Serves:5 max

Ingredients

Layer A

- 3/4 cup grass-feed butter

- 1/4 cup coconut oil, melted

- 1/3 cup cacao powder

- 8 drops stevia

- 1/4 teaspoon vanilla paste

- pinch Himalayan salt

Layer B

- 2 cups of dried, unsweetened, raw coconut

- 2/3 cup coconut butter, softened

- 8 drops stevia

- 1-2 teaspoons almond extract

Layer C

- 1/3 cup almonds, (roasted and chopped)

- 1/3 cup cashew nuts, (roasted and chopped)

- 1/3 cup walnuts, (roasted and chopped)

- Ganache (coconut cream and dark chocolate)

Directions:

1. For layer A whisk all ingredients together and pour into oiled, parchment lined pan. Set in refrigerator aside making topping.

2. The bottom layer should be set up before adding the next layer.

3. For layer B place coconut in medium bowl.

4. Whisk coconut butter, stevia and almond extract.

5. Pour over coconut and mix well. Pat over first layer, top with chopped nuts and ganache.

6. Refrigerate to set.

31.   Princess Strawberry Shortcake

Serves: 3 max

Time: 45 minutes

Ingredients

SHORTCAKE

- 1½ cups almond flour

- ½ cup coconut flour

- ½ teaspoon baking powder

- ½ teaspoon almond extract

- ¼ cup coconut milk

- 4 tablespoons coconut oil

- 5 drops stevia

- 1 pint fresh strawberries

COCONUT WHIPPED CREAM

- 1 can full fat coconut milk, refrigerated overnight.

- 2-3 drops stevia

- 1 vanilla bean extract

Directions:

For Shortcake

1.   Preheat oven to 350˚F

2.   In a large mixing bowl, whisk together the almond and coconut flour and baking powder. Stir in almond extract, milk, and stevia.

3.   Drop in the solid coconut oil and quickly crumble through the mixture.

4.   Once oil is distributed throughout dough in smaller than pea size pieces, begin to form crumbly dough into a ball.

5.   Flour the counter with some more coconut flour and dump the dough out of the bowl. Roll dough out until about ¼ inch thick. Cut out 3" circles and place on a greased cookie sheet. (Should make about 6 pieces.)

6.   Bake shortcake in the oven for 10-15 minutes or until golden brown around the edges. Let cool on a rack on the counter.

7.   Meanwhile, slice the strawberries. Set aside.

For Coconut Whipped Cream

1.   Refrigerate can of coconut milk, 8 hours or overnight.

2.   Place metal mixing bowl and beaters in the refrigerator or freezer 1 hour before making whipped cream.

3.   Open can of coconut milk, do not to shake it. Scoop coconut cream solids into cold mixing bowl.

4.   Beat coconut cream using electric mixer with chilled beaters on medium speed; turn to high speed. Beat until stiff peaks form, 7 to 8 minutes. Add stevia and vanilla extract to coconut cream; beat 1 minute more. Taste and add more stevia if desired. Assemble strawberry shortcakes by layering cake with strawberries and coconut whipped cream.

32. California Roll

Ingredients:

Dressing

- 1 cup cashews (roasted and chopped)
- 1 tbs light olive oil
- 1.5 tbs yellow mustard
- 6 drops stevia
- 1 tsp apple cider vinegar
- 1/2 tsp ground ginger
- salt to taste
- water to thin

Wraps

- 2 large spinach tortillas
- 1/2 cup shredded lettuce, or to taste
- 1 1/2 cups shredded almond cheese
- 1 avocado - peeled, pitted, and diced
- 4 slices cooked bacon, chopped
- 1 red onion, finely chopped
- 1 tomato, chopped
- 2 cooked chicken breasts, cut into chunks

Directions:

1.   Add cashews, stevia, mustard, light olive oil, vinegar, and ground ginger to a food processor.

2.   Pulse, adding water until you have a smooth sauce.

3.   Salt to taste.

4.   Cook tortillas in the microwave until warm and pliable, about 30 seconds.

5.   Spread 1 tablespoon cashew dressing down the center of each tortilla.

6.   Spread lettuce, almond cheese, avocado, red onion, tomato, and chicken, respectively, in the center of each tortilla.

7.   Fold opposing edges of the tortilla to overlap the filling.

8.   Roll 1 of the opposing edges around the filling into a wrap.

33.   Heavenly Crab Cakes

Serves: 2-3 max

Time: 30 minutes

Ingredients

For Crab:

- 1 lb of fresh crab meat

- 1 egg, whisked

- 1/3 cup of almond flour

- 1/3 cup of green onions, finely chopped

- 1/3 cup of red bell peppers, finely chopped

- 1 small red onion(chopped)

- 3 cloves garlic(minced)

- 2 tbs chopped flat-leaf parsley

- 2 tsp coconut amino

- 1/4 tsp salt

- ¼ tsp pepper

- 1 tsp lemon juice

- coconut oil

For sauce:

- 2 garlic cloves, pressed.

- 1/4 teaspoon kosher salt.

- 1/2 teaspoon paleo mayo

- 2 tablespoons olive oil.

- 1 tablespoon fresh lemon juice.

Directions:

1. In a large bowl, combine all the above ingredients together

2. Shape into patties

3. In a large skillet over medium heat, add a few tablespoons of coconut oil to fry the crab cakes

4. Place crab cakes in pan and fry for about 4-5 minutes on each side or until surface is a golden brown

5. For sauce, mix all the ingredients until smooth and serve on the patties

6. Enjoy

34. Sweet Potato Waffle

Serves: 6 max

Time: 30 mins

Ingredients

- 2 cups sweet potato (steamed & pureed)

- 2 ½ cup almond flour

- ½ cup almond milk

- 1 tsp vanilla extract

- 1 Egg

- 1 tsp Coconut Oil

- 1 tsp Salt

- 1 tsp cinnamon

- 1 tsp baking powder

Directions:

1. Preheat waffle iron

2. In a medium mixing bowl, mix together all the ingredients.

3. Scoop about ½ cup sweet potato on the waffle iron

4. Close the lid and cook for 5 minutes.

5. Remove and allow cooling

6. Serve

35. Sunshine Cup

Serves: 3 max

Time: 35 minutes

Ingredients

- 3 Tomatoes (large)
- 3 basil leaves (chopped)
- 2 tbsp shredded almond cheese
- 2 Eggs
- Sea Salt (to taste)
- Black Pepper (to taste)

Directions:

1. Preheat the oven to 350°F.
2. Scoop out inside the tomatoes like cup
3. Add the eggs and basil to a small bowl and whisk
4. Pour the egg mixture into each tomato, until half
5. Bake for 20 minutes until eggs are firm.
6. Season with sea salt and black pepper.
7. Serve immediately.

36.   Savoury Tostadas

Serves: 2 max

Time: 10 minutes

Ingredients

- 4 Eggs

- 1 tomato (chopped)

- 1 Jalapeno (diced)

- 1/4 bell pepper (diced)

- 1/4 onion (diced)

- 1/2 tsp cumin

- 1/2 tsp red pepper flake (crushed)

- 1 tbsp coconut oil

- Sea Salt and Black Pepper (to taste)

Directions:

1. Heat the coconut oil on skillet over medium heat.

2. Once the coconut oil melts, sauté the bell peppers, and onions.

3. While the onions and peppers are sautéing, add the eggs, tomato, cumin, crushed red pepper, sea salt and black pepper to a bowl. Whisk until frothy.

4. Add the eggs to the skillet with the peppers and onion.

5. Stir frequently to scramble the eggs. Cook until eggs reach desired consistency.

6. Season with salt and black pepper

7. Serve

37.   Bacon cups

Serves: 2 max

Time: 40 minutes

Ingredients

- 4 Eggs

- 2 slices bacon

- 2 Tomato slices

- 2 Bell Pepper slices

- Sea Salt (to taste)

- Black Pepper

- Coconut Oil

Directions:

1.   Preheat the oven to 400°F.

2.   Place the bacon slices on a baking sheet, arranging each slice in a circle so it cooks into a disc.

3.   Place the bacon in the oven and cook until crispy, about 15 minutes. Flip halfway through.

4.   Once bacon is done, set it aside

5.   While the bacon is cooking, start the eggs.

6.   Using a muffin tin, grease the 4 muffin cups with coconut oil.

7.   Whisk the egg and pour into muffin cups

8.   Reduce the oven to 375°F and cook until the eggs are firm, about 15 minutes.

9.   Cut around the edge of each egg, and carefully remove from the muffin tin.

10.   Assemble each sandwich with 1 egg on the bottom, then a slice of tomato, then bell pepper, then bacon, and top with another egg. Repeat for second sandwich.

11.   Season with salt and pepper.

12.   Serve immediately.

38. Paleo Belgian Waffles

Serves: 4 max

Time: 15 minutes

Ingredients

- 3 eggs

- 1/3 cup almond milk

- 1 cup almond powder

- 2 tbsp coconut flour

- 2 tsp vanilla extract

- 1 tbsp coconut oil (melted)

- 1/4 tsp sea salt

Directions:

1. Preheat waffle iron

2. In a medium mixing bowl, mix together all the ingredients.

3. Scoop about ½ cup batter on the waffle iron

4. Close the lid and cook for 5 minutes.

5. Remove and allow cooling

6. Serve

39. Baked Banana

Serves: 4 max

Time: 35 minutes

Ingredients

- 4 ripened bananas
- 4 Eggs beaten
- 1 teaspoon Cinnamon
- 7 drops stevia
- 1/2 cup sliced almonds
- 1 tbsp chopped fresh mint

Directions:

1. Preheat oven to 350˚F.

2. Mash the bananas with the eggs, cinnamon, and stevia in a large bowl. Spread in a casserole dish. Sprinkle the almonds over top.

3. Bake for 30 minutes, until almonds are toasted.

4. Remove from oven, let it cool for 5 minutes sprinkle with the mint and serve.

40. Mega Star Chocolate

Time: 30 minutes

Serves: 2-4 max

Ingredients

- 220gm cacao powder
- ¼ teaspoon stevia
- ⅓ cup coconut oil, melted
- 1-2 pomegranates, de-seeded
- 1 tsp sea salt

Directions

1. Mix well the cacao powder, stevia and coconut oil to a bowl until uniform consistency.

2. Pour mixture into a parchment

3. Pour pomegranate seeds evenly across the chocolate and push them down gently.

4. Sprinkle with sea salt.

5. Place chocolate bark in the freezer for 20 minutes.

6. Break chocolate sheet apart carefully with the pomegranate side facing down

41. Mix dessert

Serves: 2-4 max

Time: 10 minutes

Ingredients

- 2 cups young coconut meat
- 1 1/2 cups coconut water
- ¼ cup pineapple(cubed)
- 1 pomegranate (seeds)
- ¼ cup jackfruit(sliced)
- ¼ cup roasted almond

Directions:

1. Blend coconut meat and coconut water until smooth.
2. Pour mixture into bowl combined well with fruits and almond.
3. Serve

42. Milky Coconut Yam Ice-Cream

Serves: 6-8 max

Time: 2 hour

Ingredients

- 300gm grated purple yam

- 150 gm young coconut meat

- 1 cup coconut milk

- 2 cups coconut cream

- a pinch of stevia

- 1 teaspoon vanilla extract

Directions

1. Steam grated yam for 15 minutes.

2. Remove and mash with a fork.

3. Combine yam, coconut cream, coconut milk, stevia and vanilla extract. Mix it until smooth.

4. Put the mixture in the fridge and let it chill for 2 hours.

5. Then, pour the mixture in a freezer-safe container and freeze, stirring every hour to break up any ice crystals.

6. Add the young coconut meat when the ice cream has a soft-serve consistency.

43.   Sapid Strawberry Coconut Cake

Serves:6-8 max

Time:1 hour

Ingredients

Crust

- 1 cup shredded coconut
- 1/2 cup almond flour
- 2/3 cup coconut oil
- 1/4 teaspoon sea salt
- 2 drops stevia

Filling

- 4 cups young coconut meat
- 2/3 cup raw cashews (soaked for at least 1 hour)
- 1/2 cup coconut oil
- 3 tablespoon lemon juice
- ¼ teaspoon stevia
- A pinch sea salt
- 1/2 teaspoon vanilla extract

Topping

- 2 packets of strawberries, sliced thin

Directions:

1.   Mix shredded coconut, almond flour, coconut oil, sea salt and stevia until well.

2.   Press into the bottom of the pan and put into the freezer for 20 minutes

3.   Then, combine coconut meat, cashews, coconut oil, lemon, stevia, salt, and vanilla. Blend on high until very creamy and smooth. Pour into the pie crust and set in freezer for another 45 minutes

4.   Slice your strawberries and line on cheesecake

5.   Keep in the freezer for a couple hours till firm

6.   Cut and Serve

44. Sunshine Seed Oat Cereal

Serves: 1 max

Time: 10 hours

Ingredients

- 1 cup almond pulp
- 3/4 cup sunflower seeds
- 3/4 cup dried shredded coconut
- 2/3 cup whole grain flour
- ¼ tsp stevia
- 2 tablespoons water
- 2 teaspoons pure vanilla extract
- Pinch of Himalayan salt

Directions

1. Mix all ingredients together.

2. Spread out on teflex sheets and dehydrate at 145°F for 2 hours.

3. Turn the temperature down to 115°F and continue to dry for 8-10 hours (or until dry and crunchy), flipping onto the mesh screen halfway through.

45. Juicy Apple Burst

Serves: 2 max

Time: 10 minutes

Time:

Ingredients

- 2 Eggs (beaten)

- 2 slices bacon (cut into small strips)

- 1 Apple (peeled and chopped)

- 5 Walnut (halves)

- 1 tbsp Grass fed butter

- 1/2 tsp Cinnamon powder

Directions:

1. In a large skillet, scramble the eggs in the grass-feed butter and keep aside

2. Add bacon and cook until medium done.

3. Add the chopped apple and cook with the bacon until the apple is slightly soft.

4. Crush the walnuts and add on the bacon and apple.

5. Return the eggs to the skillet and stir all ingredients together.

6. Add the cinnamon powder to the mixture and stir a few times.

7. Serve.

46. Coconut Ginger Shrimp

Serves: 2 max

Ingredients

- 12 Jumbo shrimp (peeled and deveined)

- 2 tbsp. Coconut oil

- 1 tbsp. Coconut milk

- 4 tbsp. Coconut (shredded, unsweetened)

- 4 tbsp. fresh ginger (grated)

- 2 cloves garlic (minced)

- 2 tbsp. chives (chopped)

- 1 tsp Black pepper

- 1 lime(juiced)

Directions:

1.   In a sauce pan, heat the coconut oil. Add the garlic, green onion, 1 tbs of the ginger, and 1 tbs of the shredded coconut. Saute briefly.

2.   Add the coconut milk, lime juice, and black pepper to the sauce pot. Cook over medium heat for a minute or two, stirring frequently.

3.   Remove the sauce pot from the heat and allow mixture to cool a bit. Pour mixture in a small bowl or dish. In a separate bowl or dish place the remaining 3 tbs of ginger and 3 tbs of shredded coconut.

4.   Coat each shrimp with the coconut oil mixture and then coat with the dry ginger and coconut. Lace the shrimp on skewers.

5.   Cook the skewered shrimp on a grill until done..

47.   Poppy Bacon Scones

Serves: 6 max

Time: 35 minutes

Ingredients

- 2 cup blanched almond flour

- 1/2 cup Coconut flour

- 1 tsp Baking powder

- 1/8 tsp Sea salt

- 4 tbsp grass-fed butter cubed

- 1/2 cup full fat coconut milk

- 2 Eggs

- 4 slices bacon cooked and crumbled

- 2 tsp Poppy seeds

- 2 tbsp minced chives

Directions:

1. Preheat oven to 375°F.

2. Combine coconut flour and almond flour in a large bowl with the baking powder and salt.

3. Mix the butter until it becomes crumble

4. Add the coconut milk and eggs to the mixture and mix well to form a dough.

5. Add the bacon and chives and mix until just combined.

6. Line a baking sheet with parchment paper.

7. scoop the dough and place on it

8. Then, brush coconut milk and top and sprinkle the poppy seeds

9. Bake for 15 minutes, until golden brown

10. Allow to cool before serving.

48. Magic Ring

Serves: 3-4 max

Time: 25 minutes

Ingredients

- 1lb Squids (cleaned and sliced into rings and tentacles)
- 2 teaspoons paprika
- 2 teaspoons salt
- 1 teaspoon black pepper
- 1 teaspoon garlic powder
- 1/4 cup Coconut flour
- 2 Eggs (beaten)
- 4 tbsp Coconut oil (for frying)

Directions:

1. Add the squid to the eggs, toss to coat.
2. In a large bowl, stir together coconut flour, salt, pepper, paprika, and garlic powder.
3. Toss to coat. Set aside
4. Add the oil to a high-sided skillet over medium-high heat.
5. Add the calamari and fry on each side until golden brown.
6. Set aside on a paper towel lined plate.
7. Serve with lemon wedges and paleo mayo

49. Crispy Vegie Bitez

Serves: 5-6 max

Time: 30 minutes

Ingredients

- ½ cup head cauliflower(cut-into-florets)

- ½ cup head broccoli(cut-into-florets)

- ¼ cup carrot(grated)

- 1 tbsp coconut oil

- 2 tsp Garlic powder

- 2 tbsp chives (chopped)

- 3 tbsp Coconut flour

- 2 Eggs (beaten)

- 1 tsp Salt

- 5 tbsp Coconut oil (for frying)

Directions:

1. Blend the cauliflower, broccoli and carrot until rice-like

2. Transfer the mixture to a mixing bowl and microwave on high for 2 to 3 minutes, until cooked through.

3. Remove the bowl from the microwave and set aside to cool for about 5 minutes.

4. Add the coconut oil, chopped chives, garlic powder, coconut flour, eggs, and salt to the mixing bowl. Mix until all the ingredients are well combined.

5. Then, form the mixture into 6 to 8 patties. Set aside.

6. Heat the coconut oil in a skillet over medium heat.

7.   Fry the patties in the coconut oil until browned, about 2 to 3 minutes per side.

8.   Remove the patties from the oil and place on a paper towel lined plate to remove any excess oil.

9   Serve

50.   Cherrylicious Pie

Time: 35 minutes

Serving: 8 max

Ingredients

- 2 refrigerated pre-made pie crusts

- 600gm fresh cherry (pitted)

- 12 drops stevia

- 2 tablespoon lemon juice

- ½ tablespoon arrowroot powder

Directions

1.   Preheat the air fryer to 320°F

2.   Press one pie crust into a pie pan, removing excess hanging over

3.   With a fork, poke the holes all over dough

4.   Place the pie pan into air fryer basket

5.   Cook for about 5 minutes

6.   Remove pie pan from air fryer basket

7.   Heat cherry, stevia and lemon juice over medium heat.

8.   Stir in arrowroot for thickness. Boil the filling for 8-10 minutes

9.   Allow it cooled

10.   Pour the cherry pie filling into pie crust

11.   Roll out the remaining pie crust and cut into ¾ inch strips

12.   Place strips going one way across top and then the opposite way for a lattice pattern

13.	Place the pie pan into air fryer basket

14.	Cook for about 15 minutes

51. Berry Merry Pie

Time: 35 minutes

Serving: 8 max

Ingredients

- 2 refrigerated pre-made pie crusts
- 2 cups fresh blueberries
- 1 tsp stevia
- 2 tablespoon lemon juice
- ½ tablespoon arrowroot powder

Directions

1. Preheat the air fryer to 320°F
2. Press one pie crust into a pie pan, removing excess hanging over
3. With a fork, poke the holes all over dough
4. Place the pie pan into air fryer basket
5. Cook for about 5 minutes
6. Remove pie pan from air fryer basket
7. Heat blueberries, stevia and lemon juice over medium heat.
8. Stir in arrowroot for thickness. Boil the filling for 8-10 minutes
9. Allow it cooled
10. Pour the blueberries filling into pie crust
11. Roll out the remaining pie crust and cut into ¾ inch strips
12. Place strips going one way across top and then the opposite way for a lattice pattern

13.   Place the pie pan into air fryer basket

14.   Cook for about 15 minutes

52. Mango Tango Pie

Time: 35 minutes

Serving: 8 max

Ingredients

- 2 refrigerated pre-made pie crusts

- 4 mango(sliced)

- 1 tbsp stevia

- 2 tablespoon lemon juice

- ½ tablespoon arrowroot powder

Directions

1. Preheat the air fryer to 320°F

2. Press one pie crust into a pie pan, removing excess hanging over

3. With a fork, poke the holes all over dough

4. Place the pie pan into air fryer basket

5. Cook for about 5 minutes

6. Remove pie pan from air fryer basket

7. Heat mango, stevia and lemon juice over medium heat.

8. Stir in arrowroot for thickness. Boil the filling for 8-10 minutes

9. Allow it cooled

10. Pour the mango filling into pie crust

11. Roll out the remaining pie crust and cut into ¾ inch strips

12. Place strips going one way across top and then the opposite way for a lattice pattern

13. Place the pie pan into air fryer basket

14. Cook for about 15 minutes

53.   Apple Cinnamon Pie

Time: 50 minutes

Serving: 8 max

Ingredients

- 2 refrigerated pre-made pie crusts
- 9 royal gala apple(cubed)
- 1 tsp cinnamon
- 1 tbsp stevia
- ½ tablespoon arrowroot powder

Directions

1. Preheat the air fryer to 320°F
2. Press one pie crust into a pie pan, removing excess hanging over
3. With a fork, poke the holes all over dough
4. Place the pie pan into air fryer basket
5. Cook for about 5 minutes
6. Remove pie pan from air fryer basket
7. Heat apple, stevia and cinnamon over medium heat.
8. Stir in arrowroot for thickness. Boil the filling for 8-10 minutes
9. Allow it cooled
10. Pour the apple filling into pie crust
11. Roll out the remaining pie crust and cut into ¾ inch strips
12. Place strips going one way across top and then the opposite way for a lattice pattern

13.   Place the pie pan into air fryer basket

14.   Cook for about 15 minutes

54. Pine-O-Tasty Pie

Time: 35 minutes

Serving: 8 max

Ingredients

- 2 refrigerated pre-made pie crusts

- 8 oz pineapple(crushed)

- ¾ cup desiccated coconut

- 1 tbsp lemon juice

- 1 tbsp stevia

- ½ tablespoon arrowroot powder

Directions

1. Preheat the air fryer to 320°F

2. Press one pie crust into a pie pan, removing excess hanging over

3. With a fork, poke the holes all over dough

4. Place the pie pan into air fryer basket

5. Cook for about 5 minutes

6. Remove pie pan from air fryer basket

7. Heat pineapple, lemon juice, stevia and over medium heat.

8. Sprinkle over coconut

9. Stir in arrowroot for thickness. Boil the filling for 8-10 minutes

10. Allow it cooled

11. Pour the pineapple filling into pie crust

12.   Roll out the remaining pie crust and cut into ¾ inch strips

13.   Place strips going one way across top and then the opposite way for a lattice pattern

14.   Place the pie pan into air fryer basket

15.   Cook for about 15 minutes

55. Goblin Omelet

Time: 15 minutes

Servings: 4 max

Ingredients:

- 4 large eggs

- 2 tbsp coconut cream

- 2 tbsp grass-feed butter

- ¼ cup green onion(chopped)

- Salt and pepper to taste

Directions:

1. Melt butter in the Instant Pot on the sauté setting and add raw eggs.

2. Whisk and stir in coconut cream, salt and pepper

3. Sauté for 2 minutes

4. Sprinkle remaining ingredients on top

5. Close lid and cook at high pressure for 5 minutes.

6. Use a quick pressure release

56.   Vege Galore Omelet

Time: 20 minutes

Servings: 4 max

Ingredients:

- 4 large eggs

- 2 tbsp coconut cream

- 2 tbsp grass-feed butter

- ¼ cup green onion(chopped)

- ¼ cup kale leaves(chopped)

- ¼ cup cherry tomatoes, halved

- Salt and pepper to taste

Directions:

1. Melt grass-feed butter in the Instant Pot on the sauté setting and add kale.

2. Cook for 1-2 minutes until it becomes soft

3. Add green onions and cherry tomatoes sauté for 2 minutes

4. Add the egg whisk and stir in

5. Then, add in coconut cream, salt and pepper

6. Close lid and cook at high pressure for 8 minutes.

7. Use a quick pressure release

57.   Delicia Mushroom Cheese Omelet

Time: 20 minutes

Servings: 4 max

Ingredients:

- 4 large eggs   ,

- 2 tbsp grated almond cheese

- 1 tbsp coconut oil

- 2 tbsp coconut milk

- ¼ cup spinach(chopped)

- ¼ cup mushroom(sliced)

- 2 tbsp green onions(sprinkle)

- Salt and pepper to taste

Directions:

1.   Heat coconut oil in skillet add spinach and mushroom

2.   Add some salt and pepper to taste

3.   Cook 1-2 minutes until it becomes soft

4.   Whisk the egg and pour on the vegetables

5.   When, the egg is almost cook sprinkle grated almond cheese, green onions and add 2 tbsp coconut milk. Allow the cheese to melt faster

6.   Serve

58. Coconut Cheeky Omelet

Time: 30 minutes

Servings: 4 max

Ingredients:

- 4 large eggs

- 2 tbsp grated coconut

- 100gm chicken breast(shredded)

- 1 tbsp coconut oil

- 2 tbsp coconut milk

- Salt and pepper to taste

Directions:

1. Heat coconut oil in skillet add chicken, salt and pepper

2. Cook until it turns golden brown

3. Whisk the egg and add the coconut milk and grated coconut

4. Pour the mixture on the chicken when the egg is almost set add in salt and pepper to taste

5. Serve

59. Juicy Apple Omelet

Time: 10 minutes

Servings: 4 max

Ingredients:

- 4 large eggs

- 1 apple(diced)

- ½ tsp of cinnamon

- 15 gm almond (chopped and roasted)

Directions:

1. Heat coconut oil in skillet add apple and cook for 20 seconds

2. Add a ½ tsp cinnamon

3. Cook until it turns golden brown

4. Whisk the egg and pour on the apples

5. When, the egg is almost set sprinkle the chopped roasted almond

6. Serve

60. Tasty Glazed Meatballs With Coconut Sauce

Serves:3-4 max

Time:40 minutes

Ingredients:

Meatballs

- 1 pound organic ground beef (grass fed)

- 1 pineapple (diced)

- ½ cup parsley

- ½ teaspoon ground pepper

- 4 cloves garlic (chopped)

- 1 medium onion (finely chopped)

- 1 teaspoon salt

- 1 egg

- ¼ cup arrowroot flour

Sauce

- 1 clove garlic (peeled)

- 1 jalapeno chilies (chopped)

- 1/2 teaspoons fine sea salt (plus more to taste)

- 1 tablespoon coconut oil

- 1 bunch scallions (thinly sliced, ~8 scallions)

- 1/2 cups chopped cilantro (finely)

- 14 ounces coconut milk

- 3 tablespoons lemon juice (freshly squeezed, plus more to taste)

Directions

1. Preheat oven to 400°F

2. To make a sauce add organic chilli sauce, coconut amino, pineapple juice, ginger garlic paste and paprika in a saucepan. Heat for 7 minutes in a low heat

3. Combine beef, pepper, garlic, onion, parsley, salt, egg, and arrowroot starch in a bowl

4. Make ball sized meatballs with mixture and place on baking sheet

5. Bake for 20-30 minutes or until it turns golden brown

6. In a skillet cook the pineapple for 2-3 minutes over medium heat

7. Then, mix the sauce and the meatballs

8. Stir for 4 minutes until the sauce is well coated with meatballs

9. Serve

61.   Tasty Glazed Meatballs with Sunflower Seed Sauce

Serves:4-5 max

Time:40 minutes

Ingredients:

Meatballs

- 1 pound organic ground beef (grass fed)

- 1 pineapple (diced)

- 1 cup desiccated coconut

- ½ cup parsley

- ½ teaspoon ground pepper

- 4 cloves garlic (chopped)

- 1 medium onion (finely chopped)

- 1 teaspoon salt

- 1 egg

- ¼ cup arrowroot flour

Sauce

- 3 cup sunflower seed (crushed)

- 1 tablespoon coconut amino

- ¼ cup coconut milk

- ¼ cup coconut sugar

Directions

1.   Preheat oven to 400°F

2. Combine beef, pepper, garlic, onion, parsley, salt, egg, and arrowroot starch in a bowl

3. Make ball sized meatballs with mixture and place on baking sheet

4. Bake for 20-30 minutes or until it turns golden brown

5. In a skillet cook the pineapple for 2-3 minutes over medium heat

6. To make a sauce, blend the sauce until consistently

7. Stir for 4 minutes until the sauce is well coated with meatballs

8. Serve

62.   Fruity Planet balls

Serves: 3-4 max

Time: 40 minutes

Ingredients:

- 1 pound organic ground beef (grass fed)

- 1/2 cup organic chili sauce

- 1/2 teaspoon ground pepper

- 1 teaspoon ground garlic salt

- 1/2 teaspoon chili powder

- 1/2 teaspoon paprika

- 1 egg

- 1/4 cup arrowroot flour

Grape jelly

- 1 cup grapes

- 4 tablespoon chia seeds

- 1tablespoon lemon juice

- ½ teaspoon stevia

Directions:

1.   Preheat oven to 350°F

2.   Combine beef, pepper, garlic salt, egg, and arrowroot starch in a bowl

3.   To make grape jelly in a saucepan under medium heat add grapes cook until it breaks into syrup for 8 minutes

4.   Mash the fruit until smooth and add stevia and lemon juice. Stir in chia seed.

5.   Make golf ball sized meatballs with mixture and place on baking sheet

6.   Bake for 20-30 minutes or until browned

7.   Transfer meatballs to crockpot and add chili sauce, grape jelly, chili powder and paprika

8.   Cook on low for 2-4 hours, checking periodically. Do not overcook or meatballs and sauce will burn

9.   Serve with broccoli

63.   Savory Meatballs With Sauce

Serves:3-4 max

Time:40 minutes

Ingredients:

Meatballs

- 1 pound organic ground beef (grass fed)

- 1 bell pepper (finely chopped)

- ½ cup parsley

- ½ teaspoon ground pepper

- 4 cloves garlic (chopped)

- 1 medium onion (finely chopped)

- 1 teaspoon salt

- 1 egg

- ¼ cup arrowroot flour

Sauce

- ¼ cup chicken broth

- ½ cup coconut amino

- 1 tomato (pureed)

- 1 tablespoon coconut milk

- 1 tablespoon grass-feed butter

- ½ teaspoon paprika

Directions

1. Preheat oven to 400°F

2. To make sauce add the coconut amino, chicken broth, tomato puree, and a pinch of salt and pepper. Stir for a few minutes, then add the grass-feed butter and let it thicken and become glossy. Add coconut milk

3. Combine beef, bell pepper, pepper, garlic, onion, parsley, salt, egg, and arrowroot starch in another bowl

4. Make ball sized meatballs with mixture and place on baking sheet

5. Bake for 20-30 minutes or until it turns golden brown

6. Then, mix the sauce over the meatballs

7. Stir for 4 minutes until the sauce is well coated with meatballs

8. Serve

64. Green Meatballs With Spicy Tomato Sauce

Serves:3-4 max

Time:40 minutes

Ingredients:

Meatballs

- 1 pound organic ground beef (grass fed)

- 3 table spoon fresh cilantro(chopped)

- 5 tablespoon parsley(chopped)

- ½ teaspoon ground pepper

- 4 cloves garlic (chopped)

- ½ ginger (chopped)

- 1 medium onion (finely chopped)

- 1 teaspoon salt

- 1 egg

- ¼ cup arrowroot flour

Sauce

- ¼ cup bone broth

- ½ cup coconut amino

- 1 lemon(juiced)

- 1 cup tomato (pureed)

- 1 tablespoon grass-feed butter

- 2 cloves garlic(chopped)

- 1 teaspoon red pepper flakes

- Pinch of cinnamon

- Pinch of pepper and salt

Directions

1.   Preheat oven to 400°F

2.   To make sauce add the coconut amino, bone broth, tomato puree, red pepper flakes, cinnamon and a pinch of salt and pepper. Stir for a few minutes, then add the lemon juice and grass-feed butter let it thicken and become glossy.

3.   Combine cilantro, parsley, garlic, onion, ginger, salt, beef, pepper, egg, and arrowroot starch in a bowl

4.   Make ball sized meatballs with mixture and place on baking sheet

5.   Bake for 20-30 minutes or until it turns golden brown

6.   Transfer the meatballs to the pan with the sauce and let it simmer for 20 minutes.

7.   Sprinkle with fresh parsley and serve

65. Tasty Spiced Walnut Crunchy Pie

Time:45 minutes

Serves: 4 max

Ingredients:

- 1(9-inch) prepared pie dough, store-bought or homemade, at room temperature

- ¼ cup coconut oil

- 1 tablespoon grass-feed butter

- ½ cup walnut (chopped)

- ¼ cup pecan (chopped)

- ¼ cup walnut (halves)

- 2 large eggs

- ¼ cup maple syrup

- 1 tablespoons xylitol

- 2 tablespoons cashew butter

- ¾ teaspoon vanilla extract

- ½ ground cinnamon

- 1/8 teaspoon ground nutmeg

- Pinch of ground cloves

- ½ teaspoon salt

Directions:

1. Place the prepared pie dough onto a floured smooth surface top

2.   Place an 8-inch place face down on top of the pie dough and using it as a template, cut around its edges to make an 8-inch pie shell

3.   Discard the extra dough

4.   Place the dough into a pie pan and fold the edges under itself

5.   In a small pan, add the butter and chopped walnuts on medium heat

6.   Cook for about 6-8 minutes, stirring occasionally

7.   Remove from the heat and place the walnuts mixture into the pie shell

8.   In a bowl, add the eggs, maple syrup, xylitol, cashew butter, vanilla extract, cinnamon, nutmeg and salt and beat till well combined

9.   Carefully pour the mixture over the toasted walnuts

10.   Top with the remaining walnut halves in a decorative pattern

11.   Preheat the air fryer to 320°F

12.   Place the pie into an air fryer basket

13.   Cook for about to 25minutes

66.   Cutie Pie

Time: 55 minutes

Servings:6 max

Ingredients

For crust

- 1 ½ cups almond flour

- 1 teaspoon xylitol

- 1 tablespoon grass-feed butter

- ¼ cup chilled water

- Salt, to taste

For filling

- 4 granny smith apples, peeled and chopped finely

- 1 teaspoon lemon zest (grated finely)

- 1 tablespoon stevia

- 2 tablespoons almond flour

- 1 teaspoon ground cinnamon

- ¼ teaspoon ground nutmeg

- Salt, to taste

- 2 tablespoons fresh lemon juice

- 2 tablespoon grass-feed butter

For topping

- 1 egg (beaten)

- 1 teaspoon ground cinnamon

Directions:

For pastry

1. Preheat oven 350°F

2. Combine the almond flour, xylitol and salt.

3. Whisk the grass feed butter until the mixture forms soft dough.

4. Then, add cold water if the dough is dry

5. Divide the dough into 2 rounds, flattened it like a wheel and wrap the dough using cling wrap and chilled it for 25 minutes

For Filling

1. Melt grass-feed butter in a large sauté pan set over medium-high heat and add apples to the pan. Stir to coat fruit with grass-feed butter and lemon juice occasionally

2. Meanwhile, whisk stevia, almond flour, salt, and spices. Sprinkle the mixture over the apples, and stir to coat them.

3. Cook the apple filling for 6-8 minutes until it becomes softens.

4. Then, remove the filling from pan and let it cool

For pie

1. Spoon in the apple pieces and sauce into the pie crust.

2. Cover the pie with the strips of pastry, creating the lattice.

3. Press a fork along the edge to push the pastry down.

4. Bake for 25 minutes.

5. Serve hot or cold.

67. Sweet Potato Beet Crispy Chips

Serves: 4 max

Time: 40 minutes

Ingredients

- 1 Sweet potato (sliced)

- 1 Beet (sliced)

- A pinch sea salt

- Drizzle of EVOO

Directions:

1. Preheat oven to 375˚F.

2. Using a mandolin slicer, slice both the sweet potato and the beet very thin.

3. Line baking sheet with parchment paper and lay sweet potato and beet one thin layer

4. Bake for 30 minutes a, flip the beets and sweet potatoes every 10 minutes.

5. Once crisp, remove from oven, allow to cool slightly, sprinkle lightly with olive oil, and dust with coarse ground sea salt.

6. Enjoy immediately preventing loss of the "crispiness".

68.   Heavenly Mushroom Chips

Time: 1 hour 10 minutes

Serves: 3 max

Ingredients:

- 450gm king oyster mushrooms

- 2 tablespoons coconut oil

- Kosher salt

- Freshly ground pepper

Directions:

1.   Preheat the oven to 300°F

2.   Cut the mushrooms in half lengthwise and sliced

3.   Arrange the slices in a single layer on the parchment-lined baking sheets. Make sure the mushrooms are dried and strain water from the mushrooms

4.   Brush coconut oil on both sides of the mushroom slices, and season with salt and pepper to taste.

5.   Bake for 1 hour until the chips are golden brown and crispy.

69.   Erotic Tortilla Chips

Ingredients

- 1 cup almond flour

- 1 egg white

- 1/2 tsp salt

- 1/2 tsp chili powder

- 1/2 tsp garlic powder

- 1/2 tsp cumin

- 1/4 tsp onion powder

- 1/4 tsp paprika

Directions

1.   Preheat the oven to 325°F.

2.   In a large bowl, combine all of the ingredients until they form even dough.

3.   Roll out the dough between two pieces of parchment paper, as thinly as possible. Remove the top layer of parchment paper.

4.   Cut the dough into desired shapes for chips.

5.   Move the dough, with the parchment paper, onto a baking sheet.

6.   Bake for 15 minutes, until golden brown.

7.   Remove from the oven and let cool 5 minutes.

8.   Use a spatula to remove the chips from the paper.

9.   Serve with guacamole or salsa.

70.   Deluxe Apple Chips

Serves: 4 max

Time: 1 hour 35 minutes

Ingredients:

- 3 red Cameo apple (thin round-sliced)
- ¼ tsp ground cinnamon

Directions:

1. Preheat your oven to 300° F.
2. Line two baking sheets with parchment paper and set aside.
3. Cut the apples into thin slices.
4. Spread the apple slices on the baking sheets
5. Sprinkle some cinnamon on top and place in the oven.
6. Place in the oven to dry for 45 minutes, then flip the slices and cook for 45 minutes.
7. Let the chips cool down and serve.

71. Apple Nutty Bites

Serves:2-3 max

Time:25 minutes

Ingredients

- 2 apple, cored and thinly sliced

- 1 tablespoon grass-feed butter(melted)

- 4 tbsp pecans(chopped)

- 4 tbsp almonds, sliced

- 1 tbsp roasted coconut shreds

- 1 tbsp dark chocolate chips

- 2 tbsp dried cranberries

Directions:

1. Spread the grass-feed butter over one side of each apple slice.

2. Top each apple slice with nuts, dried cranberries and dark chocolate

3. Mix well until it well combined

4. Served

72.   Divine Parsnips Chips

Time:40 minutes

Serves:2 max

Ingredients

- 500g Parsnips (thin-sliced)

- 1/4 Cup Coconut oil (melted)

- 8 drops stevia

Directions:

1. Preheat the oven to 350°F

2. Line up the parsnips in a single layer on the baking sheets

3. Pour over the coconut oil and distribute evenly.

4. Drizzle over the stevia and stir to combine well.

5. Place in the oven and cook for 15 minutes.

6. Remove from the oven and toss the parsnips over to allow the other side to brown.

7. Place back in the oven and cook for a further 15 minutes until golden brown.

8. Remove from the oven and allow to cool for 5 minutes

9. Serve

73.   Tempting Sweet Potato Chips

Ingredients

- 2 large sweet potatoes (peeled and thin-sliced)

- 1 tbsp coconut oil(melted)

- 1 tsp sea salt

- 2 tsp dried rosemary(minced)

Directions

1.   Heat oven to 375°F

2.   Slice sweet potatoes until thin

3.   Toss sweet potatoes in a bowl with coconut oil and salt and rosemary until it well combined.

4.   Place on a non-stick baking sheet and place into the oven.

5.   After 10 minutes, take the pan out and flip the chips.

6.   Place back in the oven and cook for a further 15 minutes until golden brown.

7.   Remove from the oven and allow to cool for 5 minutes

8.   Serve.

74.   Lovely Roasted Almond

Serves:2-3 max

Time: 45 minutes

Ingredients:

- 600gm raw almonds(boiled)

- 2 tbsp fresh rosemary(minced)

- 1 ½ tsp salt

- 2 tbsp coconut oil

Directions:

1.   Combine almonds in a bowl with coconut oil and rosemary well

2.   Bake at 350° for 15 minutes, until a nutty aroma wafts out of the oven

3.   Remove almonds from oven and cool for 20 minutes

4.   Toss with salt

5.   Serve

75. Colors Fruit Mania

Time: 25 minutes

Serves: 5 max

Ingredients:

- 1 cup strawberries(sliced)

- 3 mandarin oranges(peeled)

- 1 mango, (diced)

- ½ cup pineapple chunks, diced

- ¼ cup red onion, chopped

- ¼ cup green onion, sliced

- ¼ cup cilantro, minced

- 1 tbsp lime juice

- ¼ tsp stevia

Directions:

1. Combine strawberries, oranges, mango, and pineapple in a large bowl.

2. Add red onion, green onion, and cilantro. Stir evenly

3. Mix lime juice and stevia well

4. Pour over the mixture and stir evenly.

5. Keep chilled and covered in the refrigerator for 15-20 minutes

6. Serve

76.   Sweet n Savory crisp

Time:45 minutes

Serves:4 max

Ingredients

- 2 sweet potato (peeled and diced)
- 3 Small Parsnips (peeled and diced)
- 4 cloves of garlic
- 1/2 red capsicum (diced)
- 1 cup almond meal
- 4 tbsp chai seeds
- 1 tbsp cumin seeds
- 1 tsp smoked Paprika
- 1 tbsp small shallots (chopped)
- 1tsp sea salt
- 2 tbsp Olive Oil

Directions:

1.   Pre-heat oven 350°F

2.   Blend raw diced sweet potato, parsnips, red capsicum, shallots, garlic and olive oil until finely mash.

3.   Then, add the rest of ingredients. Blend it until well combined.

4.   Place a sheet of cling wrap and ensure it is flat. A square shape would be desired. Place another layer of cling wrap over the top. With a rolling pin softly and evenly roll "dough" out into a rectangle shape and thin.

5.   Remove the cling wrap on top and cut the dough in rectangle shape using knife

6.   Then, greased two large oven cookie trays.

7.   Flip over the dough from the cling wrap

8.   Cut the dough into triangle shapes with a knife on baking tray.

9.   Place the chips in oven and bake

10.   Flip the chips after 7 minutes. After that every 4 minutes flip it again for 25 minutes.

11.   Baked further 10 minutes until golden color.

12.   Serve and enjoy

77.   Spiced Pumpkin Spread

Time: 2 hours 5 minutes

Serves:4 max

Ingredients

- ½ cup raw cashews

- ½ cup pumpkin (deseeded and cubed)

- 2 tbsp almond butter

- 2 tbsp lemon juice

- 1 tbsp extra virgin olive oil

- ¼ tsp salt

- ¼ tsp cumin

- ¼ tsp paprika

- ⅛ tsp cayenne

- ½ tsp pumpkin pie spice

- 1 garlic clove

Directions:

1.   Soak raw cashews in water for 4 hours

2.   Drain and wash the cashews.

3.   Blend the cashews and pumpkin until smooth

4.   Add the rest of the ingredients and blend it again until smooth.

5.   Drizzle a little bit of olive oil on top before serving.

6.   Use it as a dip for vegetables or crackers

78. Rockmelon Hummus

Serves: 6 max

Time: 20 minutes

Ingredients

- 1/2 cup whole cantaloupe

- 3 oz. sliced prosciutto(stripped)

- 1/3 cup apple cider vinegar

- 2 teaspoons extra virgin olive oil

- 1 tablespoon fresh chopped mint leaves

- fresh ground black pepper

Directions

1. Slice cantaloupe half into 6 wedges. Wrap each piece of melon with a strip of prosciutto, securing with a toothpick.

2. Heat the apple cider vinegar in a small skillet over medium-high heat.

3. Simmer about 3- 5 minutes.

4. Drizzle serving plate with apple cider vinegar and olive oil.

5. Place wrapped melon onto plate and sprinkle with mint and pepper.

6. Serve.

79.   Rich Squash Bacon Bitez

Time: 45 minutes

Serves:4-6 max

Ingredients

- 2 lbs. butternut squash, cut into cubes;

- 15 slices of bacon (cut in half)

- 1 tsp. chili powder

- 1 tsp. garlic powder

- 1 tsp onion powder

- 1 tsp. paprika

- Freshly ground black pepper (to taste)

Directions:

1.   Preheat your oven to 350 ˚F.

2.   Place the squash in a bowl and sprinkle with chili powder, garlic powder, paprika, and black pepper.

3.   Wrap bacon slices around the squash cubes and place on a baking sheet.

4.   Place in the preheated oven and bake for 20 minutes. Flip the bites over and bake for another 20 minutes.

5.   Set the oven to broil for 2 to 3 minutes for crunchier

6.   Serve

80. Luscious Carrot Cake Pancakes

Serves: 2 max

Time: 20 minutes

Ingredients

- 1 cup carrots, shredded

- 3 eggs

- ½ cup almond meal

- ½ cup coconut milk

- ¼ cup walnuts, chopped

- 2 tablespoon coconut oil

- 2 tablespoon coconut flour

- ½ teaspoon baking powder

- ¼ teaspoon salt

- ¼ tsp cinnamon

- ¼ tsp ginger powder

- ¼ tsp nutmeg

- 2 tbsp of raisins

- 1 tablespoon coconut butter (for serving)

Directions:

1.   Mix all dry ingredients together in a large bowl: almond meal, coconut flour, baking soda and powder, and spice together.

2.   Add wet ingredients to dry ingredients: carrots, eggs, coconut milk, coconut oil, and raisins. Mix thoroughly.

3.   Heat a large skillet up under medium-high heat and use coconut oil to grease the surface

4.   Pour batter into small pancakes onto hot griddle. Flip on both sides for 3 minutes.

5.   Top pancakes off with coconut butter.

81. Grilled Citrus Calamari

Serves: 4 max

Time: 30 minutes

Ingredients

- 2 lbs. calamari cleaned tubes and tentacles

- 1 lemon, sliced;

- 1 lime, sliced;

- 1 orange, sliced;

- 2 tbsp. fresh parsley, minced;

- 1/4 cup olive oil;

- 3 tbsp. lemon juice;

- 2 garlic cloves, minced;

- Sea salt and freshly ground black pepper

Directions:

1. Preheat grill to medium heat.

2. Slice the calamari tubes into thin rings.

3. Place all the ingredients in a large bowl and season to taste.

4. Toss everything gently, until well coated.

5. Grill the calamari and citrus fruit using a grilling basket or pan until fully cooked, about 4 to 5 minutes.

82.   Yummy Baked Turkey and Brussel Sprouts

Time: 30 minutes

Serves: 2 max

Ingredients

- 500gm Brussels sprouts

- 2 turkey breasts

- Olive oil, to taste

- 1 tbsp fresh rosemary (chopped)

- 1 tbsp fresh thyme (chopped)

- 2 cloves garlic (minced)

- 1 tsp ginger (minced)

- Salt, to taste

- Pepper, to taste

Directions:

1.   Preheat oven to 425°F

2.   Cut the Brussel sprouts season with olive oil, salt, pepper, rosemary, thyme, and garlic.

3.   Place the Brussels on the baking pan lined with parchment paper.

4.   Next, season both sides of the turkey with olive oil, salt, pepper, and the remaining rosemary, thyme, and garlic over parchment paper.

5.   Seal parchment paper to keep turkey moist, and place on the baking pan.

6.   Bake for 20-25 minutes, until turkey is fully cooked and Brussels

7.   Serve with cauliflower rice or brown rice

83. Wonderful Baked Sweet Potato Beet Chicken

Time: 30 minutes

Serves: 2 max

Ingredients

- 250gm sweet potatoes(cubed)
- 250gm beetroot(cubed)
- 2 chicken breasts
- Olive oil, to taste
- 1 tbsp fresh rosemary (chopped)
- 1 tbsp fresh thyme (chopped)
- 2 cloves garlic (minced)
- 1 tsp ginger (minced)
- Salt, to taste
- Pepper, to taste

Directions:

1. Preheat oven to 425°F
2. Season the beet and sweet potato with olive oil, salt, pepper, rosemary and thyme
3. Place the beet and sweet potatoes on the baking pan lined with parchment paper.
4. Next, season both sides of the chicken with olive oil, salt, pepper, and the remaining rosemary, thyme, and garlic over parchment paper.
5. Seal parchment paper to keep chicken moist, and place on the baking pan.
6. Bake for 20-25 minutes, until chicken is fully cooked and sweet potatoes

7.   Serve with cauliflower rice or brown rice

84.   Heavenly Sweet Corn & Mushroom Turkey

Time: 30 minutes

Serves: 4 max

Ingredients

- 500gm organic frozen sweet corn

- 650gm turkey breasts

- 2 shallots(sliced)

- Salt, to taste

- Pepper, to taste

- 350gm mushrooms, sliced

- 2 tbsp coconut oil

For the sauce:

- 3 cloves garlic, minced

- 1 tablespoon ginger, minced

- 2 teaspoons coconut oil

- ⅓ cup coconut amino

- 6-8 drops stevia

- 1 cup bone chicken broth

- ¼ cup coconut flour

Directions:

1.   In a large pan, heat 1 tablespoon of coconut oil over medium heat. Once the oil is hot, add turkey breast season with salt and pepper, and sauté until cooked through and browned.

2.   Remove cooked turkey from pan and set aside.

3.   In the same pan, heat 1 tablespoon of coconut oil, add mushrooms. When the mushrooms start to soften, add sweet corn and stir-fry until the corn is soften. Remove cooked mushrooms and sweet corn from the pan and set aside.

4.   Then, sauté garlic and ginger until fragrant. Add the remaining sauce ingredients and stir until smooth.

5.   Return the turkey and vegetables to the saucy pan, stir until heated through.

6.   Serve with brown rice or cauliflower rice

7.   Enjoy

85. Jingle Turkey Delight

Serves: 2 max

Time: 30 minutes

Ingredients

- 1 cup sweet potato

- 250gm asparagus

- 2 turkey breasts

- Olive oil, to taste

- 2 tablespoons fresh rosemary, chopped

- 2 tablespoons fresh thyme, chopped

- 4 cloves garlic, minced

- Salt, to taste

- Pepper, to taste

Directions:

1. Preheat oven to 425°F

2. Cut vegetables, season with olive oil, salt, pepper, rosemary, thyme, and garlic.

3. Place veggies each in a separate corner of a baking pan lined with parchment paper.

4. Next, season both sides of the turkey with olive oil, salt, pepper, and the remaining rosemary, thyme, and garlic over parchment paper.

5. Seal parchment paper to keep turkey moist, and place on the baking pan.

6. Bake for 30 minutes, until turkey is fully cooked and vegetables

7. Serve with cauliflower rice or brown rice

86. Romantic Beefvegsaurus

Serves: 4 max

Time:30 minutes

Ingredients

Vegetables

- 1cups cherry tomatoes

- 1 large carrot(sliced)

- 1 red bell pepper (sliced)

- 1 green bell pepper (sliced)

- 1 medium-size red onion(sliced)

- 200gm asparagus, trimmed and cut in half

- 3-4 tablespoons olive oil

- Salt, to taste

- Pepper, to taste

- 4 garlic cloves

- 4 sprigs of thyme

- 3 sprigs rosemary

Steak

- 1 pound rib eye

- 1 tablespoon olive oil

- 1 garlic clove

- Salt

- Pepper

Directions:

1. Preheat oven to 400°F.

2. Place cherry tomatoes, carrots, yellow bell pepper, red onion, and asparagus evenly on a baking tray.

3. Season with olive oil, salt, and pepper to taste

4. Add garlic cloves and sprigs of thyme on top of the vegetables.

5. Roast vegetables for 15 minutes.

6. Bring back the tray and push vegetables to the side to make room for the steak.

7. Place the steak in the middle of the pan and season both sides with salt and pepper.

8. Top the steak with a sprig of thyme and a clove of garlic.

9. Place back in oven for 10 more minutes or until desired doneness is reached.

10. Allow the steak to rest for 5 minutes.

11. Plate the vegetables and top with cut steak.

12. Enjoy!

87.   Caulihashbites Delight

Serves: 2-4 max

Time: 50 minutes

Ingredients

- 1 large head cauliflower(grated)

- 2 eggs

- ½ cup almond cheese(grated)

- ⅓ cup chives (thinly sliced)

- 3 cloves garlic (minced)

- 2 tbsp coconut oil

- 1 teaspoon dried basil

- 1 teaspoon salt, divided

- ½ teaspoon black pepper

Directions:

1.   Preheat oven to 400°F

2.   Transfer the cauliflower bits to a bowl and sprinkle over a ½ teaspoon of the salt. Mix the cauliflower to incorporate the salt and let sit for 20 minutes to draw out the water

3.   Transfer the soaking cauliflower to another bowl lined with a large towel. Wrap the towel closed and squeeze so that all of the excess liquid is strained.

4.   Transfer the cauliflower back into the first bowl used and mix with the cheese, chives, garlic, olive oil, basil, black pepper, and remaining ½ teaspoon of salt.

5.   Turnover a large roasting tray and line with parchment paper

6.   Divide the cauliflower mixture into 6 even portions, place on the tray, and shape into hash browns.

7. Bake for 35-40 minutes, until golden brown.

8. Let the hash browns cool for about 15 minutes until they have set.

9. Serve with desired dipping sauce.

10. Enjoy!

88.   Zombie Hashbites

Serves: 2-4 max

Time: 50 minutes

Ingredients

- 1 large head broccoli (grated)

- 2 eggs

- ½ cup almond cheese(grated)

- ⅓ cup chives (thinly sliced)

- 3 cloves garlic (minced)

- 2 tbsp coconut oil

- 1 teaspoon dried basil

- 1 teaspoon salt, divided

- ½ teaspoon black pepper

Directions:

1.   Preheat oven to 400°F

2.   Transfer the broccoli bits to a bowl and sprinkle over a ½ teaspoon of the salt. Mix the cauliflower to incorporate the salt and let sit for 20 minutes to draw out the water

3.   Transfer the soaking broccoli to another bowl lined with a large towel. Wrap the towel closed and squeeze so that all of the excess liquid is strained.

4.   Transfer the broccoli back into the first bowl used and mix with the cheese, chives, garlic, olive oil, basil, black pepper, and remaining ½ teaspoon of salt.

5.   Turnover a large roasting tray and line with parchment paper

6.   Divide the broccoli mixture into 6 even portions, place on the tray, and shape into hash browns.

7.	Bake for 35-40 minutes, until golden brown.

8.	Let the hash browns cool for about 15 minutes until they have set.

9.	Serve

89. Tango Sweetporto Hashbites

Serves:2-4 max

Time:50 minutes

Ingredients

- 1 lb sweet potato (steamed)
- 3 eggs
- ½ cup almond cheese(grated)
- ⅓ cup chives (thinly sliced)
- 4 cloves garlic (minced)
- 2 tbsp coconut oil
- 1 teaspoon dried basil
- 1 teaspoon salt, divided
- ½ teaspoon black pepper

Directions:

1. Preheat oven to 400°F

2. Remove the skin of the sweet potatoes and mash well and mix with the cheese, chives, garlic, olive oil, basil, black pepper, and remaining ½ teaspoon of salt.

3. Turnover a large roasting tray and line with parchment paper

4. Divide the sweet potato mixture into 6 even portions, place on the tray, and shape into hash browns.

5. Bake for 35-40 minutes, until golden brown.

6. Let the hash browns cool for about 15 minutes until they have set.

7. Serve

90. Pleasant Chocolate Almond Cake

Time: 1 hour

Serves: 6-8 max

Ingredients

For Cake:

- ½ cup bitter cocoa powder

- 1 teaspoon stevia

- ⅛ teaspoon pure almond extract

- 3 tablespoons extra virgin olive oil

- 2 large eggs

- 2 pinches sea salt

- 2 tsp baking powder

For Garnish:

- ¼ cup sliced almond

Directions:

1. Add one cup of water in steam basket and set aside.

2. Lightly coat a 4-cup capacity heat-proof bowl with olive oil and set aside.

3. Into the processor add the cocoa powder, stevia, almond extract, olive oil, eggs and salt. Puree the contents of the processor at high speed until well combined, then add the baking powder and process for about a minute.

4. Using a spatula plop the contents of the processor into the heat-proof bowl.

5. Lower the un-covered heat-proof bowl onto the steamer basket.

6. Close and lock the lid of the pressure cooker.

157

7. Electric pressure cookers, cook for 20 minutes at high pressure.

8. When time is up, open the cooker by releasing the pressure.

9. Remove the cake and let cool for about 5 minutes before unmolding the cake onto serving dish. Let the cake cool uncovered another 10 minutes. 10. Finally, sprinkle ¼ cup sliced almond and serve

91. Crazy Deli Carrot Walnut Cupcake

Time: 40 minutes

Serves: 4 max

Ingredients

For Cake:

- 1 teaspoon stevia

- 2 eggs

- 1/4 cup water

- 1/3 cup olive oil

- 1 1/2 cups almond flour

- 1 teaspoon vanilla

- 1 teaspoon baking powder

- 1 teaspoon cinnamon

- 1 cup carrots (grated)

- A pinch sea salt

- ¼ cup roasted walnut(chopped)

For Garnish:

- 1 cup grated almond cheese

Directions:

1. In a bowl, mix stevia, eggs, water and olive oil together.

2. Add the almond flour, vanilla, baking powder, salt and cinnamon. Blend just long enough to blend all ingredients.

3. Stir the grated carrots and chopped walnuts until evenly distributed.

4.   Take pressure cooker and place a steel bowl inside.

5.   Place the cake try carefully on the top of that bowl

6.   Cook for 1 minute in high flame (Do not put whistle while baking cake). Reduce the flame and bake for 50-60 minutes.

7.   The cake is done when firm in the middle. Check by inserting a fork in the center. If done, the fork should come out clean.

8.   Sprinkle with grated almond cheese on top

9.   Cut and serve

92. Healthy Date Cupcake

Time: 55 minutes

Serves: 8 max

Ingredients

For Cake:

- 2 eggs

- ¾ cup olive oil

- 1 1/2 cups coconut flour

- 1 teaspoon vanilla

- 1 teaspoon baking powder

- 1 teaspoon coco powder

- 1 cup dates(pitted)

- A pinch sea salt

Directions:

1.   Blend dates, eggs and olive oil smoothly

2.   Then, mix the coconut flour, vanilla, baking powder, salt and coco powder.

3.   Blend the both mixture for 2-3 minutes

4.   Take pressure cooker and place a steel bowl inside.

5.   Place the cake try carefully on the top of that bowl

6.   Cook for 1 minute in high flame (Do not put whistle while baking cake). Reduce the flame and bake for 50-60 minutes.

7.   The cake is done when firm in the middle. Check by inserting a fork in the center. If done, the fork should come out clean.

8. Cut and serve

93. King Indulgence Cake

Time: 1 hour

Serves: 5-6 max

Ingredients

For Cake:

- 1 cup almond powder
- ¼ cup bitter cocoa powder
- 2 cups banana(mashed)
- 1 teaspoon stevia
- 2 tablespoon coconut milk
- ½ cup grass-feed butter
- 2 large eggs
- ¼ teaspoon sea salt
- 2 tsp baking powder
- ¼ cup sliced almond
- ¼ cup chopped walnut

Directions:

1. In a bowl, mix stevia, eggs and grass-feed butter together.
2. Add the almond powder, cocoa flour, vanilla, baking powder, salt and coconut milk.
3. Stir the mashed banana, sliced almond and chopped walnuts until evenly distributed.
4. Take pressure cooker and place a steel bowl inside.
5. Place the cake try carefully on the top of that bowl

6.   Cook for 1 minute in high flame (Do not put whistle while baking cake). Reduce the flame and bake for 50-60 minutes.

7.   The cake is done when firm in the middle. Check by inserting a fork in the center. If done, the fork should come out clean.

8.   Cut and serve

94.   Sweet And Sour Pulled-Chicken Delight

Serves:2-4 max

Time:45 minutes

Ingredients:

- 8 – 10 chicken breast

- 1 tablespoon (15ml) olive oil

- 10 dried red chili

- 3 garlic cloves, minced

- 1 -2 stalks green onion, (green part finely chopped for garnish, white part cut into 1.5 inch pieces)

- 1 (10g) slice ginger, roughly chopped

- ½ teaspoon stevia(optional)

Sauce:

- ¼ cup (65ml) coconut amino

- 1 teaspoon black pepper

- 1 teaspoon lemon juice

- ½ teaspoon stevia

- 1 teaspoon (5ml) coconut oil

Directions:

1.   Firstly, heat up your pressure cooker (Instant Pot: press Sauté button). While the pressure cooker is heating, pour in 1 tbsp (15ml) olive oil.

2.   Add 10 dried red chili, minced garlic, white part of green onions, and chopped ginger into the pressure cooker, and allow it to slowly release fragrance. Sauté for roughly 3 minutes.

3.   Add sauce mixture and chicken breast into the pressure cooker. Close lid and pressure cook at High Pressure for 12 minutes + 12 minutes Natural Release. Release the remaining pressure and open the lid carefully.

4.   Place chicken breast in a large mixing bowl. Remove chicken skin if desired. Shred chicken drumsticks with a fork. Remove the bones.

5.   Remove the red chili. Heat up your pressure cooker (Instant Pot: press Sauté button), and bring the sauce back to a boil. Taste the sauce and add in roughly ½ tsp of stevia to sweeten the sauce if desired.

6.   Mix 2 tbsp of arrowroot starch with 2 tbsp of water and stir the mixture into the sauce one third at a time until desired thickness.

7.   Place the shredded chicken back into the sauce and mix well.

8.   Finally, place pulled chicken onto lettuce. Garnish with finely chopped green onion.

9.   Serve

95.   Sweet Sour Chicken Delight

Time: 1 hour 45 minutes

Servings: 6-8 max

- 3-4 boneless chicken breasts
- 2 large eggs
- 1 tsp coconut amino
- 1 cup arrowroot starch
- 1 tsp salt
- A dash of pepper
- 1/4 cup coconut oil
- ½ teaspoon stevia
- 4 tbs ketchup
- 1/2 cup distilled white vinegar
- 1 tbsp coconut amino
- 1 tsp olive oil
- 1 tsp garlic chopped

Directions:

1. Preheat the oven to 375 degrees.
2. Cube the chicken and set it aside in a large bowl.
3. Mix the eggs and coconut amino together in a small bowl.
4. Pour the egg mixture over the chicken and stir until covered.

5.   Mix together the arrowroot starch, salt, and pepper and pour over the chicken. Stir until the chicken is well coated with arrowroot starch.

6.   Heat 1/4 cup of oil in a large skillet. Brown the chicken, but don't cook it through. Whisk together the coconut amino.

7.   Once the chicken is browned, place it in a greased baking dish. Pour the sauce over the chicken evenly.

8.   Bake for one hour, stirring the chicken every 15 minutes. Serve with fried rice and enjoy.

96. Hot Crockpot Chicken

Servings:4-6 max

Time:

Ingredients:

- 4 boneless chicken breasts

- 4 cups organic salsa

- 2 cups kale

- 1 cups almonds

- 2 cups corn kernels (optional)

- 1 tablespoon coconut amino

- Water or chicken broth as needed

Directions:

1. Firstly, add the kale and 2 cups of the salsa. Place the chicken breasts in next and cover with the remaining 2 cups of salsa.

2. On top of that, add the coconut amino, almond and corn. Turn the crock on low heat and cook for 6-8 hours, stirring every now and then.

3. If it starts to get too thick, you can add a little water or chicken broth to thin it out

4. Serve with soaked brown rice.

97. Goblin Deli Coconut Curry

Time: 50 minutes

Serves :6 max

Ingredients

- 1.5 pounds (680 grams) chicken breast
- 2 tablespoons green curry paste
- 1 tablespoon extra-virgin coconut oil
- ½ teaspoon grey sea salt
- 800ml coconut milk
- 2 teaspoons coconut amino
- 2 tomatoes, diced
- 2 cups chopped green cabbage
- 1 zucchini, diced
- 4 green onions, green part only
- 1 medium spaghetti squash
- 4 cups raw spinach
- ½ cup packed fresh cilantro leaves
- 40 grams fresh mint sprigs, leaves removed and stems discarded

Directions:

1) Add chicken, curry paste, coconut oil and sea salt to a large saucepan. Saute on medium heat until outer pieces are white and interior is still pink.

2) Add coconut milk and coconut amino. Cover, increase heat to medium-high and bring to a boil. Once boiling, reduce heat to low and simmer for 15 minutes.

3)   Meanwhile, cook your spaghetti squash. Regardless of the method you choose, cut the squash in half lengthwise. Steam by Instant Pot for 10 minutes on the "steam" setting.

4)   For the curry, add tomatoes, green cabbage, spinach, mint, zucchini and onions. Cover and cook on low for another 10 minutes.

5)   Pour the coconut curry over top the squash bowls, add a dollop of pate and serve.

98.   Tasty Lemongrass Coconut Chicken

Time:1 hour 10 minutes

Servings:4-6 max

Ingredients:

- 1 thick stalk fresh lemongrass, papery outer skins and rough bottom removed, trimmed to the bottom 5 inches

- 4 cloves garlic, peeled and crushed

- 1 thumb-size piece of ginger, peeled and roughly chopped

- 5 tablespoons coconut aminos

- 1 teaspoon five spice powder

- 1 cup coconut milk (+¼ cup optional)

- 10 drumsticks, skin removed

- 1 teaspoon Diamond Crystal kosher salt

- ½ teaspoon freshly ground black pepper

- 1 teaspoon coconut oil

- 1 large onion, peeled and thinly sliced

- ¼ cup fresh cilantro, chopped

- Juice from 1 lime (optional)

Directions:

1)   Peel, trim, and smash the piece of lemongrass

2)   Combine the lemongrass, garlic, ginger, coconut aminos, and five-spice powder into a blender or food processor.

3)   Pour in the coconut milk and blitz until a smooth sauce forms

4)   Put the chicken drumsticks (without skin) into a large bowl and season with salt and pepper.

5)   Plug in your Instant Pot and press the "Saute" button to heat up the insert. (If you're using a stovetop pressure cooker, crank your burner to medium.)

6)   Drop in a teaspoon of coconut oil. When it melts, add the sliced onions

7)   Stir-fry the onions until they're translucent (3-5 minutes).

8)   Add the drumsticks to the pot and pour the marinade on top

9)   Press the "Cancel/Warm" button on the Instant Pot and lock the lid with the top dial pointed towards the sealed position

10)   Press the "Poultry" button and walk away. (If you're using a stovetop pressure cooker, lock the lid and increase the heat to high to bring the contents to high pressure. Once high pressure is reached, decrease the heat to low or enough to maintain high pressure. Set a timer for 15 minutes as your chicken cooks under high pressure.)

11)   When the stew finishes cooking, turn off the pressure heater (or turn off the heat) and release the pressure valve. Once the pressure drops, unlock the lid and taste for seasoning.

12)   Add a few splashes of coconut amino, a dash of salt, or a grind or two of black pepper

13)   Garnish with freshly chopped cilantro and a squeeze of fresh lime juice. Dig in!

99.   Pina Colada Chicken Mania

Time: 30 minutes

Yield: 4 servings

Ingredients

- 2 pounds Organic chicken thighs, cut into 1" chunks

- 1 cup fresh or frozen pineapple chunks

- 1/2 cup coconut cream

- 1 teaspoon cinnamon

- 1/8 teaspoon salt

- 2 tablespoons coconut aminos

- 1/2 cup chopped green onion (garnish)

Directions:

1)   Place all ingredients, except green onions, into Instant Pot.

2)   Close lid.

3)   Press Poultry button.

4)   Pot will automatically set itself for 15 minutes, high pressure.

5)   Allow to cook.

6)   Once cooking has stopped, turn off Instant Pot.

7)   Let pressure release naturally for 10 minutes.

8)   Carefully open lid and remove from pot.

9)   Stir.

10)   If you'd like to thicken the sauce a bit, simply stir in a teaspoon of arrowroot starch mixed with a tablespoon of water.

11)   Then, press the Saute button.

12)   Cook until sauce thickens to your liking.

13)   Turn off Instant Pot. Serve with green onion garnish.

100. Sweetheart Mango Chicken

Ingredients

- 1 tablespoon grass-feed butter

- 8 chicken breast

- 1/2 red onion, chopped

- 1 mango, cut into 1/2 inch chunks

- 4 cloves garlic, chopped

- Juice of 1 lime (about 2 tablespoons)

- 1/4 cup + 1 tablespoon coconut aminos, divided

- 1 piece of ginger, chopped fine

- 1/4 cup chopped cilantro

- 15 drops stevia

- 1/2 cup chicken broth

- 2 tablespoons lemon juice

- 1/2 teaspoon salt

- 1 green onion, sliced (green part only)

Directions:

1) With lid off, press sauté button on Instant Pot

2) Place cooking fat in pot.

3) Heat until melted.

4) Place chicken thighs, skin side down into pot.

5) Brown for about 3 minutes.

6)   Flip thighs over, and brown for about 2 minutes. Depending on the size of your chicken breast. Remove chicken and set aside.

7)   Add onion, mango and garlic to pot. Cook until onions are clear and mango has started to brown slightly.

8)   Turn off Instant Pot (press Cancel button).

9)   Place chicken breast back into pot, nestled into mango and onion mixture.

10)   Add lime juice, 1/4 cup coconut aminos, ginger, cilantro, stevia, chicken broth, and 1 tablespoon apple lemon juice to pot.

11)   Place lid on Instant Pot. Press Poultry button, then Pressure button twice, for high pressure setting. Timing will set automatically for 15 minutes.

12)   Once pressure cooking is done, and Instant Pot goes into Warming mode, turn pot off.

13)   Turn pressure valve to venting.

14)   Be sure all pressure is released from pot before opening lid.

15)   Open lid.

16)   Remove chicken breast from pot. Set aside.

17)   Add 1 tablespoon coconut aminos, 1 tablespoon lemon juice and salt to pot.

18)   Press Saute button.

19)   Cook sauce until it reduces into a thick sauce, about 10-15 minutes.

20)   Turn pot off.

21)   Serve chicken thighs with sauce ladled on top.

22)   Add green onion slices for garnish.

101. Sweetie Fruity Chicken Delight

Time:35 minutes

Serves:4 max

Ingredients

- 1 small head cabbage, cored and shredded

- 2 pounds boneless, skinless breasts

- 2 apples, cored and sliced

- 1/2 cup chicken broth

- 1 cup fresh or frozen cranberries

- 1 tablespoon apple cider vinegar

- 10-15 drops stevia

- 1 teaspoon cinnamon

- 1 teaspoon ground ginger

- 1/2 teaspoon salt + more, to taste

Directions:

1) In Instant Pot

2) Place all ingredients, in order above, into Instant Pot.

3) Close lid.

4) Press Poultry button.

5) Set time for 20 minutes.

6) Instant Pot will start cooking process.

7) When done cooking, press off button.

8) Allow pressure to release naturally for 10 minutes.

9) Open lid.

10) Serve.

102. Lemon Garlic Chicken

Serves:4-6 max

Time:30 minutes

Ingredients:

- 1-2 pounds chicken breasts

- 1 teaspoon sea salt

- 1 onion, diced

- 1 tablespoon coconut oil

- 5 garlic cloves, minced

- 1/2 cup organic chicken broth

- 1 teaspoon dried parsley

- 1/4 teaspoon paprika

- 1 large lemon juiced (or more to taste)

- 3-4 teaspoons arrowroot flour

Directions:

1)   Turn your Instant Pot onto the saute feature and place in the diced onion and cooking fat

2)   Cook the onions for 5-10 minutes or until softened. You can also choose to cook until they start to brown

3)   Add in the remaining ingredients except for the arrowroot flour and secure the lid on your Instant Pot

4)   Select the "Poultry" setting and make sure your steam valve is closed

5)   Allow cook time to complete, release steam valve to vent and then carefully remove lid

6)   At this point you may thicken your sauce by making slurry. To do this remove about 1/4 cup sauce from the pot, add in the arrowroot flour, and then reintroduce the slurry into the remaining liquid

7)   Stir and serve right away. This also reheats well as leftovers

103. Bufflicious Chicken

Time: 1 hour

Serves : 4-6 max

Ingredients:

- 1 pound organic pasture raised chicken breast (I used frozen)

- 1 onion, diced

- 3 tablespoons grass-feed butter

- 3 tablespoons coconut amino

- 16 ounces sweet potatoes, diced

- 1/2 teaspoon (or more) onion powder

- 1/2 teaspoon (or more) garlic powder

- Sea salt and pepper to taste

Directions:

1) Using the "Saute" feature on your Instant Pot, cook the onion in 1 tablespoon of grass-feed butter.

2) Once nicely browned, place your chicken, sweet potatoes, remaining butter, coconut amino, and spices into the pot.

3) Secure the lid and use the "Poultry" feature. Select the "Manual" setting, using high pressure Cook for 30 minutes.

4) Make sure the steam vent is closed and allow cooking for allotted time.

5) Once complete, quick release the steams vent and then remove the lid and serve.

6) Add 1-2 tablespoons of arrowroot flour to thicken the sauce and then reintroduce to the hot Instant Pot and stir.

104. Tasty Coconut Lemon Chicken Curry

Time: 4hour

Serves: 4-6 max

Ingredients

- 1 can coconut milk

- 1/4 cup lemon juice

- 1 tbsp curry spice

- 1 tsp turmeric powder

- 1/2 tsp sea salt

- 6 ethically raised chicken breasts

- 1 bunch coriander(chopped)

Directions:

1) Turn your slow cooker or crock pot onto high heat

2) Add all the ingredients to the slow cooker

3) Cook for 4 hours

4) Serve and enjoy

105. Luscious Chicken

Time: 32 minutes

Serves: 4-6 max

Ingredients

- 2-3 lbs boneless skinless chicken thighs (cut into bite-sized pieces)

- 1 Tbsp grass-feed butter

- 1½ large onions (chopped)

- 2½ - 3⅓ tsp salt

- 2 Tbsp fresh garlic (minced)

- 2 Tbsp fresh ginger (grated)

- 2 tsp turmeric

- 2 tsp paprika

- 1½ tsp cayenne powder

- 1½ - 2 cups stewed tomatoes

- 370 ml tomato paste

- 2 cans coconut milk

- 2 tsp garam masala

- ½ cup sliced almond

- ½ cup cilantro

Directions

1) If your pressure cooker has a sauté setting (as does the Instant Pot), use it to melt ghee.

2) Add 2 tsp salt and onions. Cook until onions are soft and translucent.

3) Add in garlic, ginger, turmeric, paprika and cayenne. Mix in and cook until fragrant.

4) Add stewed tomatoes and the watery portion of coconut milk, mixing thoroughly with spices (getting all of the spices stuck to the bottom off the pan).

5) Add chicken and stir well.

6) Assuming you've selected to use bite-sized pieces of chicken, the time to cook the chicken will be fast: 8-10 minutes depending on the pressure your cooker uses. With the Instant Pot it took 8 minutes of pressurized cooking time.

7) Once cooked, stir in coconut cream, tomato paste, gram masala and most of the cilantro. Add more salt if needed.

8) Top with sliced almonds and garnish with more cilantro.

106. Deli Tender Garlic Chicken

Time: 30 minutes

Servings: 4-6 max

Ingredients:

- 1 pound chicken breast

- 1/2 teaspoon sea salt

- 1 large onion, diced

- 2 1/2 tablespoon grass-feed butter

- 5 garlic cloves, (minced)

- 1/2 cup warm water

- 2 tablespoon chicken broth

- 1 teaspoon dried tarragon

- 3/4 large lemon juiced

- 3-4 teaspoons arrowroot starch

1) Sauté the onions in the Instant Pot with the grass-feed butter.

2) Add all the other ingredients except for the arrowroot starch.

3) Put in the chicken into the bottom of the pot.

4) Place some of the onions and ingredients over the chicken.

5) Close the Instant Pot, close the vent, turn off the Sauté setting.

6) Turn the Instant Pot on again by pressing the Poultry button.

7) Once you hear the 2 beeps, it is starting the cooking process and you can now walk away.

8)   Return when it beeps (about 15 minutes later) and release the vent valve. When the metal button is down, it is safe to open the lid.

9)   Take out 1/2 a cup of the broth and add it to the arrowroot starch in a mixing cup. Stir together well.

10)   Pour the mixture in to the Instant Pot and combine it well with everything else.   The contents of the pot will thicken.

107. Gorgeous Chicken Cacciatore Delight

Time: 30 minutes

Serves:4-6 max

Ingredients:

- Extra Virgin Olive Oil

- 3 Shallots, Chopped

- 4 Garlic Cloves, Crushed

- 1 Green Bell Pepper, seeded & diced

- 1/2 cup organic chicken broth

- 8-10 oz mushrooms, sliced

- 5-6 Boneless Skinless Chicken Breasts

- 2 Cans Organic Crushed Tomatoes

- 2 Tbsp Organic Tomato Paste

- 1 Can Pitted Black Olives

- Fresh Parsley

- ½ tsp Red Pepper to taste

- Sea Salt & Black Pepper to taste

Directions

1)   Heat the oil in a 4-quart or larger cooker. Add the shallots and bell pepper and cook over medium-high heat, stirring frequently, until the shallots soften slightly, about 2 minutes

2)   Stir in the broth and boil for 2-3 minutes. Scrape up any browned bits sticking to the bottom of the cooker.

3)   Stir in the mushrooms and garlic. Set the chicken on top. Cover the chicken with crushed tomatoes. Do not stir. Plop the tomato paste on top.

4)   Lock the lid in place.

5)   Over high heat bring to high pressure.

6)   Reduce the heat just enough to maintain high pressure and cook for 8 minutes.

7)   Turn off the heat.

8)   Allow the pressure to come down naturally. Remove the lid.

9)   Stir in the olives, parsley, red pepper flakes, salt and pepper.

108. Cajun Cauliflower Chicken

Time: 30 minutes

Serves: 4 max

Ingredients

- 1½ - 2 pounds rope sausage

- 1 Tablespoon Cajun seasoning (or to taste)

- 1 tsp. sea salt

- 4 Tbsp. grass-feed butter

- 2 cups cauliflower rice

- 3½ cups broth

- 1½ cups bell peppers, diced 2 small summer squash, seeded and diced

- 2 cups scallion greens or onions

- 1 bunch cilantro

Directions:

1) Mix seasoning and salt.

2) Sprinkle sausage with the seasoning mixture.

3) Heat butter in open pressure cooker on medium-high heat or in the Instant Pot on the saute feature.

4) Add sausage; cook and stir 3 minutes or until browned. Add onions if using; cook and stir 3 minutes or until softened.

5) Add broth and bring to a boil. Stir in rice, bell peppers, squash, greens, scallion greens. Close lid.

6)   Then, bring pressure cooker to full pressure on high heat. Cook 5 minutes. Remove from heat. Let stand 5 minutes. Release pressure and let sit 3 more minutes. Remove lid. Stir and serve. Top with chopped cilantro and Cajun seasoning.

109. Brown Rice Ginger Mushroom Chicken Congee With Scallop

Serves: 7 cups

Time: 1 hour 15 minutes

Ingredients:

- 1 rice measuring cup brown rice(180ml)

- 7 cup water

- 7 conpoy (dried scallops)

- 500gm steamed chicken breast(scraped)

- 1 tablespoon ginger (chopped)

- 50gm mushroom shitake(sliced)

- Salt to taste

Directions:

1. Firstly, rinse rice under cold water

2. Add 7 cups of water and ginger, mushroom, steamed chicken and conpoy into the pot.

3. Close lid and cook at high pressure for 30 minutes in an Electric Pressure Cooker.

4. Turn off the heat and Natural Release for 15 minutes. Manually release the remaining pressure by carefully turning the venting knob to the venting position. Open the lid carefully.

5. Add salt to taste.

6. Turn on the heat (Instant Pot: press sauté button) and stir the congee until the desire thickness.

7. Serve warm.

110. Tender Succulent Stewed Chicken

Servings: 8

Time: 1 hour 10 mins

Ingredients

- 3 lbs stew chicken breast (remove skin)

- 1/2 tsp salt

- 1/2 tsp black pepper

- 2 tbsp almond flour (optional)

- 2 tbsp grass-feed butter

- 1/2 onion, (diced)

- 2 cloves garlic, (minced)

- 2 tbsp tomato paste

- 3 cups bone broth

- 3 carrots (cut into chunks)

- 3 parsnips (cut into chunks)

- 3 celery stalks, (cut into chunks)

- 1.5 lbs sweet potato (cut into chunks)

- 3 sprigs fresh thyme (chopped)

- Salt and pepper to taste

- 1 small handful parsley, (chopped)

Directions

1. Combine the chicken, salt, pepper, and almond flour; toss to dust the chicken evenly.

2.   Add the grass-feed butter and warm until melted and shimmering, about 3 minutes.

3.   Add chicken and sauté until browned about 20 minutes.

4.   Then, add the onion and sauté until softened, about 4 minutes, then add the garlic and tomato paste. Sauté until aromatic, about 30 seconds, then add the broth.

5.   Bring to a simmer, scraping up any browned bits from the bottom of the pot. Add the chicken (and any accumulated juices), carrots, parsnips, celery, sweet potatoes, and thyme. Wait until it depressurizes, about 20 minutes

6.   After depressurizing, remove the lid and carefully remove the short and place on a plate, loosely cover with tin foil.

7.   Pour the braising liquid into a blender and blend until smooth, then transfer back to the pressure cooker. Bring to a simmer over medium heat about five minutes.

8.   Then add salt and pepper to taste

9.   Plate your dish by pouring the liquid into a shallow bowl and placing the ribs on top.

10.   Serve hot.

111. Zesty Herb Chicken Avocado Salad

Serves: 2-3 max

Time: 15minutes

Ingredients:

Marinade/Dressing

- 2 tablespoons olive oil

- juice of 1 lemon (1/4 cup fresh squeezed lemon juice)

- 2 tablespoons water

- 2 tablespoons balsamic vinegar

- 2 tablespoons fresh chopped parsley

- 2 teaspoons dried basil

- 2 teaspoons garlic, minced

- 1 teaspoon dried oregano

- 1 teaspoon salt

- cracked pepper, to taste

Salad

- 50gm chicken breasts

- 4 cups Romaine lettuce leaves, washed and dried

- 1 zucchini, diced

- ½ cup cherry tomatoes, (halves)

- 1 red onion, sliced

- 1 avocado, sliced

- ⅓ cup pitted Kalamata olives sliced

- Lemon wedges, to serve

Directions:

1.   Whisk together all of the dressing ingredients in a bowl.

2.   Pour ½ dressing to marinade chicken for two hours in the refrigerator.

3.   Then, prepare all of the salad ingredients and mix in a large salad bowl.

4.   Once chicken is ready, heat 1 tablespoon of oil in a grill pan or a grill plate over medium-high heat. Grill chicken on both sides until browned and completely cooked through.

5.   Allow chicken to rest for 5 minutes; slice and arrange over salad. Drizzle salad with the remaining dressing.

6.   Serve with lemon wedges.

112. Luxurious White Creamy Chick Stew

Time: 50 minutes

Serves 4-6

Ingredients

- 6 cups water

- 500g chicken breast, (steamed and scraped)

- 2 cups chicken broth

- 1 cup white onion, (diced)

- 2 cups white turnips (chopped)

- 1 cup or 2 carrots, (chopped)

- 1 cup baby corn

- 2 cups or 1 medium-ripe plantain, (peeled and halved)

- 2 garlic cloves, (peeled and chopped)

- 1 tsp sea salt, divided

- 1 bay leaf

- 1/2 tsp dried basil

- 1/2 tsp cinnamon (or a stick of cinnamon)

- 500mL coconut milk

- 1/4 cup coconut flour

- 8-10 drops stevia

- 2 cups broccoli, (cut into large florets)

Directions:

1. Select 'Sauté' function and adjust to 'more'

2. Add 6 cups water and bring to boil

3. Add chicken and allow to boil for 3 minutes before draining and setting aside

4. Add chicken broth, vegetables (except broccoli), 1/2 tsp sea salt, herbs and cinnamon

5. Stir to combine, cover, set valve to 'sealing' and select 'Manual' function for 15-20 minutes

6. Once cooking time is up, unseal lid by quick release and remove meat and vegetables from the pot and set aside, leaving broth in the pot

7. Select 'Sauté' function and add coconut milk, coconut flour, and stevia stirring to mix

8. Add broccoli florets and allow to simmer until cooked and gravy is thickened

9. Discard bay leaf and cinnamon stick (if using)

10. Return chicken and vegetables to gravy and stir gently to mix

11. Season with remaining 1/2 tsp sea salt or to taste and serve hot

113. Green Caribbean Dip Recipe

Serves: 6 max

Time: 30 minutes

Ingredients:

- 400gm artichoke hearts

- 3 cups baby spinach (blanched)

- 1/2 white onion (minced)

- 6 cloves garlic, minced

- 5 thick slices of bacon (cut into small pieces)

- ½ cup coconut milk

- Sea salt and freshly ground pepper

Directions:

1. Sauté the bacon bits in a skillet over a medium- heat until brown.

2. Add in the onion and garlic and sauté for 2 to 3 minutes.

3. Add in the artichokes and spinach and cook for an additional 3 minutes.

4. Remove from the heat and let it cool.

5. Pour in the coconut milk and combine well.

6. Refrigerate for at least 30 min, and serve with fresh vegetables.

114. Crushy Mushy Apple Ketchup

Serves: 6 max

Time: 1 hour 40 minutes

Ingredients:

- 25 red tomatoes (diced)
- 8 apples (peeled, seeded, and diced)
- 2 pears (peeled, seeded, and diced)
- 4 onions (diced)
- 2 bell peppers (seeded and diced)
- 1 cup apple cider vinegar;
- 1 teaspoon stevia
- 2 tbsp. pickling spices
- Sea salt

Directions:

1. Place the pickling spices in a piece of cheesecloth and tie tightly closed.

2. Combine all the ingredients, including the cheesecloth-wrapped spices, in a large saucepan placed over a medium-high heat.

3. Bring the ketchup to a boil, stirring frequently.

4. Lower the heat to medium and let simmer for about 1 hour, uncovered, stirring occasionally.

5. Remove the cheesecloth-wrapped spices. Pour into hot sterilized jars. Let cool and refrigerate.

115. Chunky Egg Salad Dip

Serves: 4 max

Time: 45 minutes

Ingredients:

- 4 hard-boiled eggs, peeled and coarsely chopped;

- ½ cup. paleo mayonnaise

- 1 tsp. Dijon mustard

- 2 tsp. fresh chives (minced)

- 2 tsp. fresh dill (minced)

- ¼ tsp. fresh basil (minced)

- ¼ tsp. garlic powder

- ¼ tsp onion powder

- 1 tsp. apple cider vinegar

- Sea salt and freshly ground black pepper

Directions:

1. Mash the eggs in a big bowl using a fork

2. Add all the remaining ingredients to the eggs and stir until everything is well combined

3. Season the salad to taste, stir and refrigerate.

4. Serve chilled, with vegetables for dipping.

116. Paleo Mayo

Serves: 1 cup

Time: 20 minutes

Ingredients

- 2 egg yolks;

- 1 cup olive oil

- 1 tsp Dijon mustard

- 4 tsp fresh lemon juice

- 1 pinch of salt

Directions:

1.   Place the egg yolks, 1 tsp of the lemon juice, the mustard and the pinch of salt in a bowl or in the bowl and whisk it by slowly drizzle the oil in.

2.   Continue pouring in the oil slowly, but steadily. An emulsion will eventually start to form and pour in the oil more quickly.

3.   The mayonnaise should be quite thick when all the oil is incorporated and add the remaining lemon juice and blend it in with the mayonnaise.

4.   Serve

117. Tomatillo Salsa Recipe

Serves: 4 max

Time: 10 minutes

Ingredients:

- 1/2 cup onion (chopped)

- 1 1/2 pound green tomatillos (husk removed)

- 1/2 teaspoon ground cumin

- 1/2 cup cilantro (chopped)

- 2 tbsp lime juice

- 2 jalapeño peppers, seeded and chopped;

- Salt and pepper to taste.

Directions:

1. Cut the tomatillos lengthwise and roast them either on the grill or for about 6 minutes under the broiler until the skin is a little dark.

2. Put the roasted tomatillos, onion, cilantro, cumin, lime juice and jalapeño in a blender

3. Blend or process until smooth puree.

4. Place in the refrigerator to cool and enjoy.

118. Versatile Lemon Vinaigrette

Serves: 2-5 max

Time: 25 minutes

Ingredients:

- ¾ cup lemon juice

- 2 tsp Dijon mustard(optional)

- 1 garlic clove(minced)

- ¾ cup extra-virgin olive oil

- 2 tsp fresh oregano(minced)

- Sea salt and freshly ground black pepper to taste

Directions:

1. In a small bowl, whisk all the ingredients except the oil.

2. Then, add the oil slowly while whisking vigorously until it emulsified. Refrigerate for 10 minutes

3. Shake well before using.

119. Strawberry Citric Vinaigrette

Serves: 4 max

Time: 25 minutes

Ingredients:

- 1 cup strawberries

- 1/4 cup apple cider vinegar

- 1/4 cup extra-virgin olive oil

- 1 tbsp Dijon mustard

- 1 clove garlic (minced)

- 1/4 tsp salt

- 1/4 tsp pepper

Directions:

1. Preheat your oven to 425° F.

2. Rinse the strawberries and remove the stems. Line a baking sheet with foil, folding the edges up so that you create a small wall on all sides to prevent any juices from running out.

3. Place in the oven and roast for 15- 20 minutes

4. Then, add all the ingredients to a blender.

5. Ensure the juices draws out of the berries while roasting.

6. Purée the mixture until smooth and consistent.

7. Serve cold and keep refrigerated.

120. Ruby Cranberry Relish

Time: 15 minutes

Serves: 3-5 max

Ingredients:

- 2 cups raw cranberries;
- 2 apples, skinned and cored;
- 1 large seedless orange (peel slices)
- 15 drops stevia

Directions:

1. Blend the cranberries, apples, and orange until obtain a relish consistency place In a bowl
2. Then, add the stevia and combine well.
3. Transfer to a bowl, refrigerate and serve when needed.

121. Flaming Sardine Spread

Serves: 3- 4 max

Time: 45 minutes

Ingredients:

- 1 bulb garlic (head removed)

- 1 small onion(halves)

- 1 red chili(chopped)

- 12 sardine fillets

- 2 tbsp capers

- 1 tbsp parsley

- 2 tbsp apple cider vinegar

- 4 tbsp lemon juice

- 12 tbsp extra-virgin olive oil

- A few extra dashed of olive oil for roasted garlic

- Sea salt and freshly cracked black pepper to taste

Directions:

1.   Preheat your oven to 400°F.

2.   Cut off the very top portion of the bulb; place the bulb on a sheet of aluminum foil, drizzle with olive oil and sprinkle with salt and pepper.

3.   Place foiled garlic and onion on a baking sheet and bake for 35 minutes, until the bulb is tender.

4.   Remove the bulb from the oven, open the foil immediately and let it cool.

5.   Once they have cooled, pop each individual clove out.

6.   Then, add the roasted garlic and onion, sardines, parsley, chili, lemon juice, capers and apple cider vinegar into a small blender and blend until a smooth paste

7.   Taste and add some salt and pepper to taste.

8.   Continue blending and slowly pour in the olive oil when a smooth sauce will begin to take shape.

9.   Serve immediately

122. Smashed Cauliflower

Serves: 4 max

Time: 45 minutes

Ingredients:

- 6 cups cauliflower florets

- 4 bacon slices (cooked and crumbled)

- 2 green onions (sliced)

- 2 garlic cloves (minced)

- 2 tsp grass-feed butter

- Sea salt and freshly ground black pepper;

Directions:

1. Boil water in saucepan

2. Add the cauliflower and simmer 15 minutes.

3. Drain the water and return the cauliflower to the saucepan.

4. Add the grass-feed butter and season to taste.

5. Purée the cauliflower with a hand mixer until smooth.

6. Serve the mashed cauliflower topped with the green onions and bacon.

123. Zesty Carrot Confire

Serves: 4 max

Time: 3 hours

- 2 pounds carrots (1 inch pieces)
- Zest of 1 lemons;
- 8 tbsp lemon juice
- 4 cloves garlic (finely minced)
- 3 sprigs thyme
- 2 cups grass-feed butter

Directions:

1. Preheat oven to 275° F.

2. Arrange the carrots on baking tray

3. Mix the zest, lemon juice, garlic, thyme and grass-feed butter.

4. Pour the mixture on the carrots by completely covered.

5. Put in the oven for about two and a half hours.

6. Remove from oven. At this point, the carrots will be soft

7. As an optional step before serving, brown the carrots in a large skillet with the fat mixture that was used to cook them. This will create a crispy exterior and a tender interior.

124. Smashed Carrots Beet

Serves: 4 max

Time: 35 minutes

Ingredients:

- 1 lb. carrots, peeled and chopped;

- 1 lb. rutabaga, peeled and chopped;

- 4 tbsp. grass-feed butter

- 1 tbsp. fresh parsley, minced;

- Sea salt and freshly ground black pepper to taste;

Directions:

1. Place the carrots and rutabaga in a large saucepan and cover with water.

2. Bring to a boil and reduce to a simmer; then cover and let simmer for 20 minutes until soft.

3. Drain the water.

4. Mash the carrots and rutabaga with a potato masher; add the grass-feed butter and season to taste.

5. Serve and sprinkle with fresh parsley on top.

125. Petozuuchu Mango Salsa

Time: 20 minutes

Serves: 4

Ingredients

- 1 large ripe peach(cubed)
- ½ cup tomato cherry(sliced)
- 1 medium onion(chopped)
- 1 medium zucchini(chopped)
- 1 ripe mango (cubed)
- ½ tsp minced garlic
- ¼ tsp black pepper
- ¼ tsp salt
- 3 tbsp lemon juice
- 1 tbsp cilantro

Directions:

1. Transfer all the fruits and vegetable to the bowl
2. Combine well with the salt, pepper and lemon juice.
3. Add more salt and pepper if required
4. Serve

126. Spiced Baba Ganoush

Time: 40 min

Serves: 3

- 3 medium eggplant
- 4 garlic cloves, medium sized
- ¼ cup almond butter
- 3 tbsp lemon juice, freshly squeezed
- 2 tbsp olive oil
- 1/8 tsp cayenne (optional)
- 2 tbsp fresh parsley(chopped)
- 1 tsp black pepper
- 1 tsp sea salt

Directions:

1. Preheat oven to 425°F. Place the eggplant on a baking sheet and roast until eggplant is soft for 40 minutes.

2. Peel off the outer skin of the eggplant and place the flesh in a blender.

3. Add the garlic, almond butter, lemon, olive oil, salt, pepper and cayenne to the food processor and blend until mixture is smooth and creamy.

4. Drizzle olive oil on top and sprinkle fresh parsley and sea salt if desired.

127. Versatile Roasted Cauliflower Dip

Time:35 mins

Serves: 4

Ingredients

- 1 cauliflower (stems removed and boiled)

- 4tbsp extra virgin olive oil

- 2 cloves of garlic

- 3 tbsp grated almond cheese

- 1 tsp grounded white pepper

- Salt to taste

Directions:

1. Preheat the oven at 400° F

2. Place the boiled cauliflower on a baking pan and season with salt to taste, 2 tbsp of olive oil and crushed garlic cloves.

3. Bake for 15 minutes; Then, broil until golden brown.

4. Blend the cauliflower and garlic along with the grated almond cheese, 2 tbsp of olive oil,

3 tbsp of water and grounded white pepper until smooth and consistent.

5. Serve

128. Orange Tomato Salsa

Time:15 minutes

Serves:1 cup

Ingredients:

- 1 pound tomatillos (husked, rinsed, and halved)

- 3/4 cup shallots (minced)

- 1 tbsp coconut amino

- 3 cloves garlic(minced)

- 2 medium seedless oranges(cubed)

- 1 tbsp olive oil

- 1/4 cup finely chopped fresh cilantro leaves and tender stems

- 1 tablespoon lime juice

- 2 tbsp apple cider vinegar

- 1 tsp Kosher salt, to taste

- 1 tsp pepper

Directions:

1) Heat olive oil in saucepan over medium heat. Saute garlic and shallots until soft

2) Add tomatillos, orange, lime juice, coconut amino, apple cider vinegar, salt and pepper.

3) Simmer over low heat to 10 minutes, stir well

4) Serve

129. Roasted Nutty Chia Guacamole

Time: 40 mins

Serves: 2

Ingredients

- 50gm cashew nuts (roasted)

- 50 gm almond(roasted)

- 1 ripe avocado

- 2 tbsp diced onion

- ½ tsp lime juice

- 1 tsp chia seeds

- salt to taste

Directions:

1)   Add the roasted almond, cashew nuts, avocado, lime juice and chia seeds to the food processor and puree until smooth.

2)   Serve

130. Vegan Cashew Cheese Recipe

TIME: 7 mins

Serves: 1-2 max

Ingredients

- 200gm baby carrots

- 1 cup of cashew nuts (soaked overnight)

- 2 tbsp almond starch

- 2 tablespoons nutritional yeast

- ¼ tsp of Himalayan pink salt

- 1tsp of Black pepper

- 2tbsp lemon juice

- ¼ of water

Directions:

1) Pour of the ingredients into a food processor and pulse on high speed until soft and creamy.

2) Serve with sliced carrot sticks

131. Mangolicious Chutney

Time: 40 mins

Serves: 4-5

Ingredients

- 2-3 large mangoes (cubed)

- 1 teaspoons fresh ginger (finely minced)

- ½ cup chopped onions

- ½ -teaspoon garlic minced

- 1 medium Jalapenos pepper(diced)

- 1 bell pepper(diced)

- ½ teaspoon ground coriander

- ½ teaspoon ground cardamom

- ¼ teaspoon ground cloves

- ½ tsp cumin

- ¼ teaspoon ground nutmeg

- Salt to taste

- 1 teaspoon stevia

- ½ cup apple cider vinegar

- ½ cup water

Directions:

1) Combine mangoes, ginger, garlic, onions, bell pepper, jalapenos, spices, stevia and apple cider vinegar in a large stainless steel sauce- pan.

2)   Bring to a boil, then cook, uncovered for about 20 minutes or more, until tender and the sauce thickens.

3)   Remove let it cool, refrigerate and start using- with last more than a month in the fridge, covered

132. Tomatolicious Relish

Time: 35 mins

Serves: 4-5

Ingredients

- 500gm ripe tomatoes

- 1 teaspoon fresh ginger (finely minced)

- ½ cup chopped onions

- ½ -teaspoon garlic minced

- 1 red chili(chopped)

- ½ teaspoon ground coriander

- ½ teaspoon ground cardamom

- ¼ teaspoon ground cloves

- ½ tsp cumin

- ¼ teaspoon ground nutmeg

- Salt to taste

- 1 teaspoon stevia

- ½ cup apple cider vinegar

- ½ cup water

Directions:

1)   Combine mangoes, ginger, garlic, onions, chili, spices, stevia and apple cider vinegar in a large stainless steel sauce- pan.

2)   Bring to a boil, then cook, uncovered for about 20 minutes or more, until tender and the sauce thickens.

3)   Remove let it cool, refrigerate and start using- with last more than a month in the fridge,
covered

133. Beecapple Dip

Time: 15min

Serves: 8

Ingredients:

- 2 medium sized beetroots (cubed)
- 1 carrot (chopped)
- 1 Fiji red apple (cubed)
- 1 cup macadamia nuts
- 2tbsp extra virgin olive oil
- 1 pinch of salt
- ¼ cup water

Directions:

1) Place the beetroot, carrot and apple pieces in small pot.

2) Add water a bit and bring to the boil over a medium heat. Scrape the sides of the pot to prevent from sticking.

3) While beets, carrot and apple 'cook', puree the macadamia nuts and oil with a handheld blender or pop in a

4) Puree until the mixture has a smooth consistency.

134. Grilled Spiced Eggplant Dip

Time: 50 minutes

Serves: 4-6 max

Ingredients

- 1 large eggplant

- 1 head garlic

- 1 medium onion

- 1 ginger

- 1/2 cup diced roasted red peppers

- 3 tablespoons olive oil

- 2 tablespoons lemon juice

- 1 tablespoon chopped coriander

- Sea salt and fresh ground pepper to taste

Directions:

1) Preheat grill to 400 °C

2) Slice top off of garlic, onion and peel the ginger drizzle with olive oil, and sprinkle with sea salt. Wrap in foil and place on grill over indirect heat.

3) Roast until soft and caramelized, 35minutes.Set aside

4) Place eggplant on grill and roast with lid closed, turning occasionally, until eggplant is soft, 30 - 45 minutes.

5) Cut eggplant in half and place in colander to drain and cool.

6) Peel and dice eggplant.

7) Blend the garlic and onion smoothly.

223

8)   Combine eggplant, onion garlic ginger mixture, peppers, 3 tablespoons olive oil, lemon juice, basil, salt, and pepper. Taste and adjust seasonings.

9)   Garnish with an extra drizzle of olive and coriander

135. Opassiche Salsa

Time: 12 minutes

Serves :10

Ingredients:

- 2 cups cherries (stemmed and pitted)

- 1 cup passion fruit(pulp)

- 1 cup peach (peeled and chopped)

- 1 cup red onions (finely chopped)

- 1 cup green bell pepper (finely chopped)

- 1 whole jalapeno (finely chopped)

- ½ tsp salt

- ½ tsp lemon juice

- ¼ cup cilantro (finely chopped)

Directions:

1) Coarsely grind cherries in the food processor with the chop option.

2) Now, combine all the ingredients in a mixing bowl and mix gently with a spoon.

3) Serve

136. Simple Minty Corn Dip

Serves: 3-4max

Ingredients:

- 3 cups organic frozen corn kernels

- ½ organic lemon zest

- 4 tbsp. lemon juice

- 1 large clove garlic(minced)

- ¼ cup packed mint leaves

- 2 tbsp. extra virgin olive oil

- 1-2 tbsp. almond butter

- ¼ tsp. sea salt

Directions:

1) Boil the corn kernels and add some salt into it for 2-3 minutes. Plunge them into an ice bath or very cold water to halt the cooking process. Set aside.

2) Mix other ingredients well until it well combined

3) Blend the corn and the mixed ingredients until smooth and consistent

4) Serve and consume immediately

137. Savory Salmon Melon

Time: 1 hour

Serves: 2 max

Ingredients:

For Fish

- 1" thick watermelon

- 1 tablespoon olive oil

- Sea salt

- 2 salmon flank

- 1 tsp salt

- 1 tsp ground cumin

- 1 tsp paprika powder

- 1 tsp onion powder

- ½ tsp ancho chili powder

- 1 tsp black pepper

For Sauce:

- ¼ cup sweet chili sauce

- 1 teaspoon Sirach sauce

- 2 tablespoons coconut amino

- 2 tablespoons balsamic vinegar

- 1 tablespoon dark coconut oil

Directions:

1. Rub the salmon with salt, chili powder, cumin, paprika, onion and black pepper

2. Refrigerate for 30 minutes

3. Heat olive oil in skillet to medium heat

4. Add watermelon and flip for 2 minutes until its caramelize.

5. Keep heat on and add fish to skillet used for watermelon; leave residual juices and oil in there.

6. Sauté for approximately 5 -6 minutes until fish is lightly browned on the outside, firm and flaky.

7. In a small bowl, whisk together chili sauce, Sirach sauce, coconut amino, balsamic vinegar, and oil. Pour over fish during last 2 minutes of cooking to glaze salmon and warm up.

8. Serve the fish on watermelon and spoon the sauce from pan to the fish.

138. Tropical Grilled Swordfish

Time: 2 max

Serves: 30 minutes

Ingredients:

- 2 wild swordfish steaks

- 1 avocado, diced

- 1 mango, diced

- 1 tbsp. cilantro, chopped

- 2 tsp olive oil

- ½ lemon(juice)

- 1 tsp salt

- 1 tsp ground cumin

- 1 tsp paprika powder

- 1 tsp onion powder

- 1 tsp black pepper

- 1 grapefruit peeled and sliced (optional)

- 1/2 cup balsamic vinegar (optional)

Directions:

1.   Season the fish with cumin, onion powder, paprika powder, garlic powder, black pepper and salt

2.   Preheat an outdoor grill for medium-high heat and lightly oil grate.

3.   Grill the fish for 6-8 minutes

4.   Dice the mango and avocado in small cubes.

5.   Toss mango and avocado with chopped cilantro and lime juice, and 1/2 tablespoon of oil.

6.   To serve, place the fish on grapefruit slices and top with salsa.

139. Flaming Cod with Ribbon Salad

Time: 30 minutes

Serving size:1 max

Ingredients

- 1 fillet of cod, cut into serving size pieces

- Salt and pepper

- 1 tsp oregano

- 1 small ginger (paste)

- 3 cloves garlic (minced)

- 2 tbsp olive oil

- 2 zucchinis, cut into ribbons

- ¼ yellow bell peppers (thinly sliced)

- ¼ red bell peppers (thinly sliced)

- ¼ cup balsamic vinegar

- 1 tbsp coconut amino

- 6 drops stevia

- 1 tbsp olive oil

Directions

1.   Season the cod pieces with salt, pepper, oregano and the ginger and garlic and set aside.

2.   Steam the zucchini and peppers for 3 minutes, rinse with cold water, drain and pat dry, then place in a mixing bowl.

3.   Whisk together the fresh ginger, vinegar, coconut amino, lemon juice, stevia and olive oil, then pour over the zucchini and peppers, blending well. Refrigerate until ready to serve.

4.   Fry the cod in the olive oil until cooked and serve with the zucchini salad.

140. Wonder Tomatillo Salsa with Halibut Delight

Serves:4 max

Time:30 minutes

Ingredients

For fish

- 4 halibut fillets
- 1 tablespoon olive oil
- kosher salt
- fresh cracked black pepper
- Zest of 2 lemons
- 1/4 cup freshly squeezed lemon juice
- 3 tablespoons olive oil

For sauce

- 1 cup cherry tomatoes
- 6-8 medium tomatillos
- 2 large tomatoes
- 2 large, firm peaches, (halves)
- 2 jalapeño peppers
- 3 cloves garlic
- 1 small red onion
- ¼ cup chopped, fresh cilantro, more for garnish
- 2 tablespoons fresh parsley (chopped)

- 2 tablespoons lime juice

- 3/4 teaspoon salt

- ½ teaspoon cayenne pepper

Directions

1. Place the vegetables under baking tray roast until its turn golden brown for 10 minutes

2. Allow the roasted ingredients to cool slightly and place in a food processor with the lime juice, chopped cilantro, parsley, salt and cayenne pepper.

3. Dice red onion, tomatillos, tomato and peach. Add to the smooth salsa along with one clove of minced garlic, and minced fresh jalapeño pepper.

4. Chill, garnish with fresher cilantro and serve.

5. Heat olive oil in skillet to medium heat

6. Sauté fillets until golden and cooked through, about 5-7 minutes per side.

7. Remove from heat; transfer fillets to a platter. Cover with aluminum foil to keep warm.

8. Add olive oil, to pan and melt. Let it cook a minute or two on lower heat until it begins to bubble. Add the lemon juice and zest and remove pan from heat. Pour sauce over fillets.

141. Coconut Fish Curry Delight

Time:20 minutes

Serves:4 max

Ingredients:

- 2 tsp coconut oil

- 1 large onion, chopped

- 2 cloves garlic, minced

- 1 tbsp fresh ginger, minced

- 1 tsp garam masala

- 1 tsp ground coriander

- 1 tsp ground cumin

- 1/2 tsp turmeric

- 4 tbsp curry powder

- 1 tbsp cayenne powder

- 1 cup tomatoes(halves)

- 1 can coconut milk

- 1/2 - 2 jalapeno peppers, sliced and to taste

- salt, if needed

- 2 lb firm white fish

- 2 tbsp fresh cilantro, chopped

Directions:

1. Heat the coconut oil, add the onion and cook until slightly brown

2.   Stir in the garlic, ginger, curry powder, garam masala, coriander, cumin, turmeric and cayenne powder.

3.   Cook for 2 minutes until the spices are very fragrant.

4.   Then stir in the tomatoes, coconut milk and jalapeno pepper.

5.   Bring the mixture to a simmer, then reduce the flame to low, cover the pot and cook for about an hour. Taste and add salt, if needed.

6.   Cut the fish into bite sized pieces and add to the curry. Cook for another 3-6 minutes or until the fish is cooked through.

7.   Remove from heat and sprinkle with the cilantro.

142. Crusted Halibut Fillets

Serves:2max

Time:25 minutes

Ingredients

- 1lb halibut fillets

- 1cup almond flour

- ¼ teaspoon sea salt

- ¼ teaspoon ground black pepper

- 1 egg beaten

- 1 tablespoon coconut oil

Directions:

1. Season the fish with almond flour with sea salt (optional) and freshly ground black pepper; stir to combine.

2. Dip each fillet in egg and then in almond flour mixture. Coat each fillet completely.

3. In skillet, heat coconut oil over medium-high heat.

4. Fry fillets in coconut oil for 2-3 minutes per side, or until fish flakes easily with a fork.

143. Baked Salmon Avocadolicious

Time:25 minutes

Serves:2 max

Ingredients:

- 2 salmon flank

- ½ cup ground almond

- ½ teaspoon coriander (chopped)

- ½ teaspoon cumin

- 1medium lemon(s), juiced

- ¼ teaspoon sea salt

- 1/8 teaspoon ground black pepper

- 3 tablespoon fresh cilantro

- 1 tablespoon coconut oil

Directions:

1. Preheat the oven to 350 F.

2. Combine almond meal, coriander and cumin in a small bowl.

3. Sprinkle the salmon with the lemon juice and season with salt and pepper.

4. Coat each salmon with the ground almond

5. Place skin side down on a broiler pan, greased lightly with coconut oil.

6. Bake for 12-15 minutes or until salmon flakes easily with a fork.

7. Top with freshly chopped cilantro before serving.

144. Spiced Baked Tuna Mushroom Cup Delight

Ingredients

- 2medium mushrooms Portobello

- 2 can sustainably source tuna in water

- 1 small onion(chopped)

- 1 chili(chopped)

- 2 cloves garlic(chopped)

- ¼ tsp cayenne pepper

- ¼ tsp garlic powder

- ¼ tsp ground black pepper

- 2 tbsp capers, rinsed

- 2 tsp fresh dill, chopped

- 1 tbsp coconut oil

- 1 avocado (sliced)

Directions

1. Preheat oven to 450°F.

2. Mix tuna, garlic, onion, chilli, cayenne, garlic powder, black pepper, dill (optional) and capers together in a bowl, then stuff into portobello caps.

3. Place caps on a lightly greased baking sheet and bake for 15-20 minutes (or until tops are browned and portobello cap has softened slightly).

4. Top with sliced avocado and serve warm.

145. Krunch Baked Salmon Kale Salad

Ingredients:

- 1 bunch kale, chopped

- ¾ lb salmon fillet

- 4 slices bacon, cooked and crumbled

- ½ medium yellow onion (thin-slice)

- ¼ cup almonds, (roasted and sliced)

- ¼ cup cashew nuts (roasted and halves)

- ¼ cup olive oil

- 2 tbsp lemon juice

Directions:

1. Preheat oven to 425°F.

2. Season both sides of fresh salmon filets with sea salt and black pepper

3. Place the filets on a wire rack over a baking sheet and place in the oven.

4. Bake 15-18 minutes until salmon flakes easily with fork

5. Set aside to cool and the break into flakes.

6. Put the kale in a large bowl and massage the greens for a 1-2 minutes to break up the fibers.

7. Add the cooked and cooled salmon, cooked bacon, onions, cashew nuts and almonds to the bowl and toss. Whisk the oil and lemon juice together and toss with the salad before serving.

146. Crazy Coconut Milky Salmon Delight

Serves: 2 max

Time: 40 minutes

Ingredients

- 1 lb salmon

- ¼ tsp sea salt, (optional)

- ¼ tsp ground black pepper

- 2 tsp coconut oil

- 1 onion (diced)

- 2 cloves garlic (minced)

- 1 lemon, (zest and juice)

- ½ cup coconut milk

- 2 tbsp basil(chopped)

Directions:

1. Preheat oven to 350° F.

2. Place salmon in a shallow baking dish and sprinkle both sides with sea salt and freshly ground black pepper.

3. Heat a medium sauté pan over medium heat. When pan is hot, add coconut oil, garlic and onions. Sauté until garlic and shallots soften, about 3-5 minutes.

4. Mix lemon zest, lemon juice, coconut milk and boil

5. Reduce heat and add basil.

6. Pour over salmon and bake uncovered for about 10-20 minutes

147. Salmon Baked Sweet Potato

Cooking time: 50 minutes

Serves: 5-7 max

Ingredients

- 2 pounds Sweet potatoes – (peeled and chopped)
- 3oz chopped smoked salmon
- 2 tbsp spring onions(minced)
- 1 tbsp capers
- ½ cup shredded almond cheese

Directions:

1. Insert the steamer rack into the Instant pot

2. Add about 1 cup of water into the Instant pot

3. Add sweet potatoes

4. Close lid and turn the sealing vent to "sealed"

5. Click the "manual" button and reduce the time to 10 minutes

6. While the sweet potatoes is cooking, mix almond cheese with 3oz chopped smoked salmon add some pepper to taste.

7. Add 1 tablespoon capers and minced red onion. Spoon onto baked potatoes.

148. Salmon Avocado Cheesy Bites Delight

Serves: 4 max

Time: 1 hour

Ingredients:

- 1 pound sweet potatoes (1 – 1½ inch cubes)
- 2 tablespoons of grass-feed butter
- Freshly ground black pepper
- ¼ cup minced Italian parsley
- 1 tbsp lemon juice
- 1 cup almond cheese(grated)
- 150gm bacon bits
- Spring onions(garnish)
- 2 medium avocados, peeled, pitted, and diced
- 2 tablespoons coconut yogurt
- 1 ounces smoked salmon(chopped)

Directions

1. Preheat oven to 400°F
2. Slice the potatoes and place on the parchment paper in the baking tray
3. Melt the grass-feed butter and brush onto the sweet potatoes
4. Bake the potatoes until crispy about 15-20 minutes
5. Then, sprinkle with cheese and bacon bites
6. Bake for 10 more minutes

7.   Mix avocado, coconut yogurt, lemon juice, pepper and parsley until well mashed.

8.   Add piece of smoked salmon, another dollop of avocado sauce, and a sprinkle with spring onions.

149. Yummy Salmon Frittata

Time: 30 minutes

Serving: 2

Ingredients

- 1 tablespoon coconut oil

- 1 zucchini (julienned)

- 2 tablespoon chives (chopped)

- 3oz salmon (smoked and chopped)

- 1 onion(chopped)

- 3 cloves garlics (chopped)

- 4 eggs

- ¼ teaspoon fresh basil (chopped)

- ¼ teaspoon red pepper flakes (crushed)

- Salt and freshly ground black pepper (to taste)

Directions:

1) Preheat the oven to 355°F

2) In a skillet, add olive oil on medium heat

3) Add chopped zucchini and cook about 3-4 minutes

4) In a bowl, whisk the eggs.

5) Add smoked salmon, zucchini, basil, red pepper flakes, salt, black pepper and beat well

6) Bake in preheated 355°F oven until set but still moist in centre for 30 minutes.

7) Serve hot.

150. Zesty Salmon Frittata

Time: 30 minutes

Serving: 2

Ingredients

- 1 tablespoon coconut oil

- 1 zucchini (julienned)

- 250gm chicken breast (chopped)

- 200gm sweet potato(grated)

- 1 small head broccoli (chopped small)

- 4 eggs

- ¼ teaspoon fresh basil (chopped)

- ¼ teaspoon red pepper flakes (crushed)

- Salt and freshly ground black pepper (to taste)

Directions:

1) Preheat the oven to 355°F

2) In a bowl, whisk the eggs.

3) In a skillet, add coconut oil on medium heat

4) Saute chicken about 3-4 minutes. Followed by broccoli for 5 minutes.

5) Add red pepper flakes, salt, black pepper and beat well

6) Bake in preheated 355°F oven until set but still moist in center for 30 minutes.

7) Serve hot.

151. Hot Fish Fingers

Serves: 4 max

Time:20 minutes

Ingredients

- 1 lb dory fish
- 2 Eggs (whisked)
- 2 cup Almond flour
- 1 tsp onion powder
- 1 tsp garlic powder
- 1 tsp oregano
- 1 tsp salt
- ½ tsp pepper
- 2 cup Coconut oil

Directions:

1. Crack 2 eggs into a bowl, and gently whisk until they combine.
2. Put almond flour and mix in seasonings in a bowl
3. Heat coconut oil on the stove.
4. Batter the fish and fry until golden brown.

152. Fish-O-Chunky Omelet

Time:20 minutes

Servings:4 max

Ingredients:

- 4 large eggs

- 2 oz tuna(drained)

- 2 tbsp coconut cream

- 1 tbsp olive oil

- 30gm broccoli(florets)

- ¼ cup kale leaves(chopped)

- ¼ cup cherry tomatoes, halved

- Salt and pepper to taste

Directions:

1. Heat olive oil in skillet add broccoli, kale and cherry tomatoes.

2. Add some salt and pepper to taste

3. Cook 1-2 minutes until it becomes soft

4. Whisk the egg and coconut cream and pour on the vegetables

5. When the egg is almost cook add in the drained tuna and some salt and pepper to taste

6. Serve

153. Yummy Salmon Cauliflower Rice

Servings:4 max

Time:10 minutes

Ingredients

- 1 salmon fillet
- 1cup Cauliflower Rice
- 1 tbsp coconut oil
- 2 tbsp grass-feed butter
- ¼ tablespoon chopped fresh Parsley
- ¼ tablespoon chives
- 1teaspoon sea salt (real salt)
- 1/4teaspoon black pepper
- 1 cup chicken broth
- 1 medium lemon, juiced
- ½ cup tomato cherry
- ½ bell pepper(sliced)
- 4 cloves garlic (minced)

Directions:

1. Preheat oven to 425˚F
2. Coat salmon fillets with coconut oil
3. Add salt, pepper and lemon chives on salmon and flip the fish for 2-3 minutes.
4. Set aside

5.   Melt the grass-feed butter and add chopped garlic, bell pepper and cherry tomatoes and cook till tender, salt as needed and cook 2 minutes

6.   Add additional 1 Tbsp of grass-feed butter to pan and add cauliflower rice

7.   Toss to combine and coat

8.   Add two cups of chicken broth to pan and raise heat to high

9.   cook until broth boils off and rice is tender

10.   Once cauliflower rice is tender add all herbs, lemon zest and juice from ½ lemon

11.   Salt and pepper to taste

12.   Toss to combine and let sit on low heat for 10 minutes

13.   Meanwhile Add skillet of salmon to oven and bake for 10-15 minutes depending on thickness of cut

14.   Pull out and serve salmon over cauliflower rice and vegetables

154. Emerald Mousse with Smoked Salmon

Serves: 6 max

Time: 20 minutes

Ingredients:

- 1 lb. asparagus, trimmed;

- 8 oz. smoked salmon, thinly sliced;

- ¼ tsp Fresh rosemary (to garnish)

- ¼ tsp Fresh thyme(to garnish)

- 1/4 cup coconut milk;

- 2 tbsp. gelatin powder;

- 1/2 tsp. garlic powder;

- Sea salt and freshly ground black pepper;

Directions:

1. Boil the asparagus and add some salt into it.

2. Cook until very soft, about 8 to 10 minutes.

3. Drain the water, keeping 1/4 cup of the warm water in a separate bowl.

4. Mix the gelatin powder to the warm water and stir until well dissolved.

5. Puree the asparagus until smooth using an immersion blender, adding some fresh water if too thick.

6. Add the coconut milk and garlic powder; season to taste with salt and pepper; blend again until well combined.

7. Pour in the gelatin water; whisk until well blended.

8. Place the mixture into individual serving glasses and refrigerate 2 to 3 hours; until set.

9.   Top each glass with the smoked salmon and fresh rosemary and thyme.

155. Grilled Zesty Salmon Stick

Time:25 minutes

Serves:4 max

Ingredients:

- 1 1/2 lb. salmon fillet, skinless (sliced 1 inch thick)

- 1-2 limes, thinly sliced;

- 1 lemon, thinly sliced;

- 4 tbsp. olive oil

- 2 tbsp. fresh oregano(chopped)

- 1 tsp. ground cumin

- Sea salt and freshly ground black pepper;

- Wood skewers

Directions:

1. Preheat grill to medium heat.

2. Thread the salmon, lime, and lemon onto a skewer, alternating.

3. Brush the skewers with olive oil.

4. Season the skewers with oregano, cumin, sea salt and black pepper.

5. Cook the skewers for 8 to 10 minutes, flip every 2 minutes.

156. Marvellous Grilled Herb Fish

Serves: 3 max

Time:40 minutes

Ingredients:

- Two 3/4 lb whole medium trouts, scaled, gutted and cleaned,

- 1 tbsp grass-feed butter

- 1 bunch fresh flat leaf parsley;

- 1 bunch fresh dill;

- Zest of one lemon;

- 2 lemons, one sliced and the other halved;

- Salt and pepper to taste;

Preparation

1. Preheat the broiler.

2. Rub the trouts with butter and season with salt and pepper.

3. Stuff the cavity with the chopped parsley, dill and lemon slices.

4. Put the fish on a baking rack on a pan for the drippings.

5. Sprinkle the lemon zest on top of the fish and add generous knobs of butter on the fish to form a golden crust.

6. Grill at about 6 inches from the heat source for about 6 minutes on each side.

7. Squeeze the roasted lemons on the fish

8. Serve

157. Extravagance Strawberry Chocolate Bar

Time: 1 hour

Serves: 6

Ingredients:

- 6 eggs

- 1 tsp vanilla bean paste

- 6 drops stevia powder

- 1/4 cup virgin coconut oil

- 1/2 cup coconut flour

- 2 teaspoons baking flour

- 1/2 cup frozen strawberries

- ¼ cup dark chocolate(cubed)

- 50 gm shredded coconut

Garnish

- 20gm shredded coconut

- 10 strawberries

Directions:

1.   Preheat oven to 180˚C

2.   Mix the eggs, vanilla bean and stevia until light and creamy.

3.   Pour in the melted coconut oil and mix well.

4.   Add the coconut flour, shredded coconut, baking powder and mix until combined.

5.   Fold in strawberry and diced dark chocolate.

6.   Pour the mixture onto baking mould and sprinkle the shredded coconut on the top.

7.   Bake for 25-30 minutes

8.   Cool down for 5 minutes

9.   Decorate with extra shredded coconut and strawberry. Cut into square, serve and enjoy

158. Almond Crispy Bar

Time: 1 hour

Serves: 6

Ingredients:

- 6 eggs

- 1 tsp vanilla bean paste

- 8 drops stevia

- 1/4 cup virgin coconut oil

- 1/2 cup almond meal

- 2 teaspoons baking flour

- ½ cup roasted almond slices

- ¼ cup dark chocolate(cubed)

Garnish

- ¼ cup almond slices

Directions:

1. Preheat oven to 180°C

2. Mix the eggs, vanilla bean and stevia until light and creamy.

3. Pour in the melted coconut oil and mix well.

4. Add the almond flour, baking powder and mix until combined.

5. Fold in roasted almond and diced dark chocolate.

6. Pour the mixture onto baking mould and sprinkle the almond slices

7. Bake for 25-30 minutes

8.   Cool down for 5 minutes

9.   Decorate with almond slices

10.   Cut into square, serve and enjoy

159. Gorgeous Berry Chocolate Bar

Time: 50 minutes

Serves: 16 bars

Ingredients:

Bottom layer

- 1 tsp vanilla bean paste
- 8 drops stevia powder
- ¼ tsp salt
- 1/4 cup virgin coconut oil
- 1/2 cup coconut flour
- 2 teaspoons almond flour

Top layer

- 20gm shredded coconut
- ½ cup strawberries
- ½ cup blueberries
- ¼ cup dark chocolate(cubed)
- ½ cup coconut milk

Directions:

1. Preheat oven to 350°F

2. Mix the coconut flour, almond flour, baking powder, vanilla bean, stevia and melted coconut oil until crumbly

3. Press the crumb mixture evenly into the bottom of greased pan.

4.   Bake at 350°F for 15 minutes until golden brown around the edges. Let cool completely.

5.   Add finely chopped chocolate in a large bowl.

6.   Boil and pour hot coconut milk over chocolate and let stand 1 minute, then stir until smooth and creamy.

7.   Pour warm chocolate mixture over cooled crust. Decorate the berries on top as desired.

8.   Chill for at least one hour.

9.   Cut into square, serve and enjoy

160. April Crisp Bars

Serves:10 bars

Time:45 minutes

Ingredients

- 145 gm almond flour

- 150gm grass-feed butter

- 8 drops. stevia

Slice top

- 200 g of apricot(cubed)

- 100 g roasted almond slices

- 50 g of almond flour

- 3 eggs

- 6 drops stevia

- 4 tbsp water

Directions:

1. Preheat oven at 180˚C.

2. In a bowl, mix well grass-feed butter, stevia and almond powder

3. Press the crumb mixture evenly into the bottom of greased pan.

4. Baked for 15 minutes.

5. Meanwhile, add the cubed apricot and mix them in bowl with roasted almond slices, stevia, almond flour

6. Add 3 tbsp of water to the egg mix if it is too dry.

7. Spread the egg mixture onto the baked crust

8. Return in the oven for 20 minutes.

9. Let it cool and cut into squares

10. Serve

161. Healthy Blueberry Bars

Serves:10 bars

Time:45 minutes

Ingredients

- 145 gm almond flour

- 150gm grass-feed butter

- 8 drops stevia

- 80gm rolled oats

Slice top

- 200 g of blueberries

- 50 g of almond flour

- 3 eggs

- 6 drops stevia

- 4 tbsp water

Directions:

1. Preheat oven at 180˚C.

2. In a bowl, mix well grass-feed butter, rolled oats, stevia and almond powder

3. Press the crumb mixture evenly into the bottom of greased pan.

4. Baked for 15 minutes.

5. Mix in bowl with stevia and almond flour

6. Add 3 tbsp of water to the egg mix if it is too dry.

7. Fold the mixture with blueberries

8. Spread the mixture onto the baked crust

9. Bake for 20 minutes.

10. Let it cool and cut into squares

11. Serve

162. Rocky Nuts Bars

Serves:10 bars

Time:45 minutes

Ingredients

- 150gm grass-feed butter
- 150gm dark chocolate(melted)
- 6 drops stevia
- ¼ tsp vanilla extract
- 2 cup pecans(chopped)
- 1 cup walnut(chopped)
- 1 cup macadamia(chopped)

Directions:

1. Preheat oven at 180˚C.
2. In a bowl, mix well grass-feed butter, melted dark chocolate, vanilla extract and stevia
3. Fold the mixture with mixed nuts
4. Spread the mixture onto mould
5. Put in refrigerate for 20 minutes.
6. Cut into squares
7. Serve and enjoy

163. Supreme Red Velvet Cake

Time:1 hour

Serves:10 max

Ingredients

- 2 1/4 cups coconut flour

- 2 tablespoons cocoa powder

- 1 teaspoon salt

- 1/2 cup grass-feed butter, softened

- ¼ tsp stevia

- 1 tsp vanilla extract

- 2 large eggs

- 1 cup fresh beetroot puree

- 1 cup coconut milk

- 1/2 tsp baking soda

For icing

- 40 oz almond cheese

- 2 tbsp almond milk

- 8 drops stevia

Directions:

1. Preheat oven 180°C

2. Grease the cake mould with grass-feed butter

3.   In a medium-size bowl, combine the flour, cocoa and salt. Stir the ingredients together slowly and then set aside.

4.   In a large bowl, mix well grass-feed butter, stevia and vanilla extract together until smooth.

5.   Add the eggs and beetroot puree and beat on low until fully mixed.

6.   Alternate adding 1/3 of the flour mix and 1/3 of the coconut milk to the butter mixture, beating on low until the ingredients are combined.

7.   Use a wooden spoon to stir in the baking soda.

8.   Pour the batter into the cake mould and bake for approximately 35 minutes

9.   Allow the cakes to cool for 15 minutes and then remove them from the pans and let them cool completely.

10.   Blend the icing ingredients until smooth

11.   Frost the cake with sugar-free almond cheese icing.

164. Absolute Tasty Carrot Loaf

Serves: 4

Time:1 hour

Ingredients:

- 1 cup carrot (grated)

- 1 1/2 cups almond flour

- 1/4 cups coconut flour

- 1 teaspoon baking soda

- 1/2 teaspoons salt

- 3 eggs

- 10 drops stevia

- 1/4 cups coconut oil (melted)

- 2 tablespoons almond butter

- 1/2 teaspoons cinnamon

Directions:

1.   Preheat the oven to 350°F. Line a loaf pan with parchment paper. Squeeze any excess moisture out of the grated carrot.

2.   Whisk together the almond flour, coconut flour, baking soda, and salt in a medium bowl.

3.   In a separate bowl, add the eggs, stevia, coconut oil, almond butter, and cinnamon. Use a hand blender to combine. Add the dry ingredients into the wet and stir to combine.

4.   Fold in the shredded carrots

5.   Pour the batter into the loaf pan.

6.   Bake for 45 minutes

7.   Remove from the oven and let cool completely

8.   Cut and serve

165. Fluffy Coconut Loaf

Serves: 12

Time: 45 minutes

Ingredients:

- 1/2 cups coconut flour

- 1/4 teaspoons salt

- 1/4 teaspoons baking soda

- 1 cup desiccated coconut

- 6 eggs

- 1/2 cups coconut milk

Directions:

1. Preheat oven to 350°F.

2. In a medium sized bowl sift together the dry ingredients.

3. Slowly add the wet ingredients into the dry ingredients and stir until smooth.

4. Grease a small bread pan and fill about 2/3 of the way full with batter.

5. Bake for 45 minutes

6. Let it cool

7. Cut into slices and serve

166. Tasty Bananuts Bread

Serves: 12

Time: 1 hour

Ingredients:

- 1/2 cups coconut flour

- 1/2 cups almond meal

- 1/4 teaspoons salt

- 1/4 teaspoons baking soda

- 1 tsp baking powder

- 1 cup toasted pecans

- 1 tsp ground cinnamon

- 4 eggs

- 4 bananas(mashed)

- 10 drops stevia

- 1/2 cups pumpkin seed

Garnish

- 2 tbsp pumpkin seed

- 3 tbsp roasted pecans

Directions:

1. Preheat oven to 350°F.

2. In a medium sized bowl sift together the dry ingredients.

3. Slowly add the wet ingredients into the dry ingredients and stir until smooth.

4. Grease a small bread pan and fill about 2/3 of the way full with batter.

5. Sprinkle with pumpkin seed and toasted pecans

6. Bake for 45 minutes

7. Let it cool. Cut into slices and serve

167. Mangolicious Bread

Time: 1 hour 10 minutes

Serves:10

Ingredients:

- 2 cups mango(cubed)
- 1/3 cups coconut oil
- 4 eggs
- 1 tsp vanilla extract
- 1/2 cups coconut flour
- 1 tsp baking soda
- 1/4 tsp sea salt
- 1/3 cups desiccated coconut

Directions:

1. Preheat the oven to 350°F

2. Add all the ingredients together in a medium bowl except cubed mangoes and desiccated mix until combined well

3. Fold the batter with cubed mangoes and desiccated coconut

4. Pour into a lightly greased bread pan.

5. Bake for about 50 minutes or until centre is set and top is golden.

6. Enjoy

168. Silky Blueberinana Loaf

Serves: 10 max

Time: 45 minutes

Ingredients:

- 3 bananas

- 1 cup blueberries

- 4 eggs

- 2 cup almond flour

- 8 drops stevia

- 1/3 cup grass-feed butter, softened

- 1 tsp baking soda

- 1/2 tsp vanilla extract

- A pinch salt

Directions:

1. Preheat oven to 425°F

2. In a medium bowl, mash well the banana and mix the grass-feed butter, eggs, stevia, vanilla extract

3. In a large bowl mix well the almond flour, baking soda and salt

4. Then, add the wet ingredients and mix the batter until it consistent

5. Fold with the blueberries

6. Pour batter into one bread pans

7. Bake in oven for 30 minutes or until top the centre is cooked and the crust is golden brown

8.   Remove from oven, and allow to cool

9.   Cut and serve

169. Yum-yum Chocolathy Haloween Bread

Time: 1 hour 5 minutes

Serves:10

Ingredients

- 3/4 cup coconut oil
- 10 drops stevia
- 5 eggs
- 1 1/2 teaspoons vanilla extract
- 1 teaspoons cinnamon
- 3/4 teaspoon fresh nutmeg
- 1 teaspoons baking powder
- ¾ teaspoon sea salt
- 1 cup pumpkin puree
- 2 cup coconut flour
- 3/4 cup dark chocolate cacao nibs

Directions:

1. Preheat oven to 355°F.
2. Grease a loaf pan and set aside
3. Using spoon, mix together coconut oil, eggs, vanilla extract and stevia
4. Add in nutmeg, baking powder, salt and pumpkin puree.
5. Stir in cacao nibs until just mixed.
6. Bake for 55 minutes until an inserted fork comes out mostly clean.

7.   Allow to cool, slice, and serve.

170. Glowing Beetroot Flat Bread

Time: 2 hours 20 minutes

Serves: 25

Ingredients

- 1 cup beetroot (peeled and diced)

- ½ cup water

- 2 cups coconut flour

- 1 tsp grass-feed butter

- 1 tsp salt

- 1 tsp ground black pepper

- 1 tsp coconut oil

Directions:

1. Grind the chopped beetroot with half a cup of water to a fine paste.

2. Take a bowl and add in the coconut flour. Add in the salt, cracked pepper and grass-feed butter. Add in the beet puree. Mix well and knead for a couple of minutes to form a cohesive dough.

3. Apply a teaspoon of coconut oil on the surface and spread it on the surface.

4. Cover the dough with a lid. Allow the dough to rest for a couple of hours or overnight.

5. Divide the dough small size balls. Set an iron pan on medium high heat. Let it become hot.

6. Roll the dough into a 3-4 inch round on a flat smooth surface using a rolling pin.

7. Place the flat bread on the hot griddle. Let it cook for 10-15 seconds until bubbles start to form on top. Flip the flat bread and cook for 30 seconds more.

8. Flip one more time and press on top. Flat bread should beautifully fluff up.

171. Traffic Flat Bread

Time: 2 hours 20 minutes

Serves: 25

Ingredients

- 1 cup beetroot (peeled and diced)

- ½ cup spinach puree

- ½ cup carrot puree

- ½ cup water

- 3 cups coconut flour (divided 3)

- 1 tsp grass-feed butter

- 1 tsp salt

- 1 tsp ground black pepper

- 1 tsp coconut oil

Directions:

1. Grind the chopped beetroot with half a cup of water to a fine paste.

2. Take 3 bowls and add in the coconut flour. Add in the salt, cracked pepper and grass-feed butter. Add in the beet puree in bowl A, spinach puree in bowl B and carrot puree bowl C. Mix well and knead for a couple of minutes to form a cohesive dough.

3. Apply a teaspoon of coconut oil on the surface and spread it on the surface.

4. Cover the dough with a lid. Allow the dough to rest for a couple of hours or overnight.

5. Divide the dough small size balls. Set an iron pan on medium high heat. Let it become hot.

6. Roll the dough into a 3-4 inch round on a flat smooth surface using a rolling pin.

7.   Place the flat bread on the hot griddle. Let it cook for 10-15 seconds until bubbles start to form on top. Flip the flat bread and cook for 30 seconds more.

8.   Flip one more time and press on top. Flat bread should beautifully fluff up.

172. Healthy Broccoli Tortillas

Serves: 6

Time: 35 minutes

Ingredients:

- 3/4 head broccoli

- 2 large eggs

- 1/4 cup chopped fresh cilantro

- 2 tbsp lemon juice

- ¼ tsp salt

- ¼ tsp pepper

Directions:

1. Preheat the oven to 375°F. and line a baking sheet with parchment paper.

2. Trim the broccoli, cut it into small, uniform pieces, and pulse in a food processor in batches until you get a couscous-like consistency. The finely riced broccoli should make about 2 cups packed.

3. Microwave the riced broccoli for 2 minutes, then stir and microwave again for another 2 minutes. Place the broccoli in a fine cheesecloth and drain the water

4. In a medium bowl, whisk the eggs. Add in broccoli, cilantro, lemon juice, salt and pepper. Mix until well combined.

5. Shape 6 small "tortillas" on the parchment paper.

6. Bake for 10 minutes, carefully flip each tortilla, and return to the oven for an additional 7 minutes, until completely set.

7. Allow the tortilla to cool

8. Heat a medium-sized skillet on medium. Place a baked tortilla in the pan, pressing down slightly, and brown for 2 minutes on each side.

173. Royal Sunkin Bread

Time: 1 hour 5 minutes

Serves:10

Ingredients

- 3/4 cup coconut oil

- ¼ teaspoon stevia

- 5 eggs

- 1 1/2 teaspoons vanilla extract

- 1 teaspoons cinnamon

- 3/4 teaspoon fresh nutmeg

- 1 teaspoons baking powder

- ¾ teaspoon sea salt

- 1 cup pumpkin puree

- 2 cup coconut flour

- 3/4 cup sunflower seed

Directions:

1. Preheat oven to 355°F.

2. Grease a loaf pan and set aside

3. Using spoon, mix together coconut oil, eggs, vanilla extract and stevia

4. Add in nutmeg, baking powder, salt and pumpkin puree.

5. Stir in sunflower seed until just mixed.

6. Bake for 45 minutes until an inserted fork comes out mostly clean.

7.   Allow to cool, slice, and serve

174. Heavenly Dried Cranberry Zucchini Loaf

Serves: 4

Time: 55 minutes

Ingredients:

- 1 cup zucchini(grated)

- 1 1/2 cups almond flour

- 1/4 cups coconut flour

- 1 teaspoon baking soda

- 1/2 teaspoons salt

- 3 eggs

- 10 drops stevia

- 1/4 cups coconut oil (melted)

- 2 tablespoons almond butter

- 1 cup dried cranberries

- 1/2 teaspoons cinnamon

Directions:

1.   Preheat the oven to 350°F. Line a loaf pan with parchment paper. Squeeze any excess moisture out of the grated zucchini.

2.   Whisk together the almond flour, coconut flour, baking soda, and salt in a medium bowl.

3.   In a separate bowl, add the eggs, stevia, coconut oil, almond butter, and cinnamon. Use a hand blender to combine. Add the dry ingredients into the wet and stir to combine.

4.   Fold in the shredded zucchini and dried cranberries

5.   Pour the batter into the loaf pan.

6. Bake for 45 minutes

7. Remove from the oven and let cool completely

8. Cut and serve

175. Heavenly Dried Cranberry Pecan Loaf

Serves: 4

Time: 55 minutes

Ingredients:

- 1 cup roasted pecan nuts(chopped)

- 1 1/2 cups almond flour

- 1/4 cups coconut flour

- 1 teaspoon baking soda

- 1/2 teaspoons salt

- 3 eggs

- 10 drops stevia

- 1/4 cups coconut oil (melted)

- 2 tablespoons almond butter

- 1 cup dried cranberries

- 1/2 teaspoons cinnamon

Directions:

1. Preheat the oven to 350°F. Line a loaf pan with parchment paper.

2. Whisk together the almond flour, coconut flour, baking soda, and salt in a medium bowl.

3. In a separate bowl, add the eggs, stevia, coconut oil, almond butter, and cinnamon. Use a hand blender to combine. Add the dry ingredients into the wet and stir to combine.

4. Fold in the chopped roasted pecan nuts and dried cranberries

5. Pour the batter into the loaf pan.

6. Bake for 45 minutes

7. Remove from the oven and let cool completely

8. Cut and serve

176. Fluffy Carrot Banana Crunchy Muffin

Serves: 15 cups

Time: 35 minutes

Ingredients:

- 2 cups almond flour

- 1 cup almond flakes

- 2 teaspoons baking soda

- 1 teaspoon salt

- 1 tablespoon cinnamon

- 220gm xylitol

- 3 ripe bananas

- 3 eggs

- 1 teaspoon apple cider vinegar

- 1/4 cup coconut oil

- 1 cups carrots, shredded

Directions:

1. Combine dry ingredients.

2. Blend bananas, xylitol, eggs, vinegar, and coconut oil in a food processor.

3. Mix wet ingredients with dry and fold in carrots and almond flakes

4. Spoon into greased or lined muffin tins and bake at 350°C for 25 minutes

177. Amazing Peach Cake Cup

Time: 5 minutes

Serves: 1 max

Ingredients:

- 1 eggs

- 2 tablespoons coconut milk

- 2 tablespoons coconut flour

- 1/4 cups peach

- baking soda (pinch)

- 2 tablespoons coconut flakes

Directions:

1. In small bowl, add all ingredients except for coconut flakes and mix well.

2. Add the mixture into cup

3. Sprinkle coconut flakes on top.

4. Microwave for 3 minutes.

5. Let cool and enjoy

178. Delish Vanilla Cake

Ingredients

Time: 2 hour 25 minutes

Serves: 10

Cupcake

- 4 eggs

- 5 tablespoons coconut flour

- 1/2 teaspoons baking powder

- 1/8 teaspoons salt

- seeds from one vanilla pod

- ¾ cup xylitol

Filling

- 1 3/4 cups raw cashews (soaked overnight)

- 1/4 cups coconut oil (melted)

- 1/3 cups water

- 1/2 teaspoons lemon juice

- 4 tbsp xylitol

- seeds from one vanilla pod

- 1/8 teaspoons sea salt

- 1 sliced almonds

Directions:

1.   Make the filling a day ahead. Place all the ingredients except water in a high power blender and blend until smooth.

2.   Add the water, a tablespoon at the time until the filling become silky and you get your desired texture. Transfer the filling to a bowl, cover with plastic wrap and chill overnight.

3.   Preheat oven to 350°F.

4.   Line two 8 inch spring-form pans with parchment paper.

5.   In a large bowl cream the eggs with xylitol.

6.   Add the salt, coconut flour mixed with baking powder and seeds from vanilla pod and mix until combined.

7.   Divide the mixture between prepared pans and bake for 15-20 minutes or until a fork comes out clean when inserted.

8.   Remove cakes from the oven and set aside to cool completely.

9.   Remove the cakes from the pans and take the filling from the fridge.

10.   Whip the filling with a hand mixer until filling become fluffy.

11.   Place one of the cakes on a platter and spread 1/3 of filling evenly.

12.   Top with another cake and spread top and sides of cake with remaining filling.

13.   Sprinkle with sliced almonds if using and place in a fridge for minimum two hours before serving.

179. Sweetheart Pistachio Muffins

Time: 50 minutes

Serves: 12

Ingredients

- 300 gm coconut flour
- 100gm pistachios
- 2 tsp baking powder
- 4 eggs
- 60 ml coconut oil
- 60 ml coconut milk
- 25 g stevia powder
- 200 g frozen strawberries

Directions:

1. Preheat the oven to 180°C
2. Combine the flour and baking powder in a bowl.
3. Add the eggs, oil, coconut milk and stevia
4. Mix to form a batter
5. Pour in the frozen strawberries and pistachios
6. Filled paper-lined muffin tray.
7. Bake for 35 minutes until the crust turns golden colour

180. Very Merry Cherry Muffins

Time: 50 minutes

Serves: 12

Ingredients

- 300 gm coconut flour
- 100gm desiccated coconut
- 2 tsp baking powder
- 4 eggs
- 60 ml coconut oil
- 60 ml coconut cream
- 25 g stevia powder
- ½ tsp vanilla extract
- 200 g unsweetened frozen cherries(halves)

Directions:

1. Preheat the oven to 180°C
2. Combine the flour and baking powder in a bowl.
3. Add the eggs, oil, coconut cream, vanilla extract and stevia
4. Mix to form a batter
5. Pour in the frozen cherry and desiccated coconut
6. Filled paper-lined muffin tray.
7. Bake for 35 minutes until the crust turns golden color

181. Berry Manialuscious Muffins

Time: 50 minutes

Serves: 12

Ingredients

- 300 gm coconut flour
- 2 tsp baking powder
- 4 eggs
- 60 ml coconut oil
- 60 ml coconut milk
- 25 g stevia powder
- ½ tsp vanilla extract
- 50 g frozen cherries(halves)
- 50gm frozen strawberries
- 50gm frozen blueberries

Directions:

1. Preheat the oven to 180°C
2. Combine the flour and baking powder in a bowl.
3. Add the eggs, oil, coconut milk, vanilla extract and stevia
4. Mix to form a batter
5. Pour in the mix berries
6. Filled paper-lined muffin tray.
7. Bake for 35 minutes until the crust turns golden color

8.   Remove from oven, allow to cool and serve

182. Mafia PeachyBerry Cake

Time: 45 minutes

Serves: 12

Ingredients

- 1 ½ cup coconut flour

- 2 tsp baking powder

- ½ tsp baking soda

- 4 eggs

- 1/3 cup coconut oil

- 1/3 cup coconut milk

- 25 g stevia powder

- 1 tsp vanilla extract

- 2 peach(slices)

- 50gm frozen blueberries

Directions:

1. Preheat the oven to 180°C

2. Line a cake pan with parchment paper

3. Combine the flour, baking soda and baking powder in a bowl.

4. Add the eggs, oil, coconut milk, vanilla extract and stevia

5. Mix to form a batter

6. Pour in the tray and mix well with peach and blueberries

7. Bake for 35 minutes until at the centre cook well

8.   Remove from oven, allow to cool and serve

183. Cupid Banana Walnut Cake

Time: 45 minutes

Serves: 12

Ingredients

- 1 ½ cup almond flour

- 2 tsp baking powder

- ½ tsp baking soda

- 4 eggs

- 1/3 cup coconut oil

- 1/3 cup almond milk

- 25 g stevia powder

- 1 tsp vanilla extract

- 1 cup mashed banana

- 1 cup roasted walnut (chopped)

Directions:

1. Preheat the oven to 180°C

2. Line a cake pan with parchment paper

3. Combine the almond flour, baking soda and baking powder in a bowl.

4. Add the eggs, oil, almond milk, vanilla extract and stevia

5. Mix to form a batter

6. Pour in the tray and mix well with mashed banana and walnuts

7. Bake for 35 minutes until at the centre cook well

8. Remove from oven, allow to cool and serve

184. Custard Mango Pie

Time:50 minutes

Serves:4-6 max

Ingredients:

Filling

- 400 ml coconut milk

- 300 ml coconut cream

- 60 g shredded coconut

- 5 eggs

- ½ teaspoon stevia powder

- 3 drops vanilla extract

- 120 g coconut flour

- 20 gm grass-feed butter

- 1 fresh mango, diced

Pie crust

- 10 tablespoon coconut fat

- 3 cups flour

- 1/3 cup + 6-8 tablespoon cold water

Directions:

1. Preheat the oven at 180˚C.

2. Grease the mini pie pan.

3. Set aside.

For pie crust.

1)   In a large mixing bowl, add the flour, melted coconut fat and water. Combine well until form a dough

2)   If too sticky add slightly more flour or if too dry add more water 1 tablespoon at a time.

3)   Roll the dough as thin

4)   Then, cut out the dough in circle.

5)   Arrange onto the buttered pan.

6)   Peel and dice a mango.

7)   Add some mango dice into each pie.

For coconut custard

1)   In a sauce pan bring to boil the coconut milk and coconut cream with the vanilla extract.

2)   Meanwhile, in a bowl, whisk the eggs, coconut flour, shredded coconut and stevia.

3)   Pour the boiling coconut milk mixture onto the flour mix and whisk really quickly.

4)   Bring back to the saucepan and simmer for 1 minute.

5)   Keep whisking until the custard is thick.

6)   Pour the custard onto the custard pie already filled with diced mango.

7)   Bake for 40 minutes or until the top of each pie is yellow

185. Custard Peach Pie

Time:50 minutes

Serves:4-6 max

Ingredients:

Filling

- 400 ml coconut milk

- 300 ml coconut cream

- 5 eggs

- ½ teaspoon stevia powder

- 3 drops vanilla extract

- 120 g coconut flour

- 20 gm grass-feed butter

- 1 peach, diced

Pie crust

- 10 tablespoon coconut fat

- 3 cups flour

- 1/3 cup + 6-8 tablespoon cold water

Directions:

1) Preheat the oven at 180˚C.

2) Grease the mini pie pan.

3) Set aside.

For pie crust.

1) In a large mixing bowl, add the flour, melted coconut fat and water. Combine well until form a dough

2) If too sticky add slightly more flour or if too dry add more water 1 tablespoon at a time.

3) Roll the dough as thin

4) Then, cut out the dough in circle.

5) Arrange onto the buttered pan.

6) Add diced peach into each pie.

For coconut custard

1) In a sauce pan bring to boil the coconut milk and coconut cream with the vanilla extract.

2) Meanwhile, in a bowl, whisk the eggs, coconut flour and stevia.

3) Pour the boiling coconut milk mixture onto the flour mix and whisk really quickly.

4) Bring back to the saucepan and simmer for 1 minute.

5) Keep whisking until the custard is thick.

6) Pour the custard onto the custard pie already filled with diced peach.

7) Bake for 40 minutes or until the top of each pie is golden brown

186. Very Berry Strawberry Ice Cream

Serves: 2-3 max

Time: 1-3 hours

Ingredients:

- 2 cup frozen strawberries

- ½ cup coconut milk

- 1 tsp vanilla

Directions:

1. Place all ingredients into blender and blend until smooth.

2. Pour contents into a small pan.

3. Freeze one hour or until solid.

4. Enjoy

187. Strawberry Squeeze Ice Cream

Serves: 2-3 max

Time: 1-3 hours

Ingredients:

- 3 frozen bananas

- ½ cup frozen strawberries

- ½ cup coconut milk

- 1 tsp vanilla

Directions:

1. Cut bananas into round and place in freezer in a sealable bag. Freeze overnight.

2. Place all ingredients into blender and blend until smooth.

3. Pour contents into a small pan.

4. Freeze one hour or until solid.

5. Enjoy

188. Banana Burst Ice Cream

Serves: 2-3 max

Time: 1-3 hours

Ingredients

- 3 bananas, cut and frozen
- 1 ripe mango(cubed)
- ¼ cup coconut milk

Directions:

1. Cut bananas into slices and place in freezer in a sealable bag. Freeze overnight.

2. Place all ingredients into a blender and blend until smooth.

3. Pour contents into a loaf or small pan.

4. Freeze one hour or until solid.

5. Enjoy

189. Banana Chocolate Blast Ice-cream

Serves: 2-3 max

Time: 1-3 hours

Ingredients

- 3 bananas

- 2 tablespoon coconut yogurt

- 1 tablespoons cocoa powder

- ¼ cup coconut milk

Directions:

1. Cut bananas into slices and place in freezer in a sealable bag. Freeze overnight.

2. Place all ingredients into blender and blend until smooth.

3. Pour contents into a small pan.

4. Freeze one hour or until solid.

5. Enjoy

190. Coconut Rocky Road Ice-cream

Time:2 hour

Serves:5 max

Ingredients:

*   5 egg yolks

*   700 ml coconut cream

*   150ml coconut water

*   ¼ tsp stevia

*   1 cup coconut meat

*   1 teaspoon vanilla

Directions:

1.   Whisk the egg yolks in a bowl. Set aside

2.   In a saucepan, add the coconut cream, coconut water and sweetener. Gently heat on the stove top stirring constantly to dissolve the sweetener. Remove from the heat after it boils.

3.   Start gently whisking the egg yolks very gradually add a spoon at a time of the warm cream to the egg yolks.

4.   Stir in the vanilla then pour back into the saucepan and heat again whilst stirring, to thicken to a custard consistency.

5.   Remove from the heat and allow to cool completely. Stir through the toasted coconut meat

6.   Freeze until solid.

7.   Enjoy

191. Green Minty Chocolate Ice-cream

Serves: 2-3 max

Time 2 hours

Ingredients

- 1/3 cups avocado puree

- 65 fresh mint

- ¼ tsp stevia

- 1 teaspoon pure vanilla extract

- 500ml coconut milk

- 1/2 cups almond milk

- 1/2 teaspoons mint extract

- 1 pinch fine sea salt

- ½ cup dark chocolate chips

Directions:

1. Place all ingredients into blender except chocolate chips and blend until smooth.

2. Add chocolate chips and evenly

3. Pour contents into a small pan.

4. Freeze until solid.

5. Enjoy

192. Cherry Merry Ice-cream

Serves:1-2 max

Time:2 hours

Ingredients:

- 2 cup frozen cherries

- 2 cups almond milk

- ¼ tsp stevia

Directions:

1. Place all ingredients into blender and blend until smooth.

2. Pour contents into a small pan.

3. Freeze two hour or until solid.

4. Enjoy

193. Meachgo Ice-cream

Serves:1-2 max

Time:2 hours

Ingredients:

- 2 cup mango(cubed)

- 1 cup peach(sliced)

- 2 cups coconut milk

- ¼ tsp stevia

- ¼ tsp guar gum

Directions:

1. Place all ingredients into blender and blend until smooth.

2. Pour contents into a small pan.

3. Freeze two hour or until solid.

4. Enjoy

194. Cobupeca Ice-cream

Serves: 2-3 max

Time: 3 hours

Ingredients

- 1 cup coconut cream
- 2 tablespoons grass-feed butter
- ¼ tsp stevia
- 1 teaspoon vanilla extract
- 2 egg yolks
- 2/3 cups chopped pecans
- 1/8 teaspoons guar gum

Directions:

1. Melt the butter in a pan under low heat

2. Add the chopped pecans, coconut cream, vanilla extract, stevia, guar gum and mix well until consistent. Let it cool

3. Blend the mixture

4. Freeze for 3 hours

5. Serve

195. Mix Berrylicious

Serves: 2-3 max

Time: 2 hours

Ingredients:

- ½ cup frozen strawberries

- ½ cup frozen raspberries

- ½ cup frozen blueberry

- 1 teaspoon vanilla

- 6 drops stevia

Directions:

1. Place all ingredients into blender and blend until smooth.

2. Pour contents into a small pan.

3. Freeze two hour or until solid.

4. Enjoy

196. Zucchini Pesto

Serves:4-6 max

Time:13 minutes

Ingredients

- 1 tablespoon olive oil

- 1 onion, roughly chopped

- 1½ pounds (750g) zucchini, roughly chopped

- ¾ cup water

- 1½ teaspoons salt

- 1 teaspoon black pepper

- 1 bunch basil, leaves picked off

- 2 cloves garlic, roughly minced

- 1 tablespoon extra-virgin olive oil

Directions

- In the pre-heated pressure cooker, on medium heat add the oil and onion and saute until the onions begin to become soft (about 4 minutes).

- Add the zucchini, salt and water (1/2 cup for stovetop and ¾ cup for electric cookers).

- Close and lock the lid of the pressure cooker.

- Electric pressure cookers: Cook for 3 minutes at high pressure. Stovetop pressure cookers: Turn the heat up to high and when the cooker indicates it has reached high pressure, lower to the heat to maintain it and begin counting 3 minutes pressure cooking time.

- When time is up, open the pressure cooker with the Normal release - release pressure through the valve.

- Toss in the basil leaves and garlic.

- Using an immersion blender puree' the contents of the pressure cooker until all of the garlic and basil are fully incorporated.

- Mix with freshly strained pasta and serve immediately with a swirl of extra-virgin olive oil.

197. Zucchini Shrimp Pesto

Serves:4-6 max

Time:13 minutes

Ingredients

- 1 tablespoon olive oil

- 1 onion, roughly chopped

- 750gm zucchini, roughly chopped

- 100gm shrimp

- ¾ cup water

- 1½ teaspoons salt

- 1 teaspoon black pepper

- 1 bunch basil, leaves picked off

- 2 cloves garlic, roughly minced

- 1 tablespoon extra-virgin olive oil

- 2 tablespoon lemon juice

Directions

1.   In the pre-heated pressure cooker, on medium heat add the oil. After it heats add shrimp and onion and saute until become soft (about 4 minutes).

2.   Add the zucchini, lemon juice, salt and water (1/2 cup for stovetop and ¾ cup for electric cookers).

3.   Close and lock the lid of the pressure cooker.

4.   Electric pressure cookers: Cook for 3 minutes at high pressure. Stovetop pressure cookers: Turn the heat up to high and when the cooker indicates it has reached high pressure, lower to the heat to maintain it and begin counting 3 minutes pressure cooking time.

5. When time is up, open the pressure cooker with the Normal release - release pressure through the valve.

6. Toss in the basil leaves and garlic.

7. Using an immersion blender puree' the contents of the pressure cooker until all of the garlic and basil are fully incorporated. Mix with freshly strained pasta and serve immediately with a swirl of extra-virgin olive oil.

198. Zucchini Glazing Cherry Pesto

Serves:4-6 max

Time:13 minutes

Ingredients

- 1 tablespoon olive oil

- 1 onion, roughly chopped

- 1½ pounds (750g) zucchini, roughly chopped

- 150gm cherry tomatoes

- ½ yellow bell peppers(sliced)

- ¾ cup water

- 1½ teaspoons salt

- 1 teaspoon black pepper

- 1 bunch basil, leaves picked off

- 2 cloves garlic, roughly minced

- 1 tablespoon extra-virgin olive oil

Directions

1.   In the pre-heated pressure cooker, on medium heat add the oil. After the oil heats up add bell peppers, onion and shrimp. saute until begin to become soft (about 4 minutes).

2.   Add the zucchini, salt and water (1/2 cup for stovetop and ¾ cup for electric cookers).

3.   Close and lock the lid of the pressure cooker.

4.   Electric pressure cookers: Cook for 3 minutes at high pressure. Stovetop pressure cookers: Turn the heat up to high and when the cooker indicates it has reached high pressure, lower to the heat to maintain it and begin counting 3 minutes pressure cooking time.

5.   When time is up, open the pressure cooker with the Normal release - release pressure through the valve.

6.   Toss in the basil leaves and garlic.

7.   Using an immersion blender puree' the contents of the pressure cooker until all of the garlic and basil are fully incorporated.

8.   Mix with freshly strained pasta and serve immediately with a cherry tomatoes swirl of extra-virgin olive oil.

199. Crazy Seafoodies Zucchini

Time:30 minutes

Serves:2-3 max

Ingredients:

- 4 zucchinis (spiralized)

- 20 clams

- 5 oz. sea scallops

- 5 oz. shrimp, peeled and deveined;

- 6 oz. cooked crab meat;

- 2 tomatoes (diced)

- 1 bell pepper(diced)

- 3 garlic cloves, minced;

- 1 onion(diced)

- 2 tbsp. fresh basil, minced;

- 1 tsp. dried oregano;

- 1/2 tsp. red pepper flakes;

- 1/2 cup tomato sauce;

- 1/2 cup fish stock;

- 1-2 tbsp. coconut fat

- Sea salt and freshly ground black pepper;

Directions:

1. Melt cooking fat in a skillet over medium heat.

2.   Add the onion, bell pepper, and garlic and cook until fragrant, 4 to 5 minutes.

3.   Pour in the fish stock and bring a boil.

4.   Add in the tomato sauce, diced tomatoes, basil, oregano, and chili flakes; season to taste with salt and pepper, and give everything a good stir.

5.   Let the sauce simmer 5 to 8 minutes.

6.   Add the scallops, shrimp, and crab meat; cook 4 to 5 minutes or until shrimp redden.

7.   Add the spiralized zucchini and clams; cover and cook until clams open for 8 minutes.

8.   Serve the pasta topped with fresh basil

200. Haunted Sweet Potato Wedges

Serves:3-4 max

Time:45 minutes

Ingredients

- 3 large sweet potatoes

- ⅓ cup olive oil

- 1 teaspoon salt

- ½ teaspoon pepper

- 1 tablespoon garlic powder

- 1 tablespoon rosemary

- 1 tablespoon paprika

Directions

1. Preheat oven to 400°F

2. Thoroughly wash potatoes, cut in half, and slice into wedges

3. Toss wedges in olive oil and seasonings. Place on a baking sheet

4. Bake for 40 minutes

5. Enjoy

201. Crazy Crisp Zucchini

Time:40 minutes

Servings: 3-4max

Ingredients

- 3 large zucchinis

- 2 eggs, beaten

- 2 cups Italian breadcrumbs

- 1 teaspoon red pepper flakes

- 1 tablespoon garlic powder

- 1 tablespoon onion powder

- 1 teaspoon salt

- ½ teaspoon pepper

Directions:

1. Preheat oven to 350°F

2. Slice the ends off of each zucchini, then slice them in half and into wedges.

3. In a bowl, mix breadcrumbs, red pepper flakes, onion powder, garlic powder and salt.

4. Dip each wedge into egg mixture, then breadcrumb mixture.

5. Place on a baking sheet, skin side down.

6. Bake 15-20 minutes.

7. Enjoy

202. Magical Avocado Crisp

Servings: 3-4

Time:30 minutes

Ingredients

- 3 ripe avocados
- 2 eggs, lightly beaten
- 1 cup arrowroot flour
- 2 cups panko breadcrumbs
- Salt, to taste
- Cayenne pepper, to taste

Directions:

1. Preheat oven to 400°F

2. Slice each avocado in half, then into wedges. Scoop out of the peel.

3. Mix panko breadcrumbs with salt and cayenne. Dip each avocado wedge in flour, then eggs, then panko. Place on a parchment-lined baking sheet, and bake 12-15 minutes, flipping once.

4. Enjoy!

203. Savoury Caulicrispylicios

Serves:2-3 max

Time:25 minutes

Ingredients:

- 1 large cauliflower
- ⅓ cup olive oil
- 1 teaspoon salt
- ½ teaspoon pepper
- ½ tsp chili powder
- 1 tablespoon garlic powder
- 1 tablespoon curry powder
- 1 tablespoon dried oregano
- 1 tablespoon paprika

Directions:

1. Preheat oven to 400°F
2. Then, wash cauliflower, remove the stems and cut into ¼ inch thick
3. Toss florets in olive oil and seasonings. Layered on a baking sheet.
4. Bake 20-35 minutes.
5. Enjoy

204. Baked Rosemary Carrot Chips

Time: 20 minutes

Serves: 4 max

Ingredients

- 4 carrots (thinly coin sliced)

- 1 tbsp. olive oil

- 2 sprigs rosemary

- 1 tsp. garlic powder

- 1 tsp onion powder

- 1 tsp Salt

- ¼ tsp pepper

Directions:

1.   Preheat the oven to 425°F

2.   Toss the carrots with olive oil, rosemary, salt, and pepper.

3.   Lie on a baking sheet without letting the carrots overlap.

4.   Bake for 10 minutes

5.   Add some pepper and salt if desired

6.   Serve

205. Cheezomato Chips

Serves:5 max

Time:1 day

Ingredients

- 5 cups thinly sliced Roma tomatoes

- 2 tbsp coconut oil

- 2 tsp sea salt

- 1 tsp garlic powder

- 1 tbsp fresh chopped parsley

- 1 tbsp dried basil

- 2 tbsp grated almond cheese

Directions:

1. Gently drizzle and toss the sliced tomatoes in the coconut oil to coat slices.

2. Place ½ inch thick slices without overlapping on a baking pan.

3. Preheat oven to 200°F

4. In a small bowl whisk together the remaining ingredients.

5. Sprinkle mixture over each slice.

6. Dehydrate for 12 hours until crispy

7. Serve

206. Spicy Carrot Chips

Time: 20 minutes

Serves: 4 max

Ingredients

- 5 carrots (thinly coin sliced)

- 1 tbsp. olive oil

- 1 tsp curry powder

- 1 tsp chili powder

- 1 tsp. garlic powder

- 1 tsp onion powder

- 1 tsp Salt

- ¼ tsp pepper

Directions:

1. Preheat the oven to 425°F

2. Toss the carrots with olive oil and seasonings.

3. Lie on a baking sheet without letting the carrots overlap.

4. Bake for 10 minutes

5. Add some pepper and salt if desired

6. Serve

207. Tasty BBQ Smoked Sweet Potatoes

Serves: 4 Max

Time:35 minutes

Ingredients:

- 500gm sweet potatoes (sliced into coin)

- 1 tbsp olive oil

- 1 teaspoon smoked paprika

- 1/4 teaspoons onion powder

- 1/4 teaspoons chili powder

- 1 pinch garlic powder

- 1 pinch mustard powder (ground)

- 1 pinch salt

Directions:

1. Preheat oven to 320˚F.

2. Toss sweet potatoes in enough olive oil to coat.

3. Combine spices together well

4. Lay sweet potatoes in a single layer on cookie sheet.

5. Bake for 30 minutes.

6. Turn chips after 15 minutes and check every 5 minutes after.

208. Savory Apple Delight Chips

Time: 20 minutes

Serves: 4 max

Ingredients

- 5 apples (thinly cored and sliced)
- 1 tbsp. olive oil
- 1 tsp curry powder
- 1 tsp chili powder
- 1 tsp. garlic powder
- 1 tsp onion powder
- ¼ tsp lemon juice
- ¼ tsp pepper

Directions:

1. Preheat the oven to 425˚F
2. Toss the apples with olive oil, lemon juice and seasonings.
3. Lie on a baking sheet without letting the apples overlap.
4. Bake for 10 minutes
5. Add some pepper and salt if desired
6. Serve

209. Eggplant Curry Crunchy

Time: 20 minutes

Serves: 4 max

Ingredients

- 2 eggplants (thinly cored and sliced)
- 1 tbsp. olive oil
- 1 tsp curry powder
- 1 tsp chili powder
- 1 tsp. garlic powder
- 1 tsp cayenne powder
- 1 tsp onion powder
- ¼ tsp lemon juice
- ¼ tsp pepper
- ½ tsp ground cumin
- ¼ dried thyme

Directions:

1. Preheat the oven to 425˚F
2. Toss the apples with olive oil, lemon juice and seasonings.
3. Lie on a baking sheet without letting the apples overlap.
4. Bake for 10 minutes
5. Add some pepper and salt if desired
6. Serve

210. Flavourful Butternut Squash Chips

Ingredients

Time:2 hours

Serves:2 max

Ingredients:

- 1 butternut squash (small sliced)

- 2 teaspoons fresh sage

- 2 teaspoons thyme

- 2 teaspoons oregano

- 4 teaspoons olive oil

- 1/2 teaspoons kosher salt

Directions:

1. Preheat the oven to 250°F

2. Toss the apples with olive oil and seasonings.

3. Lie on a baking sheet without letting the apples overlap.

4. Bake for an hour, then flip the slices using tongs or a spatula.

5. Bake for another hour. Turn the slices again, lower the heat to 200°F bake for another hour. Turn off the oven and let the chips cool

6. Add some pepper and salt if desired

7. Serve

211. Burst Turkey Lasagna

Time:2 hr 30 mins

Serves: 6 max

Ingredients:

Marinara:

- 1/4 cup olive oil
- 1 small onion (diced)
- 1 tsp salt
- 1 tsp garlic(minced)
- 7 cups tomatoes diced
- 8 drops stevia

Filling:

- 1 tbsp olive oil
- 1 small onion diced
- 1 ½ lb ground turkey
- 1/2 tsp salt
- 1/4 tsp Black Pepper
- 20 Large Basil Leaves chopped

Cheese Sauce:

- 1/2 tbsp olive oil
- 1 small onion (chopped)
- ¼ tsp pepper

- ½ Yellow Summer Squash (chopped)
- ½ tsp garlic (minced)
- ¼ tsp salt
- ½ cup coconut milk (divided)
- 1 Egg
- 4 medium-sized Zucchini (thinly spiraled)

Directions:

To make the Marinara:

1. Heat the olive oil in a large saucepan over high heat.
2. Sauté the garlic, onion and salt for 1-2 minutes.
3. Add the tomatoes and stevia and reduce heat to medium.
4. Let the sauce cook down for about 20 minutes until slightly thick.
5. Check seasonings and add more salt, if needed.

To make the meat filling:

1. Heat the olive oil in a saute pan over high heat.
2. Add the ground turkey and break apart with a spatula.
3. Cook the turkey for 2 minutes then add the onion, salt and pepper.
4. Continue cooking until turkey crumbles and the onion is soft.
5. Remove the pan from heat and toss the fresh basil into the mixture.

To make the Paleo "Cheese Sauce"

1. Heat the olive oil to medium in a small saucepan.
2. Add the chopped onion, summer squash, salt, pepper and garlic to the pan and saute for about 3-4 minutes until the onion is translucent. Do not brown.

3.   Add 1/4 C. of the coconut milk to the pan and bring to a boil until more than half of the liquid is absorbed.

4.   Place the mixture in a blender with the remaining 1/4 cup coconut milk and puree until very smooth.

5.   Add the egg and puree until well blended.

To assemble lasagna:

1.   Lightly grease the inside of a crock pot.

2.   Cover the bottom of the crock pot with about 3/4 cup. of the marinara sauce, spreading it out evenly.

3.   Place about 5 zucchini 'noodles' side by side over the marinara sauce.

4.   Spoon a layer of the 'cheese sauce' over the zucchini noodles (about 1/2 C).

5.   Sprinkle about 1/2 heaping cup of the meat mixture over the sauce.

6.   Spoon about ¾ cup of the marinara sauce evenly over the meat mixture.

7.   Repeat this layering process until 5 layers (zucchini, sauce, meat, marinara) ending with the marinara sauce.

8.   Cover and cook on high for 1 1/2 hours.

9.   After 1 1/2 hours, remove the lid.

10.   Using a turkey baster or a ladle, remove all excess liquid that has pooled in the crock pot and place it in a shallow frying pan.

11.   Bring the liquid to a boil and simmer for about 5-7 minutes, or until reduced into a thick, creamy sauce.

12.   Pour the sauce over the top of the lasagna in the crock pot and serve.

212. Loaded Meatasaurus Cups

Time: 2 hour 30 minutes

Serves: 12

Ingredients

Roasted Tomato Sauce:

- 4 medium tomatoes (cut in half)

- 1 tbsp olive oil

- Salt and pepper

- ¼ tsp stevia

- 1 tbsp apple cider vinegar

- 2 tbsp tomato puree

- 2 Tbl water

- 1/8 tsp ground mustard

- 1/8 tsp garlic powder

- 1/8 tsp onion powder

- 1/4 tsp salt

Meatasaurus

- 2 cup olive oil

- 1 small onion (finely diced)

- 2 cloves garlic (minced)

- 2 carrots (grated)

- 3 button mushrooms (finely diced)

- 1 small zucchini (grated)

- 1/8 cup fresh rosemary (chopped)

- 1/8 cup parsley (chopped)

- 600gm ground turkey

- 300gm ground Pork

- ½ cup roasted tomato sauce

- 2 eggs

- 2 egg whites

- 1/4 cup coconut milk

- 1 tbsp coconut flour

- 1/4 tsp black pepper

- 1 1/2 tsp real salt

Directions:

For the Roasted Tomato Sauce

1.   Preheat oven to 375˚C

2.   Place the halved tomatoes, cut side up, on a greased baking sheet and drizzle the olive oil over the tops. Season lightly with salt and pepper.

3.   Roast the tomatoes for 2 hours on the top rack. Remove from oven and let cool slightly.

4.   Place the roasted tomatoes, stevia, apple cider vinegar, tomato paste, water, ground mustard, garlic powder, onion powder and salt in a blender and puree until smooth. Use in and on top of Meatasaurus cups.

For the Meatasaurus Cups

1.   Preheat oven to 400˚C and lightly grease a muffin tin.

2.   Heat the olive oil to high in a large saute pan.

3.   Sauté the onion, garlic, carrot, mushrooms, zucchini, and herbs to the pan for about 5 minutes, until the vegetables are soft and onions are translucent.

4.   Place the sautéed vegetables in a large bowl and let cool for 5 minutes.

5.   Add the ground turkey, pork, tomato sauce, eggs, egg whites, coconut milk, coconut flour, salt, and pepper to the vegetables and mix together very well using hands. Let sit for 5 minutes so that the coconut flour can fully absorb liquid.

6.   Divide the meat mixture into 12 portions.

7.   Shape each portion into a ball and place in well of a muffin tin. Muffins will be tall and dome shaped on top.

8.   Bake meatloaf muffins for 25 minutes until cooked through.

9.   Remove from the oven and, using a spoon, lift the meatloaf muffins out of the tin onto a platter. Scrape off any fat that may have clung to the sides of the muffins.

10.   Top each muffin with a spoonful of the remaining hot roasted tomato sauce

213. Incredible Loaded Winter Squash

Time: 45 mins

Serves: 8

Ingredients:

- 4 large winter squash (ends cut off, halved and deseeded)

- 1 lb. lean ground turkey

- ½ small onion, diced

- 2 garlic cloves, minced

- 400gm diced tomatoes

- 1 tsp salt

- 2 handfuls fresh spinach, chopped

Directions:

1. Preheat oven to 400˚F.

2. Brown meat in a large skillet over medium high heat. After meat has been cooking for about 2-3 minutes, add onion and garlic.

3. Meanwhile, microwave the squash for about 1 minute to soften the squash up a bit.

4. Once meat is almost fully cooked, add tomatoes, seasoning salt and spinach. Stir to combine and continue to cook until spinach is wilted.

5. Use a slotted (this will help drain excess liquid) spoon to spoon the turkey mixture into the squash halves. Load it as full as possible.

6. Bake stuffed squash at 400˚F for 20 to 30 minutes, until tops are browned and squash is soft.

7. Enjoy

214. Graved Delicious Turkey

Time: 50 minutes

Serves: 8

Ingredients:

- 6.5 lb. bone-in, skin-on turkey breast
- 1 tsp salt
- 1 tsp pepper
- 1 tsp garlic powder
- 1 tsp onion powder
- 1 tsp paprika
- 1 cup chicken broth
- 1 large onion, quartered
- 1 stock celery, cut in large pieces
- 1 sprig of thyme
- 3 cloves of garlic
- 3 tbsp arrowroot starch
- 3 tbsp cold water

Directions:

1. Season turkey breast with spices.

2. Stuff with onion, celery, garlic and thyme.

3. Brown turkey breast if desired with a bit of butter on sauté mode. Leave turkey breast side up when done

4.   Add chicken broth.

5.   Lock lid in place, select High Pressure and 30 minutes cooking time.

6.   When beep sounds, turn off pressure cooker and use a natural pressure release for 10 minutes, then do a quick pressure release to release any remaining pressure.

7.   When valve drops carefully remove lid. Use an instant read thermometer to check to see if the turkey is done. It should be 165°C lock the lid in place and cook it for a few more minutes.

8.   When, turkey has reached 165°C. Carefully remove turkey and place on large plate. Cover with foil.

9.   Strain and skim the fat off the broth if desired.

10.   Whisk together corn starch and cold water then add to broth in cooking pot.

11.   Select Sauté and stir until broth thickens. Add salt and pepper to taste.

12.   Remove breast from broiler and slice the turkey and serve immediately.

215. Ground Turkey Curry

Time: 30 minutes

Serves:4 max

Ingredients

- ½ onion (finely chopped)
- 1 tbsp grass-feed butter
- 1 tbsp olive oil
- 1 pound turkey, ground

Seasoning

- 1 ½ tbsp curry powder
- 1 tsp garam masala
- ¼ tsp cumin
- 1/8 tsp turmeric powder
- 1/8 tsp cayenne
- 1 tsp salt
- ½ tsp pepper
- 1 ½ cup coconut milk, light
- Cauliflower Rice

Directions:

1. Sauté onion in grass-feed butter and olive oil in a large skillet or pan over medium heat for about 5 minutes, or until onions turn translucent.

2. Add ground turkey and cook for another 7-10 minutes over medium heat, or until meat is cooked through.

3.   While meat is cooking, combine all of the seasoning ingredients (except the coconut milk) in a small bowl.

4.   Once meat is done cooking, add seasoning ingredients and coconut milk to the pan and stir until combined.

5.   Reduce heat to low and let simmer for another 10 minutes. Served with cauliflower rice

216. Zucchini Turkey Burgers

Serves: 5

Time : 35 Minutes

Ingredients:

- 1/4 cup chopped red onion

- 1 tbsp extra virgin olive oil

- 1 tbsp apple cider vinegar

- kosher salt and fresh cracked pepper to taste

- 3 medium vine ripe tomatoes(chopped)

- 2 small cloves garlic, minced

- 2 tbsp fresh basil leaves, chopped

- 3 oz almond cheese, diced

For the turkey zucchini burgers:

- 2 lbs lean ground turkey

- 1 cup zucchini, grated

- 1/4 cup seasoned whole wheat breadcrumbs

- 1 clove garlic, grated

- 1 tbsp red onion, grated

- salt and fresh pepper

For serving:

- 2 medium tomatoes, sliced into 10 thin slices

- 4 loose cups baby arugula

Directions:

1.   Combine the red onion, olive oil, apple cider, salt and pepper in a large bowl. Set aside a few minutes

2.   Then, place the chopped tomatoes in the bowl. Add the garlic, basil and additional salt and pepper, to taste and mix well and set aside. Toss in the cheese when ready to serve.

3.   Squeeze the excess moisture from the zucchini in a paper towel. In a large bowl, combine the ground turkey, shredded zucchini, breadcrumbs, garlic, onion, salt and pepper. Form into 5 equal sized patties.

4.   Heat a large skillet on medium-high heat. When hot, add olive oil. Add the burgers to the pan and reduce the heat to medium-low. Cook until browned, about 4 minutes, then flip and cook another 4 minutes, careful not to burn.

5.   To serve, arrange 3 slices of tomatoes on each dish, then place 1 cup arugula on top in the centre, then top with the burger, cheese and finish with the bruschetta serve right away.

217. Broccoli Rapini Turkey Burgers

Servings: 4 max

Time:

Ingredients:

For the broccoli rapini

- 1 bunch broccoli rapini, (washed, stems trimmed off)
- 1 tablespoon olive oil
- 3 cloves garlic, sliced thin
- kosher salt, to taste
- 1/4 teaspoon crushed red pepper flakes

For the patties

- 1 lb lean ground turkey
- 3 tbsp freshly grated almond cheese
- 1 garlic clove, crushed
- 1/2 tsp kosher salt
- 1/4 tsp fresh black pepper
- 1/4 teaspoon red pepper flakes (optional)

For the burger

- 4 slices large tomato
- 4 large lettuce leaves

Directions:

1.   Cut the remaining broccoli rapini into 2-inch pieces. Bring a large pot of salted water to a rolling boil, and then add the broccoli rapini. Blanch for about 1-1/2 to 2 minutes, drain well and set aside in a colander.

2.   Meanwhile, in a medium bowl, combine the turkey, 3/4 cup chopped broccoli rapini, almond cheese, garlic, salt and pepper. Form into 4 patties and refrigerate until ready to cook.

3.   Heat a large, deep sauté pan to medium-high heat, when hot add the olive oil and garlic and cook until golden about 1 minute, careful not to burn.

4.   Add the broccoli rapini to the pan and toss with garlic and oil, season with 1/4 tsp salt and crushed red pepper; cook about 2 to 3 minutes, or until heated through.

5.   While that is cooking, cook the burgers on a hot skillet over medium-high heat for about 7 minutes on each side, or until cooked through in the center.

6.   To serve place a lettuce leave on each plate, top tomato slice and cooked burger. Finish with the cooked broccoli rapini and optional more grated cheese if desired.

218. Turkey Kofta Kebabs

Serves: 4 max

Time:

Ingredients:

- 20 oz lean ground turkey
- 1 small onion, minced
- 2 cloves garlic. minced
- 1 tbsp ginger paste
- 1/4 cup fresh parsley, chopped
- 2 tbsp bread crumbs
- 1/4 tsp allspice
- 1/4 tsp coriander(chopped)
- 1/4 tsp paprika
- 1/4 tsp chili powder
- salt and fresh pepper (to taste)

Directions:

1.   In a large bowl combine the ground turkey, onion, garlic, parsley, breadcrumbs, spices, salt and pepper until evenly blended.

2.   Divide into a heaping 1/4 cup portions so you get 12; roll into log shaped ovals. Place on a cookie sheet and refrigerate at least 30 minutes.

3.   Soak the wooden skewers in water at least 30 minutes before grilling

4.   When ready to eat, preheat grill to high heat. Carefully insert the skewer through the formed meat.

5.   Grill for 10 to 15 minutes on indirect heat turning occasionally.

219. Turkey Sausage, Kale and White Bean Soup

Serves: 4

Time: 40 minutes

Ingredients:

- 550gm organic turkey sausage meat
- 2 tsp olive oil
- 1 clove garlic (minced)
- 1/2 bunch kale (chopped)
- 1 cup butternut squash (cubed)
- 4 cups vegetable broth
- 4 cups water
- 1 small pinch dried red pepper flakes (optional)
- salt and freshly ground pepper to taste

Directions:

1. Heat oil over medium-high heat in a medium sized pot.

2. Add sausage meat breaking it up with a spatula or wooden spoon into large chunks. When completely cooked. Sauté garlic for 2 – 3 minutes

3. Add the water, vegetable broth, butternut squash and red pepper flakes (if using) and stir thoroughly.

4. Simmer on low for 10 minutes, covered.

5. Add in kale and allow simmering for another 10 minutes covered.

6. Adjust salt and pepper to taste.

7. Serve hot.

220. Gravy Turkeylicious

Serves: 6 max

Time: 1 hour 15 mins

Ingredients

- 2kg pound bone-in turkey breast

- 1 ½ tbsp salt

- 2 tsp pepper

- 2 tablespoons coconut fat

- 1 medium onion, cut into medium dice

- 1 large carrot, cut into medium dice

- 1 celery rib, cut into medium dice

- 1 garlic clove, peeled and smashed

- 2 teaspoons dried sage

- 1½ cups bone broth

- 1 bay leaf

- 1 tablespoon arrowroot starch

Directions:

1. Season the turkey breast with salt and pepper.

2. Melt coconut fat in an Instant Pot, use the "saute" function. Brown turkey breast, skin side down, about 5 minutes, and transfer to a plate, leaving fat in pot.

3. Add onion, carrot, and celery "saute" function on Instant Pot until softened, about 5 minutes. Stir in garlic and sage and cook until fragrant, about 30 seconds.

4. Stir in broth and bay leaf, scrape up all browned bits stuck on bottom of pot.

5.   Lock lid in place and set electric pressure cooker for 35 minutes on high pressure.

6.   Transfer turkey breast to plate and tent loosely with foil, allowing it to rest.

7.   Transfer cooking liquid and vegetables to blender and puree until smooth. Return to medium high heat and cook until thickened and reduced to about 2 cups. Adjust seasoning to taste.

8.   Combine a tablespoon of arrowroot starch with a tablespoon of warm water and whisk into the gravy to thicken the gravy

9.   Slice turkey breast and serve with hot gravy.

221. Superlicious Chipotle Turkey

Time: 35 minutes

Serves: 4 serves

Ingredients

- 1 tbsp. coconut oil

- 1 lb. ground turkey

- 1 cup onion (diced)

- 4 cloves garlic (minced)

- 600gm tomatoes (diced)

- 2 small sweet potatoes (peeled and cut into small cubes)

- 2 cups chicken broth

- 2 tsp. chili powder

- 1 tsp. dried oregano

- 1 tsp. ground cumin

- ½ tsp. ground chipotle powder

- Sea salt and pepper to taste

Directions:

1. Heat oil in medium saucepan set over medium-high heat.

2. When oil starts to shimmer, add ground turkey. Break up turkey with a wooden spoon and cook 5 minutes.

3. Add onions and garlic and continue to cook an additional 10 minutes or until onions are translucent and meat is almost cooked through.

4.   Turn up the heat to high. Add tomatoes, sweet potatoes, broth and seasonings and bring to a boil.

5.   Reduce heat to medium-low and simmer uncovered 15 minutes until chili is hot and sweet potatoes are tender.

222. Tango Turkey

Serves: 4 max

Time: 45 minutes

Ingredients

- 1 lb lean ground turkey

- 2 small onions (diced)

- 1 tsp olive oil

- 2 bell pepper (diced)

- 4 cloves garlic (minced)

- 350gm tomatoes(diced)

- 100gm green chilies(diced)

- 1 cup salsa

- 1/4 cup cilantro (chopped)

- 2 cups fat free chicken stock

- 2 tsp cumin

- 2 tsp chili powder

- 1 tsp smoked paprika

- Salt and pepper to taste

Directions:

1.   Heat oil over medium high in skillet. Add in ground turkey, season with salt and pepper, and cook until no longer pink.

2.   Add in onions and garlic and cook until onion is soft, about 1-2 minutes.

3. Stir in diced tomatoes, chilies, bell peppers and cook for another 2 minutes.

4. Add in chicken stock, and salsa and stir well to combine.

5. Mix in the spices, and add salt and pepper to taste. Cover and let simmer on low for 10 minutes.

6. Top with fresh cilantro and serve.

223. Flavoursome Ground Turkey With Cabbage

Serves: 1 max

Time:25 minutes

Ingredients:

- 1/2 pound ground turkey

- 1 medium sweet yellow onion (chopped)

- 1 green cabbage (sliced)

- 10 Walnut pieces(roasted)

- 1 tbsp Coconut oil

- ½ tsp red chili powder

- 1 tsp Garlic powder

- 1 tsp onion powder

- ¼ tsp black pepper

- Salt

Directions:

1. Heat coconut oil over a medium heat in wok.

2. Add one handful of chopped onion and let cook 3 to 4 minutes, stirring occasionally.

3. Add ground turkey and, using a wooden spatula, break into small pieces and cook 7 minutes.

4. Season with of salt, garlic powder, and black pepper.

5. Add several handfuls of sliced cabbage. Season with of salt and garlic powder.

6. Add a dusting of red chili powder if you like heat. Stir meat and veggies together.

7.   Throw a handful of walnut pieces on top. Cover and let cook 5 minutes

8.   Serve.

224. Daintiness Ground Turkey Brussels Sprouts

Time: 40 minutes

Serves: 4 max

Ingredients

- 3 tablespoons coconut oil, divided

- 1 onion, diced

- 1 pound ground turkey

- 4 cloves garlic, minced

- 2 teaspoons chili powder

- 1 teaspoon salt, adjust to taste

- ½ teaspoon black pepper

- ½ teaspoon cayenne

- 1 bell pepper, diced

- ½ pound brussels sprouts, shredded

Directions:

1. Melt 2 tablespoons of coconut oil in a large skillet over medium heat.

2. Add the onion and stir-fry for 5 minutes or until the onions are soft.

3. Then add the ground turkey, garlic and spices and cook for 15 minutes.

4. Set some of the meat aside in a bowl to make room for the brussels sprouts.

5. Melt the remaining coconut oil in the skillet and add brussels sprouts and a bell pepper. Stir-fry for 5 minutes, or until the vegetables are tender.

6. Add the meat back into the pan and mix well.

7.   Serve.

225. Glory Pizza

Serves:4 max

Time: 45 minutes

Ingredients

For Crust

- 1 1/2 cup cauliflower (shredded)
- 2 Eggs
- 1 tsp Italian seasoning
- ½ tsp oregano
- ½ tsp Garlic powder
- ½ tsp Onion powder
- 1/4 tsp Salt

For Pizza

- 2 Eggs
- 1½ cups mushrooms, sliced
- 4 ounces pepperoni, quartered
- 1 tbsp Fresh Chives (chopped)

Directions:

1. Preheat oven to 375 ° F.

2. Add the ingredients for the crust to a large mixing bowl and mix until well combined.

3. Pour the crust mixture onto a baking pan lined with foil. Shape the mixture into a pizza crust shape. Use your fingers to create a raised ridge around the edge of the crust.

4.   Bake the crust in the oven for 15 minutes.

5.   While the crust is cooking heat a skillet over medium heat. Saute the mushroom and pepperoni. Remove from the skillet and transfer to a bowl and allow cool for 3-5 minutes. Beat together 2 eggs and add to the bowl with the pepperoni and mushrooms

6.   Remove the cauliflower crust from the oven. Pour the eggs, mushroom and pepperoni into the crust, being careful not to let any spill over the edges.

7.   Return the crust to the oven and bake for an additional 8-10 minutes, until the eggs have set.

8.   Remove from the oven. Garnish with chopped chives and serve.

226. Supreme Pizza

Serves:4 max

Time:55 minutes

Ingredients

- 2 cups sweet potato(shredded)

- 2 eggs(whisked)

- 1/2 tsp garlic powder

- 1/2 tsp onion powder

- 1/2 tsp Italian seasoning

- Salt & pepper to taste

- 1/3 pound ground grass-feed beef

- 1/3 cup diced onion

- 1/2 cup broccoli

- 1/2 cup cherry tomatoes(sliced)

- 4 fresh eggs (for topping pizza)

Directions:

1.   Preheat oven to 350°F. Lightly grease a pizza pan.

2.   Mix eggs, sweet potatoes, and the seasonings in a small bowl. Use the mixture to form a "crust" by spreading it out in the center of the pizza pan to create a flat round shape

3.   Bake the crust for 20 minutes.

4.   While the crust is baking, sauté the onions in a skillet over medium heat for 3-4 minutes. Next add the ground grass-feed beef to the same skillet with the onion and cook until sausage is browned.

5.   Remove pan with the crust from the oven after 25 minutes and top with the onion and beef mixture. Next add the tomatoes and broccoli. Finally crack one fresh egg on top of each quarter section of the breakfast pizza.

6.   Then, bake the pizza about 15 minutes.

7.   Cut and serve

227. Fruity Delight Pizza

Serves:2 max

Time:20 minutes

Ingredients

- 2 Tbsp. coconut flour

- 1 tsp. cinnamon

- 1 egg(whisked)

- 1/2 cup shredded zucchini

- 5 drops stevia

- 1/8 tsp. pure vanilla extract

- 1/4 cup coconut yogurt

- ¼ cup strawberries(sliced)

- ¼ cup grapes (sliced)

- ¼ cup bananas(sliced)

Directions:

1. Preheat oven to 350 ˚F

2. Combine coconut flour and cinnamon in a bowl. Add egg, stevia, vanilla extract and shredded zucchini mix well to combine.

3. Spread mixture into a pizza crust on a cooking sheet lined with parchment paper.

4. Bake for 15 minutes

5. Let cool and spread on coconut yogurt and top with fruits.

6. Enjoy

228. Farmhouse Pizza

Serves:4 max

Time: 45 minutes

Ingredients

For Crust

- 1 1/2 cup cauliflower (shredded)
- 2 Eggs
- 1 tsp Italian seasoning
- ½ tsp oregano
- ½ tsp Garlic powder
- ½ tsp Onion powder
- ¼ tsp Salt

For Pizza

- 4 Eggs
- 1 cups mushrooms, sliced
- ½ cup tomato cherry(sliced)
- ½ cup black olives(sliced)
- 1 medium onion (sliced)
- ½ cup green bell pepper (sliced)
- 1 tbsp Fresh Chives (chopped)

Directions:

1. Preheat oven to 375 ˚ F.

2. Add the ingredients for the crust to a large mixing bowl and mix until well combined.

3. Pour the crust mixture onto a baking pan lined with foil. Shape the mixture into a pizza crust shape. Use your fingers to create a raised ridge around the edge of the crust.

4. Bake the crust in the oven for 15 minutes.

5. While the crust is cooking heat a skillet over medium heat. Saute the mushroom, tomato cherries, bell peppers, olive and onion.

6. Remove from the skillet and transfer to a bowl and allow cool for 3-5 minutes. Beat together 2 eggs and add to the bowl with the sauted vegetables

7. Remove the cauliflower crust from the oven. Pour the mixture into the crust, being careful not to let any spill over the edges.

8. Return the crust to the oven and bake for an additional 8-10 minutes, until the eggs have set.

9. Remove from the oven. Garnish with chopped chives and serve.

229. Tasty Scrape Pork

Serves:4-6 max

Ingredients

- 3.5 lbs boneless pork shoulder roast
- 2 tablespoons paprika
- 2 tablespoons chili powder
- 2 tablespoons cumin
- 1 tablespoon ground black pepper
- 1 tablespoon white pepper
- 1 tablespoon oregano
- 1 teaspoon parsley
- 2 teaspoons cayenne
- 2 teaspoons dried mustard
- 2 teaspoons sea salt

Directions:

1) Combine spices and mix well.
2) Remove any string holding your pork together.
3) With your hands, rub all parts of the pork with the spice mixture - making sure to get into every crevice.
4) Wrap pork tightly with plastic wrap and let it sit overnight.
5) The next morning, unwrap the pork and set it in your slow cooker or Instant Pot.
6) Cook on low for 8 hours and serve.

230. Rainbow Pulled Pork Taco Salad

Serves:4 max

Ingredients:

- 1 batch slow cooker pulled pork
- 2 heads of romaine lettuce, shredded
- 1 sliced avocado
- 1 cup cherry tomatoes (cut into 4)
- 1 medium onion (chopped)
- 1 fresh cilantro
- 1 red bell pepper, seeds removed and sliced
- 1 green bell pepper, seeds removed and sliced
- 1 yellow bell pepper, seeds removed and sliced
- 1 carrot, sliced and cut 2 inch long
- 1 tablespoon coconut amino
- 1 tablespoon olive oil

Directions:

1) Heat a pan over medium high heat and add in olive oil.
2) Once oil is hot, add the sliced peppers and onions
3) Sauté until both the onions and peppers are relatively soft but not mushy.
4) Place shredded lettuce in a bowl and top with pulled pork, avocado, vegetables and pepper mixture.
5) Top with coconut amino

231. Tangy Wangy Delitender Pork

Serves: 6

Time: 1 hour 15 minutes

Ingredients

- 2 lbs boneless pork roast

- 1 tbsp grass-feed butter

- 12 oz fresh cranberries

- 10 oz bone broth

- 2 tbsp chopped fresh herbs (a mix of oregano, marjoram, and sage)

- 2 tbsp lemon juice

- 15 drops stevia

- ¼ tsp cinnamon

- 1/8 tsp ground cloves

- ¼ tsp granulated garlic

- Sea salt

Directions:

1) Set your Instant Pot to the sauté function. Add grass-feed butter. Salt pork generously on all sides and place in hot oil. Sear on each side, uncovered, for 2 minutes until lightly browned.

2) Set the Instant Pot to the manual pressure cooker setting for 70 minutes. Add cranberries and broth to the bottom of pot, being sure not to "wash away" the salt off the pork. Sprinkle chopped herbs, lemon juice and stevia on top and close the lid. Cook undisturbed for full 70 minutes.

3) Release the pressure using the release valve, remove the pork to a cutting board and use two fork to shred the pork.

4) Place back in the Instant Pot, sprinkle with a pinch more sea salt, and set the manual option for another 10 minutes. This allows the shredded pork to absorb the broth, increasing its moisture and flavor.

5) Remove pork and cranberries from the liquid and place in a large serving dish. Toss with the cinnamon, garlic, and cloves and serve warm.

232. Tasty Oink Cauli Gravy

Time:1 hour 15 minutes

Serves:6 max

Ingredients

- 2 to 3pound pork roast

- 1teaspoon sea salt (real salt)

- 1/2teaspoon black pepper

- 4cups chopped cauliflower

- 1medium onion, chopped

- 4cloves garlic

- 2ribs celery

- 8ounces portabella mushrooms (sliced)

- 2tablespoons organic coconut oil

- 2cups filtered water

Directions:

1) In the bottom of your pressure cooker, place cauliflower, onion, garlic, celery and water. Top with pork roast and season with sea salt & pepper.

2) Cook under pressure for 90 minutes. Quick depressurize following manufactures directions.

3) Carefully remove pork roast from the pressure cooker and place in an oven proof dish.

4) Bake at 400 °F while preparing the gravy, this helps to render the fat and crisp up the edges of the pork to be more like as if it was slow roasted.

5) Transfer cooked vegetables and broth to your blender and blend until smooth, set aside.

6) Then, cook mushrooms in coconut oil until soft, roughly 3-5 minutes. Add blended vegetables and continue to cook on the saute function until it is thickened as desired.

7) Serve mushroom gravy over shredded pork

233. Tangy Pork Chop

Time:20 minutes

Serves:4 max

Ingredients

- 4 thick-cut Pork Chops
- 1 teaspoon fennel seeds
- 1 teaspoon salt
- 1 teaspoon pepper
- 500gm head of cabbage
- 1 tablespoon olive oil
- ¾ cup meat stock
- 2 teaspoons arrowroot flour

Directions

1) Firstly, unwrap the pork chops and sprinkle with fennel, salt and pepper.

2) Prepare the cabbage by slicing the cabbage in half almost through the core, and then in thick ¾ inch slices and set aside.

3) In the pre-heated pressure cooker, on medium-high heat without the lid, add oil, and brown all of the chops

4) When all of the chops have been browned and set aside, add the cabbage slices into the empty pressure cooker.

5) On top of the cabbage arrange the pork chops brown-side up, overlapping as needed. Pour any juice from the chops and meat stock around the edges.

6) Close and lock the lid of the pressure cooker.

Electric pressure cookers: Cook for8 minutes at high pressure.

Stove top pressure cookers: Cook for 6 minutes at high pressure.

7) When time is up, open the pressure cooker with the Normal release - release pressure through the valve.

8) Using tongs, move the cabbage and pork chops to a serving platter and tent lightly with foil while preparing the gravy.

9) Bring the left-over juices in the pressure cooker to a boil and whisk-in the flour.

10) Pour thickened sauce on top of cabbage and pork chop platter and serve.

234. Sexy Graved Pork

Serves:4 max

Time:1 hour 45 minutes

Ingredients

- 900g pork shoulder
- 1 teaspoon xylitol
- 2 tbsp coconut aminos
- 1 tsp sea salt
- ⅓ cup water or bone broth
- 1 1"/ 2.5cm length fresh ginger, peeled and smashed
- A few sprigs of coriander/ cilantro leaves, to garnish

Directions

1. Fill a pot with enough water to cover the quantity of pork cubes and bring to boil over high heat

2. Add the pork and boil for 3 minutes, then drain and rinse off any scum or impurities

3. Set aside the pork cubes in a colander to drain

4. Heat the xylitol in the inner pot of the Instant Pot on 'sauté' setting

5. Add the pork cubes to the heated xylitol and brown the pork for approximately 10 minutes (use a splatter guard)

6. Add the rest of the ingredients to the pot

7. Bring to a boil, then press cancel/ keep warm

8. Seal the lid, and valve, then select 'manual' setting and adjust the cooking time to 25 minutes

9. Allow the pressure to release naturally

10. Open the lid and select 'sauté' setting

11. Bring the contents to a simmer until the sauce is sufficiently reduced and thickened to coat the pork cubes (or to your liking)

12. Serve with coriander/ cilantro leaves as a garnish

235. Browny Wonder Pork

Time:30 minutes

Servings:4-6 max

Ingredients:

- 1kg/ 2lb pork belly

- 1 teaspoon stevia

- 3 tbsp coconut aminos

- 6 cloves garlic, smashed lightly

- 1 inch ginger, peeled and thickly sliced

- 2 strips mace

- 1 clementine peel, dried (optional)

- 1 stick cinnamon or 1/2 tsp ground cinnamon

- 2/3 cup bone broth or water

- 1 tsp sea salt

Directions:

1) Firstly, in Instant Pot select 'Sauté' setting and once 'Hot' is displayed on the panel, add in all ingredients except for the pork

2) Stir in the pork pieces and seal the Instant Pot with the lid

3) Cancel the 'Sauté' setting and select 'Manual' setting

4) Cook the pork for 20 minutes

5) Once the pressure cooker beeps, uncover and remove meat from the pot and set aside

6) Select 'Sauté' setting and allow the sauce in the pot to boil until the sauce is slightly thickened

7) Slice pork cheeks into diagonal slices

8) Serve garnished with coriander leaves and sauce spooned over

236. Jawbreaker Duck

Serves:5 max

Ingredients:

- 4 duck legs with thighs;

- 4 duck wings;

- 4 cups coconut fat;

- 3 tbsp salt;

- 4 garlic cloves, very finely minced;

- 1 onion, sliced;

- 6 springs thyme;

- 3 springs rosemary;

- Pepper to taste;

Directions:

1. Mix the salt, garlic, onion, thyme, rosemary and pepper.

2. Using a dish large enough to hold all the duck pieces in a single layer sprinkle 1/3 of the salt mixture on the bottom.

3. Put the duck pieces in the dish, skin side up on the salt mixture bed.

4. Add the remaining 2/3 of the salt mixture evenly on the duck.

5. Cover and refrigerate for about 2 days.

6. When ready, preheat your oven to 225°F

7. Remove the salt from the duck and arrange the duck in a baking dish in a tight single layer.

8. Melt the coconut fat and pour on the duck. Make sure it covers the meat entirely.

9. Put in the oven for 3 hours until the meat can easily scrape from the bone.

10. The duck is now ready and can be stored in the fat where it will stay good for weeks.

237. Salad Paleo

Amaze Coconut Dill Turkey Salad

Serves:2-3 max

Time:40 minutes

Salad

- 50gm turkey breasts
- 4 cups Romaine lettuce leaves, washed and dried
- ½ cup cherry tomatoes, (halves)
- 1 red onion, sliced
- 1 avocado, sliced
- ⅓ cup pitted black olives sliced
- Lemon wedges, to serve

Dressing

- 1/2 a cup Thai coconut meat
- Juice of 1/2 lemon
- 1 tablespoon chia seeds
- 3 cups chopped zucchini
- 1/2 cup of water
- 1 tablespoon garlic powder
- 2 tablespoons onion powder
- 1 tablespoon dried dill, or fresh chopped dill
- 1 teaspoon Himalayan salt

Directions:

1. Whisk together all of the dressing ingredients in a bowl.

2. Pour ½ dressing to marinade turkey for 30 minutes in the refrigerator.

3. Then, prepare all of the salad ingredients and mix in a large salad bowl.

4. Once turkey is ready, heat 1 tablespoon of olive oil in a grill pan or a grill plate over medium-high heat. Grill turkey on both sides until browned and completely cooked through.

5. Allow turkey to rest for 5 minutes; slice and arrange over salad. Drizzle salad with the remaining dressing.

6. Serve with lemon wedges.

238. Egovado Salad

Serves:1

Time:5 minutes

Ingredients

- 1 hard-boiled egg(diced)

- 1/2 Avocado (diced)

- 2 slices bacon (crumbled)

- 2 tbsp lemon juice

- Sea salt and Black pepper (to taste)

Directions:

1. Mash the avocado.

2. Drizzle with lemon juice.

3. Add the diced egg and crumbled bacon to the mashed avocado and mix until it well combined

4. Season with sea salt and black pepper.

5. Serve immediately.

239. Sweet Potato Bacon Egg Salad

Serves:3 max

Time:15 minutes

Ingredients

Salad

- 3 Sweet potato (diced)
- 6 pieces bacon (chopped)
- 3 Eggs (cubed)

Dressing

- 1 tbsp Dill (dried)
- 2 tbsp lemon juice
- 1 tbsp Yellow mustard
- 4 tbsp paleo mayo
- ½ tsp Salt
- ½ tsp black pepper
- 1 tsp onion powder
- 1 tsp garlic powder

Directions:

1. Fry diced sweet potato until tender about 8-10 minutes.
2. While those items are cooking, add ingredients for the dressing to a medium-sized mixing bowl, and whisk.
3. Once everything is complete, add bacon, eggs, and potatoes to a large bowl, and combine well.

4. Then, top with dressing mixture. Serve

240. Tangy Shrimp Salad

Serves: 2

Cook : 40 minutes

Ingredients:

- 1 lb. shrimp, peeled and deveined;

- 5 cups mixed greens;

- 1/2 cup cherry tomatoes, (halved)

- 1 avocado, chopped;

- 1/2 red onion, (sliced)

- 1 tbsp. chili powder;

- 1/2 tbsp. paprika;

- 1/2 tsp. cumin powder;

- 1/2 cup lemon juice;

- 1/3 cup packed cilantro leaves, roughly chopped;

- 1/4 cup extra virgin olive oil;

- Sea salt and freshly ground black pepper;

- Wood skewers;

Directions:

1. In a bowl, combine the chili powder, paprika, cumin, and 1/4 cup lemon juice.

2. Place the shrimp in the chili mixture and marinate for 20 minutes.

3. Preheat grill to medium-high heat.

4. Thread the shrimps on wood or metal skewers.

5. Grill the shrimp until it turns pink for 5 minutes per side.

6. In a dressing jar, combine the cilantro, olive oil, 1/4 cup lime juice, and season to taste.

7. In a salad bowl, combine the mixed greens, tomatoes, avocado, red onion and shrimp.

8. Drizzle with vinaigrette and serve.

241. Shrimp Salad Vinaigrette Delight

Serves: 2 max

Time:25 minutes

Ingredients

Salad

- 2-3 cups Romaine lettuce
- 1 Carrot (sliced)
- 1 tbsp capers
- 1/4 cup Onions (sliced)
- 10 Shrimp (medium-sized, peeled and deveined)
- 1 tbsp grass-feed butter

Vinaigrette

- 1/3 cup evoo
- 1/4 cup Apple cider vinegar
- 1 tbsp garlic (minced)
- 5 drops stevia

Directions :

1. Prepare the salad mix (excluding the shrimp and the butter) in a large salad bowl. Set aside.

2. Blend all the vinaigrette ingredients until it becomes smooth and creamy

3. In a pan sauté the shrimp with 1 tbsp grass-feed butter for 4 minutes

4. Serve the salad and the shrimp and top with the vinaigrette.

5. Enjoy

242. Saladious

Scrapped Chicken Gem Salad with Almond Dressing Recipe

Serves: 4

Time: 20 minutes

Ingredients:

- 4 pcs chicken breast
- 1 tsp chili powder
- 1 cup pomegranate
- 1 cup fresh blueberries;
- 1 cup arugula(chopped)
- 1 cup spinach(chopped)
- 1 cup romaine lettuce(chopped)
- ½ cup almond (crushed)
- 1 tbsp Coconut fat
- Sea salt and freshly ground black pepper (to taste)

Almond Dressing

- 3 tbsp. almond butter
- 1 tbsp. olive oil
- 2 tbsp. lemon juice
- 3 tbsp. water
- 1 tbsp. ground mustard;
- 6 drops stevia

- ½ garlic clove (minced)

- Sea salt and freshly ground black pepper to taste

Directions:

1. Season the chicken breast with chilli powder, salt and pepper.

2. In a large skillet, heat coconut fat over a medium-high heat.

3. Add the chicken to the skillet cook by flip it both sides until golden for 10 minutes.

4. When the chicken is done, remove from the heat and wait for it to cool for 5 minutes

5. Then scrapped the chicken using fork

6. Combine well all the ingredients for the dressing in a bowl and season to taste.

7. In a salad bowl, combine the spinach, lettuce, arugula, pomegranate, blueberries, almonds, and scrapped chicken.

8. Pour the dressing on top and serve.

243. Delish Cardini's Salad

Serves:4 max

Time:25 minutes

Ingredients:

- 1 head Romaine lettuce;

- 2 chicken breast

- 1 avocado (sliced)

- 4 bacon slices (cooked and chopped)

- 2 eggs, (hard-boiled and sliced)

- ¼ tsp. pepper

- ½ tbsp. garlic powder

- ½ tbsp. onion powder

- ½ tbsp. dried oregano

- Sea salt and freshly ground black pepper

Caesar Dressing

- 1 cup paleo mayonnaise;

- 2 garlic cloves, minced;

- 2 tbsp. fresh lemon juice;

- 1 tbsp minced anchovy fillet(optional)

- 1 tsp. Dijon mustard;

- Sea salt and freshly ground black pepper

Directions:

1. Preheat the grill to medium-high heat.

2. Season the chicken with chili powder, garlic powder, onion powder, oregano, and salt and pepper to

3. Grill the chicken for 10 minutes both sides

4. Transfer chicken to a cutting board and slice.

5. In a medium bowl, whisk together all the ingredients for the Caesar dressing until well blended and season to taste.

6. In a bowl toss the lettuce with the bacon and avocado.

7. Top with sliced chicken and eggs.

8. Pour the dressing on top, mix and serve.

244. Healthy Monster Salad

Serves: 4

Time: 20 minutes

Ingredients:

- 2 cup arugula

- ¼ cup onion(sliced)

- 1 cup pomegranate

- 1 cup coconut meat

- 1 avocado(sliced)

- ½ cup sprouts

- ¼ cup rosemary

- 1 handful basil (chopped)

- ½ cup almond (crushed)

- Sea salt and freshly ground black pepper (to taste)

Dressing

- ¾ cup lemon juice

- ½ cup olive oil

- 1 tbsp. ginger(minced)

- 3-5 drops stevia

- 1 garlic clove (minced)

- Salt and pepper

Directions:

1. Combine well all the ingredients for the dressing in a bowl

2. In a salad bowl, combine all the ingredients and season to taste.

3. Pour the dressing on top and serve.

245. Mindfulness Salad

Serves:2-3 max

Time:30 minutes

Ingredients:

- 1 cup smoked salmon(chopped)

- 1 avocado, peeled, pitted and diced

- 2 cups baby spinach

- 2 cup arugula

- 1 cup dandelion (chopped)

- 1/2 cup fresh blueberries

- 1/4 cup almond cheese

- 1/4 cup chopped walnuts (optional)

- half a red onion, thinly sliced

Dressing

- 1/3 cup olive oil

- 2 tbsp. apple cider vinegar

- 1 tbsp. chia seeds

- 6-8 drops stevia

- 1/4 tsp. salt

Directions:
1. Combine well all the ingredients for the dressing in a bowl
2. In a salad bowl, combine all the ingredients and season to taste.

3. Pour the dressing on top and serve.

246. Glory Beauty Salad

Serves:2-3max

Time:20 minutes

For the salad:

- 2 cups baby arugula

- 1 cup kale (chopped)

- 1 large carrot, scrubbed well and shredded

- ½ medium beet, peeled and shredded

- ½ cucumber, (and thinly sliced)

- 1 small onion(chopped)

- 10 tomato cherries (halves)

- 1 firm ripe avocado (sliced)

- 2 tablespoons sunflower seeds

- 2 tablespoons raw sliced almonds

- 2 tablespoons raw shelled pumpkin seeds

For the detox dressing:

- ¾ cup lemon juice

- 4-6 drops stevia

- ½ cup olive oil

- pinch dry mustard powder

- sea salt and black pepper

- ¼ cup fresh parsley, chopped

Directions:

1. Add the kale to the water just until it turns bright green (about 1 minute). Drain.

2. Refrigerate kale until cold.

3. Combine well all the for the dressing in a bowl

4. In a salad bowl, combine all the salad ingredients and season to taste.

5. Pour the dressing on top and serve.

247. Seafood Paleo

Zesty Steamed Clams

Serves:4 max

Time: 20 minutes

Ingredients:

- 3 pounds fresh clams, (scrubbed)

- 1/4 cup grass-feed butter

- 4 cloves garlic, (minced)

- 1 cup (250 ml) dry white wine

- 1 cup bone broth

- 1 cup water

- 1 bunch green onions, (chopped)

- 3 tbsp fresh parsley stems

- 1 lemon sliced

Directions:

1. In a pressure cooker, melt butter over medium heat.

2. Add minced garlic and sauté for about 2 minutes.

3. Pour bone broth and water. Increase heat to medium-high and bring mixture to a boil. Boil for 1 minute. Stir in green onions, parsley stems and lemon slices.

4. Arrange the trivet and steamer basket in the pot. Fill the basket with scrubbed clams.

5. Close pressure cooker and lock the lid. Set the burner heat to high pressure. When cooker reaches high pressure, reduce heat to low. Set timer to cook for 4 minutes (don't overcook or the clams will be tough)

6. Open pressure cooker, using Quick Release method. Discard any unopened clams.

7. Using tongs, transfer cooked clams to serving bowl. Strain cooking liquid through cheesecloth. Discard the solids.

8. Pour cooking liquid over cooked clams.

9. Serve with lemon wedges and chopped fresh parsley.

248. Seafoodlicious Rice

Serves:4 max

Time:55 minutes

Ingredients:

Fish Stock

- 4 white cod fish heads
- 2 carrots(diced)
- 1 Celery(chopped)
- 1 Bay leaf
- Bunch of parsley with stems
- 6 Cups of water

Paella

- 4 Tbsp EVOO
- 1 Medium Yellow Onion, diced
- 1 Red Bell Pepper - diced
- 1 Green Bell Pepper - diced
- Large pinch saffron threads
- 2 Cups cauliflower rice
- 1¾ Cups filtered water
- ⅛ tsp ground turmeric
- 2 tsp Sea Salt
- 1 Cup of seafood (squid, meaty white fish, scallops)

- 2 Cups of mixed shellfish (clams, mussels, shrimp)

Directions:

Fish Stock

1. Add all the ingredients to Instant Pot

2. Set on HIGH for 5 minutes

3. When timer goes off, use NPR to release pressure

Paella

1. Set Instant Pot on "SAUTE" and heat EVOO. If using stove top pressure cooker, heat the pot on medium heat until the pot is hot and add EVOO. All the other electric pressure cooker, use the direction to heat the unit hot to add EVOO.

2. When the oil gets hot, add onions and peppers and saute until onions soften, about 4 minutes.

3. Stir in the saffron, cauliflower rice, and seafood and sauté everything together for 2 minutes.

4. Then add stock, turmeric, salt, and mix well.

5. Arrange the shellfish on top and do not mix further.

6. Close and lock the lid of the pressure cooker.

7. Cook at high pressure for 6 minutes.

8. When timer is up, use natural pressure release (NPR) method.

9. If NPR doesn't release pressure in 15 minutes, release the pressure manually by opening the vent valve.

10. After the pressure is completely released, open the lid, mix the paella well, cover and let stand for 1 minute before serving.

249. Harmony Lagareiro Octopus

Makes 8 servings

Total Time: 45 minutes

Ingredients

- 1kg octopus

- 1 cup sweet potatoes (cubed)

- 1 tbsp olive oil

- 10 cloves garlic

- 2 tsp parsley

- 1 bay leaf

- 1 tablespoon lemon juice

- salt (to taste)

Directions

1. Rinse and place the octopus in a pressure cooker with 1 cup of water.

2. Boil over medium heat then cook for 15 minutes

3. Remove the octopus and drain well.

4. Boil the sweet potatoes until soft

5. Preheat oven to 210°C

6. Smack each potato with a wooden spoon to crack and flatten.

7. Arrange octopus and sweet potatoes in a baking dish. In a small saucepan, heat olive oil, garlic, parsley, bay leaf, and lemon juice.

8. Bring to a boil over medium heat. Pour the sauce over the potatoes and octopus.

9. Place the dish in the oven and cook until well browned. Serve immediately.

250. Beaufort Stew Shrimp

Time: 42 minutes

Serves: 4-6 max

Ingredients:

- 6 chicken breast

- 2 pounds sweet potatoes

- 4 smoked Andouille sausages

- 2 - 4 ears of sweet corn

- 8 ounces fresh shrimp

- 7 teaspoons coconut aminos

- 1 teaspoon thyme

- 1 teaspoon oregano

- 2 tablespoons lemon juice

- 1 teaspoon coarse kosher salt

- ½ teaspoon coarsely ground pepper

- 2 – 3 tablespoons broth

- 1 – 2 tablespoons grass-feed butter (optional)

- 2 dried bay leaves

Directions:

1. Stir to mix the shrimp with coconut amino

2. Clean the sweet potatoes and then cut them into approximately. Submerge the potato pieces in cold water until you are ready to pressure cook them.

3. Season the chicken breast with salt, thyme, oregano, ginger, garlic and pepper and brown them in either a large skillet or your pressure cooker. Set your pressure cooker, with the lid off, to the "Browning" setting, add 1 tablespoon of grass-feed butter, and half of the chicken parts. When the chicken has been browned, turn off the machine.

4. Add the coconut amino, coarse kosher salt, coarsely ground pepper and lemon juice to the pressure cooker pot..

5. Layer the chicken in the bottom of the pot, squeezing the pieces in if need be, to try to get them in a single row if possible. Add any drippings if you browned the thighs in a skillet. Add 1 cup of water.

6. Add the sweet potatoes to the pot, tucking them into any spaces created by the chicken, adjusting them to fit as much of the potatoes into a single layer.

7. Prick the sausages with a fork repeatedly to reduce the chances of splitting. Shuck the corn, remove the silks, cut off the stalk and trim the tip if needed to fit the corn into the pressure cooker. Layer the sweet corn and sausages into the machine, and then any chicken and potatoes reserved earlier, making sure not to exceed the fill line (if need be, remove the corn, pressure cook the rest of the ingredients first, then pressure cook the corn separately 3 minutes with the boil broth).

8. Add the bay leaves, lock the lid and pressure cook at HIGH PRESSURE (10 PSI) for 4 minutes.

9. If shrimp is already cooked, turn off the "Keep Warm" function. When pressure finishes releasing, unlock the lid, discard the bay leaves, and remove the food.

10. If shrimp is cooked, place it on top of the rest of the ingredients and let the heat of the food warm it up. Turn your machine off.

11. Cut up the corn and sausages now, or serve them whole. Season the food with additional salt, oregano and pepper to taste

12. Serve

251. Bombastic Lobster

Serves:4 max

Time:40 minutes

Ingredients

For Lobsters

- 4 live lobsters

- 1/3 cup olive oil

- 2 tbsp. fresh basil, minced

- 2 tbsp. fresh chives, minced

- 1 tbsp. fresh fennel leaves, minced

- 1 tbsp fresh rosemary, minced

- 1 clove garlic, minced

- Lemon wedges, quartered

- Sea salt and freshly ground black pepper

For the Fresh Herb Butter

- ½ cup grass-feed butter

- 2 tbsp. fresh chives, minced

- 1 tbsp. fennel leaves, minced

- 1/4 teaspoon minced garlic.

- ½ teaspoon black pepper

- 1 tablespoon minced scallions (white and green parts)

- 1 tablespoon minced fresh dill.

- 1 tablespoon minced fresh flat-leaf parsley.

- 1 teaspoon freshly squeezed lemon juice.

- 1 teaspoon kosher salt.

Directions:

1. Preheat grill to a medium heat.

2. For each lobster, place the tip of a knife on the cross at the base of the head and cut the lobster in half.

3. Discard the sand sac near the head. Using the tip of the knife, carefully remove the gray intestinal vein. With a small spoon, scoop out the liver and any coral or eggs.

4. In a small bowl, combine all the remaining ingredients for the lobster, and season to taste.

5. Baste each lobster with the fresh herb oil.

6. Place the lobsters on the grill, cut side up.

7. Cover and cook for about 10 minutes.

8. In a bowl, combine all the ingredients for the herb butter.

9. Serve the lobster with the butter and fresh lemon wedges.

252. Joy Lobster Salad With Zest Herbal Ajoaceite

Serves:2 max

Time: 45 minutes

Ingredients:

- 1/4 cup paleo mayo
- 1 large garlic clove, minced
- 1/2 tsp. Dijon mustard
- 2 Tbsp. chopped fresh dill
- 1 tsp. chopped fresh chives
- 1/2 tbsp. chopped fresh parsley
- 1 tsp. freshly squeezed lemon juice
- 1 medium onion(sliced)
- 1/4 tsp. paprika
- Salt and pepper
- 1 lb. cooked lobster meat, roughly chopped
- 4 Tbsp. melted grass-feed butter
- Arugula lettuce
- Butterhead lettuce
- Red coral lettuce
- ¼ cup Pomegranate seeds
- Lemon juice
- Olive oil

Directions:

1. In a medium sized bowl with a lid combine all ingredients, except lobster, lettuce and pomegranates and mix together well.

2. Place lid on bowl and transfer to refrigerator for at least 30 minutes before using, to ensure the flavour combine

3. Meanwhile, roughly chop the lobster meat and melt 4 tablespoons of grass-feed butter, toss with the lobster meat and set aside.

4. Remove from refrigerator and add in the chopped lobster meat. Combine until lobster meat is coated well.

5. Toss the lettuce with a bit of olive oil, lemon juice, salt and pepper to taste.

6. Top with lobster and pomegranate seeds.

7. Garnish with fresh dill

8. Serve

253. Jungle Queen Salad

Serves:2-4 max

Time:30 minutes

<u>For the lobster salad:</u>

- 2 cups cooked lobster meat, chopped into bite sized pieces
- 1½ cups cauliflower florets, cooked until tender and chilled
- ½ cup paleo mayo
- 1 tsp fresh tarragon leaves, chopped

<u>To serve:</u>

- 4 radicchio leaves
- 8 fresh romaine lettuce leaves
- 2 cups arugula leaves(chopped)
- ½ cup chopped tomatoes
- 1 lemon wedges

Directions:

1. Combine the cooked lobster, cooked cauliflower, mayonnaise and tarragon in a medium bowl. Stir until well combined and creamy.

2. Lay the lettuce leaves on a platter. Divide the lobster salad mixture between the 8 leaves. Sprinkle with chopped tomatoes.

3. Serve with lemon wedges

254. Tasty Shrimp Garden Delight

Servings:4 max

Time:10 minutes

Ingredients

- 1pound frozen wild caught shrimp, 16-20 countshell & tail on

- 1cup Cauliflower Rice

- 1/4cup grass-feed butter

- 1/4cup chopped fresh Parsley

- 1teaspoon sea salt (real salt)

- 1/4teaspoon black pepper

- 1pinch crushed red pepper (to taste)

- 1 medium lemon, juiced

- 1pinch saffron

- 1 ½ cups filtered water

- 4 cloves garlic (minced)

Optional Garnishes

- Grated almond cheese

- Desiccated coconut

- Chopped fresh parsley

- Fresh lemon Juice

Directions:

1. Combine all ingredients in your pressure cooker, layering the frozen-shell-on-shrimp on the top.

2. Secure lid and cook under pressure (high if you have a choice) for 5 minutes.

3. Quickly depressurize (by turning the valve of an electric multi cooker or placing a stove top unit under cool running water)

4. The paella can be served with the shells on the shrimp or gently remove cooked shrimp from the rice and peel. Add peeled shrimp back into the rice and serve.

5. Serve each serving with a garnish of fresh parsley, desiccated coconut, grated almond cheese and squeeze of lemon juice.

255. Bold Szechwan Shrimp

Time:35 minutes

Serves:4 max

Ingredients:

- 20 medium shrimp (peeled and de-veined)
- 1/2 onion, minced;
- 1/2 bell pepper, minced;
- 5 dried red chilies;
- 1 garlic clove, minced;
- 1 thumb-size piece fresh ginger root, minced;
- 2 tbsp. coconut oil;
- 1/4 cup coconut amino
- 2 tbsp. water
- 1 tsp. apple cider vinegar
- 1 tbsp. lime juice
- 8 drops stevia
- Fresh cilantro (to garnish)

Directions:

1. In a bowl, combine the coconut amino, apple cider vinegar, lime juice, stevia and water.
2. Melt the coconut oil in a skillet over medium heat.
3. Add the ginger and garlic to the skillet; cook 1 to 2 minutes.

4. Add the onion, bell pepper, and dried red chillies to the skillet and cook until onions are soft.

5. Place the shrimp in the skillet and cook until pink.

6. Pour in the sauce and stir until well-mixed; cook until the sauce thickens to desired consistency for 5 minutes

7. Serve topped with fresh cilantro.

256. Crab Mushroom Pockets

Serves: 4 max

Time: 30minutes

Ingredients:

- 20 portabello mushrooms (cleaned and washed)

- 1 1/2 cup cooked crab(minced)

- 1/2 red onion(minced)

- 1 celery stalk(minced)

- 2 garlic cloves (minced)

- 1/2 cup almond meal

- 1 tbsp fresh parsley (minced)

- 1 egg, beaten;

- Sea salt and freshly ground black pepper

Directions:

1. Preheat the oven to 425° F.

2. Wash the mushrooms and remove the stems; keep the stems and caps.

3. Place the caps on a baking sheet with the hole face up.

4. Mince the mushroom stems, then place in a bowl.

5. Add the crab meat, red onion, celery, garlic, almond meal, fresh parsley, sea salt and black pepper to the bowl with the minced stems, toss everything until well mixed.

6. Pour the beaten egg in the bowl, and mix again until well combined.

7. Fill each muffin cap with the crab mixture, then place in the preheated oven.

8. Bake for 15 to 20 minutes. Serve

Bone Broth

257. PALEOCROCK BONE BROTH

Ingredients

1. 2 bags beef bones or 2 chicken carcasses

2. 1 large onion, sliced in half

3. 1 head garlic, sliced in half

4. 3-4 slices celery, cut into 1" pieces

5. 1 cup baby carrots

6. 1 large handful fresh thyme or sage

7. 1 tablespoon apple cider vinegar per pound of bones

8. Water

Instructions

1. Place all ingredients in a 5-7 quart slow cooker. Fill with enough water to completely immerse. Cover and cook for 12 hours on low.

2. Remove large bones with tongs, and pour the broth through a slotted spoon into freezer-safe containers or mason jars. Cool and freeze what you don't plan to use within 4 days. Frozen bone broth will last up to 6 months in the freezer. Enjoy!

258. TITILLATING 12 HOUR BROTH

Ingredients

1.   2 kg beef bones, chopped into 2 inch lengths

2.   2 carrots, roughly chopped

3.   2 onions, roughly chopped

4.   1/2 head garlic

5.   2 bay leaves

6.   1 bunch fresh parsley, whole

7.   4 litres water

Preparation

1.   Pre heat the oven to 200C.

2.   Place the bones, onions, and carrots on a roasting tray.

3.   Place in the oven for 40 minutes and transfer into a large pan.

4.   Add the herbs, and cover with the cold water.

5.   Bring to a gentle simmer and let it cook for at least 6 hours.

6.   When ready, strain the broth.

7.   You should have about 1 litre of liquid that will set to a jelly in the fridge.

8.   To serve, reheat and drink as soup or use the jelly to flavour soups, stews and sauces. You could even garnish salad with it.

9.   Add salt to taste and fresh ginger, garlic, or grated horseradish if you like.

259. BASIC BEEF BROTH

Ingredients

1. Beef Bones

2. Water

3. Carrots

4. Onions

5. 1 satchel bouquet garnish

Instructions

1. Place the bone is a large pot

2. Cover with water

3. Add onions, carrots, and bouquet garnish

4. Simmer on medium-low heat for 8 hours

260. PALEO PHOBROTH

Ingredients

1. 1 onion, halved

2. 2" fresh ginger, halved lengthwise

3. 1 teaspoon avocado oil

4. 6 cups of Bare Bones Beef Broth

5. 4 cups of filtered water

6. 2 tablespoons fish sauce

7. 1 teaspoon sea salt

Spices

1. 1 cinnamon stick

2. 6 whole star anise

3. 5 whole cloves

4. 2 cardamom pods

5. 1 tablespoon fennel seeds

Directions:

Wrap the above ingredients in cheesecloth and securely tie

1. 1.5 lbs. of sirloin, very thinly sliced

2. 3 to 4 large parsnips, peeled

Toppings

1. lime wedges

2. chilli peppers

3. basil

4. mint

5. cilantro

6. bean sprouts

7. hot sauce

coconut aminos

1.   Char your ginger and onions, by placing them on a baking sheet in the highest position of your oven (toaster oven works great for this!). Turn your broiler on high. Brush the onions and ginger with avocado oil and place them on your baking sheet. Broil for 10 minutes and then turn and continue to broil for another 5 to 10 minutes.

2.   In a large pot, add the broth, filtered water, the charred onions and ginger, fish sauce, salt and spices wrapped in cheesecloth. Cover the broth and bring to a light boil and then turn down to a simmer. Continue simmering for 1 to 1.5 hours.

3.   Towards the end of your broth's cooking time, slice the parsnips and thinly slice the meat and set in the fridge, until ready to use.

4.   Put the broth through a mesh strainer to remove the ginger, onions and spices. Return it to the pot. Taste the broth and adjust the seasoning. The broth is the star of the show, so make sure it tastes great. You can add more salt or fish sauce, if it is not salty enough. If it is too salty, you can even add a little bit of honey to balance it out.

5.   Bring your broth back to a light boil. Add the sliced meat to the strained broth and allow it to cook through. This is how I do it. Some people place the meat in individual bowls and pour the piping hot broth over it. Which I think is the more traditional method, but I prefer to cook it all in the large pot.

6.   Add parsnips to the bottom of each bowl, ladle hot piping broth and meat into each bowl. Garnish with your favourite toppings and enjoy!

261. FANTASTIC PALEO BROTH

Ingredients

1.   1 quart beef bone broth (see above notes)

2.   1 piece ginger root

3.   1 onion

4.   1 beef steak thickly cut

5.   2 whole star anise

6.   1 tsp. fennel

7.   1 tsp. coriander

8.   2 whole cloves

9.   1 stick cinnamon

10.   1 cardamom pod

11.   2 Tbsp. fish sauce I used the liquid that comes off from my homemade anchovies.

12.   Garnishes spicy peppers, lime slices, sprouts, basil leaves, etc.

Instructions

1.   Begin by making your beef bone broth as explained above. You can either add in your spices during that process or separate out some broth and continue with the recipe as follows.

2.   Simmer your broth in a pot on the stove with your spice blend added in. I usually put my spices into a cotton bag to make for easier straining later on. As you simmer the broth, skim off any foam that comes to the top.

3.   Meanwhile, wash both your ginger root and your (peeled) onion, slice them in half, and place them on a baking sheet in your oven.

4.   Broil them until they get dark on top.

5. Once your ginger and onion are ready, add them to your simmering broth to give it more flavour.

6. Keep simmering for around half an hour, or until the soup has absorbed the flavours of the spices to your liking. At this point, I like to add in the fish sauce to taste. I start by adding one tablespoon and then taste it and then add more, a little bit at a time, if I think it needs it.

7. Remove your broth from the stove and remove the ginger and onion. I like reserving the onion for adding back to the soup later on. Strain the broth if necessary to get out any of the remaining spices, and put the broth back into the pot.

8. Meanwhile, I like to sear the outside of the beef that I will be adding to the pho. Many people like to thinly slice it raw and add it to the soup that way. I prefer to sear the edges first, leaving it very rare inside.

9. When you are ready to serve the soup, add the broth to each bowl. Thinly slice the seared beef and place the thin slices on top of the soup. The heat of the soup will help lightly cook the thin slices.

10. Serve with garnishes that each person can add to their bowl of soup as desired.

262. EXTRA EASY BROTH

Ingredients

1.   4 - 8 lbs of bones, from grass fed animals (depending on the size of stock pot)

2.   2 Tbsp apple cider vinegar

3.   vegetables, carrots, onions, celery

4.   water

Instructions

1.   Roast the bones in the oven at 375 F for 1 hour. This gives a good flavour to the stock.

2.   Remove the bones from the oven and place in a stock pot.

3.   Fill the pot with water - cover the bones.

4.   Add the vegetables - avoid Brussels sprouts, cabbage, broccoli, turnips as these tend to give a bitter flavour to the broth.

5.   Bring the water to a boil and add the vinegar.

6.   Turn the pot down to a simmer.

7.   Allow the broth to simmer for 24 hours or longer.

8.   As it cooks, add water as necessary and skim off any foam.

9.   When finished, strain the broth through a wire mesh and catch the broth in mason jars.

10.   Once cooled, the fat will rise to the top and the broth should gel like gelatine.

11.   The fat can be skimmed off and used for cooking or left in the broth.

12.   The broth will keep refrigerated for 1 week and can also be frozen for months.

263. BEEFY BROTH

Ingredients

1. 1 pound / ½ kilo beef bones

2. 4 small carrots

3. 1 stick celery

4. 1 leek

5. 1 brown onion

6. 1 teaspoon thyme

7. 1 bay leaf

8. 1 tablespoon apple cider vinegar

9. 8 cups / 2 L water

Instructions

1. Place the bones in a large stock pot. Pour filtered water over the bones and add the apple cider vinegar. Bring to a boil.

2. Roughly chop and add the vegetables, except the garlic to the pot.

3. Add the herbs.

4. Simmer over low heat for 12 hours or more.

5. Remove from the heat and allow cooling.

6. Strain using a fine metal strainer to remove all the bits of bone and vegetable.

7. When cool enough, store in glass jars in the fridge for up to 5 days, or freeze for later use.

264. BONE BROTH COCKTAIL

Ingredients:

1. 3 ounces potato vodka (2 shots)

2. 1 cup Beef bone both

3. 1 cup organic tomato or vegetable juice

4. Beef bone broth frozen ice cubes or regular ice cubes

Directions:

Combine first 3 ingredients in a pitcher or drink shaker and whisk or shake well. Serve over bone broth ice cubes.

Variation:

A Broth Mary is sometimes prepared with only the broth and tomato juice as noted above; however, I think it's much more flavorful seasoning it as a Bloody Mary. Here's the recipe for that:

1. 3 ounces' potato vodka (2 shots)

2. 1 cup Beef bone both

3. 1 cup organic tomato or vegetable juice

4. 1 tablespoon fresh lemon juice

5. 1 tablespoon fresh lime juice

6. 1 to 2 teaspoons Worcestershire Sauce

7. 1 teaspoon garlic, minced (optional)

8. ½ teaspoons Tabasco

9. ½ teaspoon Celtic or Pink Himalayan salt (if juice is unsalted)

10. ½ teaspoon pepper

11. Beef Bone Broth frozen ice cubes

12.   Chipotle in Adobo, sauce only (optional, for smoky and hotter variation)

265. BEEFY BONY BROTH

Ingredients:

1.   1 ½ pounds bone-in beef short rib

2.   2 ½ pounds beef shank or oxtail

3.   2 pounds beef knucklebones or neck bones, or a combination of both (or add 1 more pound beef shank or oxtail)

4.   2 tablespoons extra-virgin olive oil

5.   2 tablespoons tomato paste

6.   ¼ cup apple cider vinegar

7.   3 carrots, peeled and coarsely chopped

8.   3 celery stalks, coarsely chopped

9.   2 onions, halved and peeled

10.   1 (14.5-ounce) can tomatoes (they can be whole, peeled or diced)

11.   1 head garlic, excess skins removed, top chopped off to expose the cloves

12.   2 bay leaves

13.   1 bunch fresh flat-leaf parsley

14.   ½ bunch fresh thyme

15.   ¼ ounce dried shiitake mushrooms

16.   1 tablespoon black peppercorns

PREPARATION

1.   Heat oven to 350 degrees. Place meat and bones in a roasting pan or on a large rimmed baking sheet. Drizzle with olive oil, turning to coat, then brush all over with tomato paste. Roast until browned, 30 to 35 minutes. They don't need to cook all the way through but to just develop some color.

2.   Put roasted meat and bones in a 12-quart stockpot and add vinegar and enough cold water to cover by 3 inches (about 6 quarts). Bring to a boil, then reduce to a low simmer, uncovered, for 2 to 3 hours. While simmering, occasionally skim fat and foam from the top using a ladle.

3.   Add all the remaining ingredients. Continue to simmer, uncovered, for a minimum of 3 hours. If using knucklebones, simmer overnight, 9 to 15 hours, so the knucklebones have sufficient time to break down.

4.   Remove meat and bones with a slotted spoon or tongs; reserve meat for another use (such as soup). Pour broth through a fine-mesh strainer into a large heatproof bowl. Once broth has cooled, store in the refrigerator in an airtight container.

266. GUT-GETTING BETTER BONE BROTH

Ingredients:

1. 4 lbs beef bones

2. 12 cups water

3. 2 T apple cider vinegar

4. 1 medium onion, roughly diced

5. 1 1/2 cups chopped carrots

6. 1 1/2 cups chopped leeks

7. 3 bay leaves

8. 3-5 sprigs fresh rosemary

9. 6 cloves garlic

10. 1 t black peppercorns

Directions

1. Preheat oven to 450 °F and line a baking sheet with aluminum foil. Place the bones on the baking sheet and roast for 40 minutes, flipping halfway through.

2. Once the bones are cooked place bones in a large stockpot and cover with water. Add the vinegar and allow to sit at room temperature for about 30 minutes.

3. Roughly chop the vegetables and add to the stockpot. Bring to a rolling boil and then lower to a simmer.

4. For the first 2-3 hours, skim any foamy layer that develops on the top and discard.

5. For beef bone broth, simmer for 48 hours, for chicken bone broth, simmer for 24 hours, for fish broth, simmer for 8 hours.

6. Allow to cool slightly and strain. Transfer the broth to an airtight container and refrigerate for 4-6 hours or overnight. This will allow the fat to rise to the top and solidify.

7. Scrape the fat off the top with a spoon. This will leave you with a gelatinous bone broth when cold.

8. Store in an airtight mason jar or freeze until ready to use. When ready to use, slowly warm the broth over a low heat to bring it back to a liquid consistency.

267. BONE BROTH SLOW COOK

Ingredients:

1.   2 carrots, peeled

2.   2 celery stalks

3.   1 medium onion, cut in half

4.   1 parsnip, cut in half

5.   3-4 lbs of beef bones

6.   2 Tablespoons of Apple Cider vinegar

7.   3-4 cloves garlic

8.   1 bay leaf

9.   Water

10. 1 teaspoon of salt

Directions:

1. Place everything in a crockpot except for salt and fill it with water until it just covers the ingredients. Season with salt (you can do more or less than the recommended 1 tsp). Cook on low heat for 8-10 hours. I recommend 10, so this is a perfect one to make overnight or while you are at work all day.

2. Strain the broth through either a strainer or cheesecloth.

3. Since bone broth can be quite fatty, I like to cool mine in the fridge overnight. Once cool, it will usually have a layer of fat on top. This is a good indication of a good broth. Remove most of the fat with a spoon and discard.

4. Bone broth can be keep in fridge for about a week or it can be frozen for about 4 months.

268. BEEFY SHANKY BROTH

INGREDIENTS:

1.   2 lbs/1 kilo beef shanks (I choose bones about 2"- 2-1/2" diameter). The meat is completely optional, but I find it a nice benefit. If you prefer to cook bones only, use 2 lbs of bones.

2.   1-2 liters cold, filtered water

3.   4 Tbsp Apple Cider Vinegar

4.   2 Bay Leaves

5.   2 Tbsp Sea Salt, divided (or 3 Tbsp Magic Mushroom Powder)

6.   2 Tbsp Tamari, Fish sauce, coconut aminos OR Worcestershire sauce (always opt for gluten free)

7.   1 tsp Garlic, granulated

8.   1 tsp dried Oregano

9.   2 tsp dried Parsley

10.   1 tsp dried Thyme

11.   1 cup Onions (white or yellow), sliced

12.   1 cup Carrot, sliced in rounds

13.   1/2 cup Celery, sliced

14.   1 Tbsp butter, ghee or coconut oil (for the seering pan)

15.   Optional: 1/2 cup sliced mushrooms (button or shitake)

INSTRUCTIONS:

Heat butter, ghee or coconut oil in a large frying pan or griddle over med-high heat. Add the beef shanks to the pre-heated pan, along with 1 Tbsp sea salt and the dried spices (garlic, oregano, parsley and thyme) and cook for 4-5 minutes per side or until a nice brown crust starts to form on the meat. Turn the meat and cook the other side for an additional 3-4 minutes.

269. QUICK AND EASY BROTH

INGREDIENTS

1. Bones from 1 or 2 chickens (feet if possible), or 2-3 lbs of beef bones

2. 1-2 onions

3. 4-5 garlic cloves

4. rosemary or thyme (optional)

5. 2 tablespoons coconut vinegar (or apple cider vinegar)

6. Salt to taste

7. Just enough water to cover all ingredients

INSTRUCTIONS

1. Place all ingredients in a large stockpot and bring to a boil.

2. Reduce to simmer and cook on low for 8 hours minimum, but as long as possible. I like to start it in the morning and let it cook all day.

3. Once done cooking, remove the bones and let cool to use again. Once cool, place in a gallon zip bag and freeze.

4. Place a fine mesh strainer over a large bowl and carefully pour the broth through the strainer. Discard all the solid bits.

5. Cover and refrigerate overnight.

6. Once fully cooled, a layer of fat will be on the top. I always remove it and throw it away, but that is optional.

7. Divide into mason jars and store in the fridge.

8. This can also be frozen. I like freezing it in a mini muffin tin, then once frozen, putting them in a quart size bag. This makes adding them to dishes very easy.

270. LEMON GINGER BROTH DELIGHT

Ingredients

1. 2 tablespoons vegetable oil

2. 1 large onion, chopped

3. 1 (3-inch) piece of ginger, chopped (no need to peel)

4. Zest from 1 lemon, peeled into strips

5. 1 whole split (two halves) organic chicken breast (about 2 pounds)

6. 10 cups water

7. 1 tablespoon apple cider vinegar

8. 2 teaspoons kosher salt

Instructions

1. Heat the oil in a large pot over medium-high heat. Add the onion, ginger, and lemon zest and cook until the onion has softened, 3 to 5 minutes. Add the chicken, skin side down, and cook until just beginning to brown, 8 to 10 minutes.

2. Add the water, apple cider vinegar, and salt and bring to a boil. Reduce the heat to the lowest possible setting, partially cover the pot, and cook for as long as you would like, but at least 3 hours.

3. Transfer the chicken to a plate. Remove the bones and skin, shred the meat, and reserve for another use.

4. Pour the broth through a fine mesh sieve (lined with cheese cloth, if you have it) into a large bowl. Discard the solids. Cool to room temperature, then transfer to quart containers and refrigerate overnight. The next day, use a spoon to skim excess fat from the surface of the broth.

5. Reheat the broth until it is piping hot, then transfer to mugs and serve.

271. HOMEMADE CHICKEN BROTHSTOCK

INGREDIENTS

1. 2 pounds chicken bones

2. water

3. 2 sprigs of fresh rosemary

INSTRUCTIONS

1. Wash chicken bones and place them in a Crockpot. Add enough water to cover the bones and fill ¾ths of the Crockpot.

2. Tear the leaves off the rosemary stalks and add to the Crockpot.

3. Simmer on low for 2 days. Once the Crockpot cools, place it in the refrigerator until the fat solidifies and rises to the top. Skim off the fat with a ladle or pour the broth through a strainer to strain the fat. Discard the fat and you have bone broth!

272. RED HOT CHICKEN BROTH

Ingredients

1. ½ red onion, sliced

2. 3 garlic cloves, minced

3. 2 Tbs schmaltz (chicken fat)

4. 1 tsp smoked paprika

5. ½ tsp anchochilli powder or chipotle

6. 1 tsp chili flakes

7. 1 tsp sea salt

8. ½ tsp fresh cracked pepper

9. 1 large sweet potato, cubed

10. 2 large carrots, cubed

11. 8 C homemade chicken stock

12. 2 kaffir lime leaves (optional)

13. 1 Tbs lime juice

14. 2½ C leftover roast chicken, pulled into bite size chunks

15. green onions for garnish

Instructions

1. Heat schmaltz in a large pot, add onion and garlic and cook until onion is translucent.

2. Add spices, salt, sweet potato, carrots and cook for about 2 minutes stirring continuously.

3. Add chicken stock, lime leaves, lime juice and chicken and allow simmering for 20 minutes.

273. SIMPLE AND ESY CHCKEN BROTHSTOCK

Ingredients

1.   3 kg chicken (Roasted chicken carcasses, chicken wings/winglet's, left over bones from chicken drumsticks)

2.   1 tbsp apple cider vinegar

3.   3 onions

4.   3 carrots

5.   2 sticks of celery

6.   1 tsp peppercorns

7.   5 garlic cloves (unpeeled)

Instructions

1.   Place the chicken into a very large stock pot and add enough cold water to cover the bones.

2.   Add the cider vinegar and leave the mixture to sit for half an hour.

3.   Roughly chop the onions, carrots and celery.

4.   Place the pan on the heat and add the chopped veg, garlic and peppercorns.

5.   Bring the water to a boil, and then reduce the heat to its very lowest setting and place on a vented lid.

6.   During the first couple of hours use a large spoon to skim off any foam/scum that rises to the top of your stock. This should reduce after the initial cooking period.

7.   Allow the stock to cook at the lowest possible heat for at least 6 hours; 12 hours would be even better.

8.   Remove from the heat and carefully pour the stock through a sieve lined with a clean J-cloth. You will need to do this slowly to ensure you don't dump all the solids back over the side of the sieve and into your stock. Even better would be do to it in 2 or 3 small portions.

9.   Return the stock to the hob, bring to the boil and boil vigorously for 10 minutes.

10.   Your stock is now ready to use in soups, risottos or to freeze for when you need it.

Notes

There is no salt in this recipe; the elongated cooking time can vastly change the water level, making seasoning hard until the stock is fully cooked. I like to freeze the stock without salt and then season it depending on the dish I use it in.

274. CHICKEN CHEEKY BROTH

Ingredients

1.   Giblets and carcasses from 2-3 chickens (I might use the carcasses from two chickens but also bones saved from a night of wings)

2.   1 Tbsp apple cider vinegar

3.   2 medium yellow onions, roots cut off and halved

4.   4-5 carrots, washed and cut in half (or about 2 cups of baby carrots)

5.   6-8 celery stalks, washed and cut into thirds

6.   6-8 cloves of garlic

7.   3 bay leaves

8.   1 tsp salt

9.   1 gallon cold water (enough to cover the ingredients)

Directions:

1.   Place chicken giblets and carcasses into a big stock pot. Add enough water to cover the bones (approximately 1 gallon) and the apple cider vinegar.

2.   Cover and bring to a boil on top of the stove, then turn down the heat to keep a low simmer for 24-48 hours. Stir once or twice in the first few hours, and then stir at least a couple of times over the next couple of days.

3.   Add the vegetables, garlic, salt and bay leaves to the pot. Increase heat to bring back up to a boil, then cover and reduce heat to maintain a simmer.

4.   Cook for 4-8 hours more, stirring every hour or so. Let simmer with lid off for the last 2-3 hours.

5.   Strain all the ingredients by pouring bone broth from one pot to another through a colander or strainer.

275. IMMEDIATE POTBROTH

Ingredients

1.   Cooked bones/carcass of chicken cow, deer, turkey, pig etc depending on what you have (I like about half of the pot to be bones/carcass. You can freeze whatever bones don't fit for another time.)

2.   1-2 chicken feet (optional depending on if you have access - it gives really good gel to the broth. Ask your chicken farmer for them!)

3.   1-2 large carrots, coarsely chopped

4.   1 medium onion coarsely chopped

5.   2-3 stalks of celery, coarsely chopped

6.   1 head of garlic, smashed

7.   1-2 TB apple cider vinegar

8.   Water enough to cover the bones

Instructions

1.   Put the bones into the pot first followed by the veggies, garlic, and apple cider vinegar. Fill the pot with water to cover the bones - be sure you don't go over the "Max" line on the pot.

2.   Let the pot sit for about 30 minutes without any heat to let the apple cider vinegar pull the minerals from the bones.

3.   Put the Instant Pot lid on and turn the vent valve to close. Push "Soup" and use the manual button to bring the time up to 120 minutes.

4.   The pot will turn "On" automatically and will take about 20 minutes to come to pressure before the 120 minutes starts counting down.

5.   After the 120 minutes of pressure cooking is done, turn the Instant Pot off and leave it be to naturally release about 15 minutes before opening the vent valve and straining your broth.

276. HYPO ALLERGENIC CHICKEN BROTH

Ingredients:

1.   2 or more pounds raw chicken bones/carcasses (from about 3 or 4 chickens)

2.   6 to 8 chicken feet

3.   One whole chicken and additional wings or thighs, optional

4.   Enough purified water to just cover the bones when they are in the pot

5. ¼ to ½ cup apple cider vinegar, depending on the size of the pot

6. 2 to 4 carrots, scrubbed and roughly chopped

7. 3 to 4 stalks organic celery, including leafy part, roughly chopped

8   1 or 2 whole cloves (optional)

9   2 teaspoons peppercorns

10.   1 bunch parsley, add in the last hour

Directions:

1.   Place all the bones in a slow cooker or large stockpot. Add the vinegar and enough purified water to cover everything by 1 inch.

2.   On medium heat, bring the water to a simmer. Use a shallow spoon to carefully skim the film off the top of the broth. Add carrots, celery, and spices and reduce the heat to low. You want the broth to barely simmer. Skim occasionally over the first 2 hours, and be sure the bones are always covered with water. You will have to add water during the cooking process. Simmer for at least 2 hours.

3.   When the broth is done, turn off the cooker or remove the pot from the heat. Using tongs and/or a large slotted spoon remove all the bones and the meat. Save the chicken for use in the broth or for another recipe. Pour the broth through a fine mesh strainer and discard the solids.

4.   Let cool on the counter before refrigerating. You can skim off the fat easily after the broth is chilled if desired. When chilled the broth should be very gelatinous.

5.   The broth will keep for 5 days in the refrigerator and 3 or more months in your freezer.

Notes:

(1) If it's hard to get chicken bones from your butcher, you may be able to get backs and necks.

(2) The number of pounds of bones will vary based on the size of your slow cooker or stock pot. You want the bones to fill the vessel so you can just cover them with water. If you have chicken bones from any leftover chicken, also add those.

(3) You use chicken feet for the cartilage which is necessary for good broth and the health benefits of gelatine, collagen and calcium.

If you use chicken feet, you need to remove the outer yellow skin if the butcher has not already done so. To do this, immerse in boiling water for about 10 to 20 seconds, and they will peel easily. If you boil them any longer, it's nearly impossible to peel them because they become rubbery. It's also easier to peel them before they are frozen. You can cut off the claws if you choose.

(4)The chicken meat is optional, but I usually add it so I have the chicken for soup or another recipe.

If you have favourite herbs, you can add them to the bone broth to enhance the flavour. Thyme is particularly nice with chicken broth. Since you might use the broth in a variety of recipes, I prefer not to salt it while cooking.

277.CHICKEN SLOW COOKER BROTH

Ingredients

1.   2-3 roasted chicken carcasses (approx. 2 lbs. of bones); include any leftover skin or pan drippings

2.   1 or 2 medium onions, unpeeled & quartered

3.   1 head of garlic, unpeeled, cut in half crosswise

4.   2 celery ribs, cut in 1 to 2 inch pieces

5.   2 carrots, cut in 1 to 2 inch pieces

6.   5 sprigs of fresh thyme

7.   5 sprigs of fresh parsley

8.   1 bay leaf

9.   1-1/2 teaspoons peppercorns

10.   2 tablespoons cider vinegar (1 tablespoon per pound of bones)

11.   2 to 2-1/2 quarts water (enough to immerse above ingredients)

Directions

Add all of the ingredients to a 6 quart (or larger) slow cooker. * Cook on low for 12 hours (or more). While still hot, use tongs or slotted spoon to remove large pieces from broth. Then pour through a wire mesh strainer to remove the remaining solid bits.

For a fat-free broth, use one of these methods for removing the fat:

METHOD 1: Pour broth into a large bowl or container, cover, and refrigerate overnight or until completely chilled. Scrape the hardened fat from the top and discard.

METHOD 2: While broth is still warm, pour it into a grease separator (available on Amazon and at cooking stores), that allows you to pour the fat-free broth from the bottom.

FREEZE IT. Broth can be refrigerated for 4 to 5 days. For extended storage, it should be frozen. It's convenient to freeze it in 1 or 2 cup portions for easy use in recipes.

USES: This broth can be used in any soups, gravies, or any recipes calling for chicken broth. It also can be drunk as is for a healthy supplement to your diet.

NOTE: This is a salt-free broth. Add salt to taste, as desired.

*If your slow cooker is smaller, you can half the recipe using 1 chicken carcass and half of the remaining ingredients.

278. CHICKEN STOCKBROTH

Ingredients

1. 1 raw whole chicken, rotisserie chicken, chicken carcass or parts

2. 2 Tbsp apple cider vinegar

3. 2 onions, chopped

4. 4 - 6 stalk celery, chopped

5. 2 carrots, chopped (optional)

6. water

Instructions

1. If using raw chicken - cover the chicken with water in either a crock pot or stock pot. Cook until tender (4 hours on high in the crock pot), remove from water, separate the meat from the bones.

2. If using a roasted chicken - separate the chicken meat from the bones.

3. Place the chicken bones in a crock pot or stock pot and cover with water. If the chicken was cooked in the crock pot covered with water, place the bones back into this water/broth.

4. Add vegetables and vinegar.

5. For crockpot - turn crock pot to high until it boils and turn to low - cook for 24 hours.

6. For stock pot - Bring to a boil and reduce the heat to simmer.

7. Cook on low for 24 hours.

8. Strain the broth and allow it to cool.

Notes

Chicken bone broth will keep refrigerated for 1 week or in the freezer for months.

279. PALEO KETO BONE BROTH

Ingredients

1.   3.3 lb oxtail (1.5 kg) or mixed with assorted bones (chicken feet, marrow bones, etc.)

2.   2 medium carrots

3.   1 medium parsnip or parsley root

4.   2 medium celery stalks

5.   1 medium white onion, skin on

6.   5 cloves garlic, peeled

7.   2 tbsp apple cider vinegar or fresh lemon juice

8.   2-3 bay leaves

9.   1 tbsp salt (I like pink Himalayan)

10.   8-10 cups water, enough to cover the bones, no more than 2/3 capacity of your pressure cooker or 3/4 capacity of your Dutch oven or 3/4 capacity of your slow cooker

Instructions

1.   Peel the root vegetables and cut them into thirds. Halve the onion and peel and halve the garlic cloves. Keeping the onion skin on will help the broth get a nice golden colour. Cut the celery into thirds. Place everything into the pressure cooker (or slow cooker) and add the bay leaves.

2.   Add the oxtail and bones. You can use any bones you like: chicken, pork or beef, with or without meat. Because I used chicken and turkey bones with some skin on, the fat ended up being quite runny. You can still use it for cooking but I binned it.

Oxtail is rich in gelatin and contains more fat. Although traditional bone broth is made just from bones, especially beef marrowbones, I found oxtail to give the best flavor to my broth. The advantage of using oxtail is that it will yield 3 superfoods: bone broth, tender oxtail meat and tallow. Tallow is great when used for cooking the same way as ghee or lard.

3.   Add 8-10 cups of water or up to 2/3 of your pressure cooker, slow cooker or Dutch oven, vinegar or freshly squeezed lemon juice and bay leaves. Make sure you use the vinegar or lemon juice – this will help release more minerals into the broth.

4.   Add pink Himalayan salt (whole or powdered). While adding vinegar to bone broth helps release the gelatin and minerals from the bones, pink Himalayan rock salt adds extra minerals, including potassium!

Pressure Cooker: Lock the lid of your pressure cooker and turn to high pressure / high heat. Once it reaches high pressure (either you have an indicator or in case of old pressure cookers, see a small amount of vapor escaping through the valve), turn to the lowest heat and set the timer for 90 minutes.

Dutch oven or Slow cooker: Cover with a lid and cook for at least 6 hours (high setting) or up to 10 hours (low setting). To release even more gelatine and minerals, you can cook it up to 48 hours. To do that, you'll have to remove the oxtail using thongs and shred the meat off using a fork. Then, you can place the bones back to the pot and cook up to 48 hours.

5.   Pressure cooker: When done, take off heat and let the pressure release naturally for about 10-15 minutes. Remove the lid.

6.   Remove the large bits and pour the broth through a strainer into a large dish. Discard the vegetables and set the meaty bones aside to cool down.

7.   When the meaty bones are chilled, shred the meat off the bone with a fork. If there is any gelatine left on the bones, you can reuse the bones again for another batch of bone broth. Just keep in the freezer and add some new pieces when making bone broth again. Use the juicy oxtail meat in other recipes (on top of lettuce leaves, with cauli-rice or as omelet filling) or eat with some warm bone broth.

8.   Use the broth immediately or place in the fridge overnight, where the broth will become jelly. Oxtail is high in fat and the greasy layer on top (tallow) will solidify. Simply scrape most of the tallow off (as much as you wish).

9.   Keep the broth in the fridge if you are planning to use it over the next 5 days. For future uses, place in small containers and freeze.

280. TURKEY STOCKBROTH

INGREDIENTS

1.   1 turkey carcass, broken into chunks to easily fit in your pot – can be raw but this is a great way to use the bones after you roast a turkey for Thanksgiving or Christmas

2.   2 medium onions, quartered (you can leave the skin on)

3.   2 celery stalks, roughly chopped

4.   2 carrots, roughly chopped

5.   1 head of garlic, cut in half (no need to peel the cloves)

6.   ½ teaspoon peppercorns

7.   Optional: 1 rosemary branch, a few sage leaves, a few sprigs of thyme

INSTRUCTIONS

1.   Put all ingredients in a large pot and cover with water till the bones are 2-3 inches under water.

2.   Bring to a simmer then reduce heat so that it stays at a very gently simmer. You don't want it to boil as it will make the stock look dirty. It won't affect the taste but it won't look as nice and clear.

3.   Continue to simmer gently, uncovered, for about 4 hours.

4.   Remove from heat and strain though a colander into a large bowl. Place a fine mesh sieve over another bowl and strain once more to remove any small particles. Season to taste with sea salt.

5.   Store in covered containers in your fridge for up to 3 days or freeze for longer storage*

NOTES

*DO NOT freeze stock in glass mason jars. The stock will expand as it freezes and break the jars. Plastic freezer bags work great for freezing stock.

281.TURKEY SLOWCOOK STOCK

Ingredients

1.   carcass of cooked turkey (12-13 lb bird), meat and skin removed

2.   1 large onion, peeled and quartered

3.   2 large carrots, washed and cut into thirds

4.   3 ribs of celery, cut into thirds

5.   6-8 cloves garlic

6.   2-3 sprigs fresh rosemary

7.   1 tablespoon apple cider vinegar

8.   1 tablespoon peppercorn

9.   cold, GOOD water

10.   salt and pepper to taste

Directions

1.   Place carcass, onion, carrots, celery, garlic, rosemary, vinegar and peppercorn in the base of a slow cooker. Fill with cold water to the top. Cook on low for 24 hours.

2.   Let cool and strain stock.

3.   Season with salt and pepper to taste.

4.   Ladle stock into glass jars, leaving 1-inch headspace to allow for expansion if freezing.

5.   Freeze stock and use for any recipe calling for stock or warm up one serving at a time a sip on the warm stock- I promise it's delicious!!

282. THANKSGIVING TURKEY BONE BROTH

Ingredients:

1.   One turkey carcass (majority of the meat removed)

2.   A large soup pot

3.   Enough water to cover at least most of the bones

4.   Salt

Directions:

1.   Place the turkey carcass in the soup pot. Cover it as much as possible with water. I like to use filtered water, just because, but you don't have to. If the carcass is too big, you can try and break it up and jam it in. If you don't have a pot big enough, buy. You won't regret it.

2.   Place the pot on the stovetop and turn the heat on high. Bring to a boil. Once it boils, skim the weird stuff off the top and turn the heat down.

3.   Let it cook. For hours. I find two to three hours is usually enough. What you want to wait for is that moment when everything just collapses and the broth is golden and fragrant and has a nice glow to it.

4.   Add salt to taste. You will need a lot. More than you think.

5.   Turn off the heat and let the soup sit until cool enough to strain. But in the meantime, enjoy eating as much as you can.

283. STANDARD TURKEY STOCK

Ingredients

1.   4 quarts cold water

2.   6 pounds total of turkey carcass, raw turkey necks, raw turkey wings and/or any other chicken or turkey parts you have been saving in your freezer such as backs.

3.   2 chicken feet, or 4 chicken wings or 1 additional turkey wing

4.   1 clove of garlic, peeled and bruised

5.   1 medium to large onion, peeled and cut in half

6.   2–3 carrots peeled and cut into 1 inch pieces (about one cup)

7.   2 celery ribs, tops and all cut into 1 inch pieces (about one cup)

8.   1 leek, white part only, cleaned of sand and cut in half vertically

9.   2 parsnips peeled and cut in half

10.   1 knob of unpeeled ginger (about 2-3 ounces)

11.   ½ bunch fresh flat leaf parsley, tied with a string

12.   2 bay leaves

13.   1 ½ teaspoon salt

14.   2 sage leaves, or 1 teaspoon dry ground sage

15.   6 whole black peppercorns

Instructions

1.   Place all ingredients into a large stock pot and slowly bring to a boil.

2.   Reduce heat and simmer for three hours. Skim foam that rises to the top as it cooks. Depending on the type and amount of the bones and meat you started with, you may need to simmer longer (up to four hours if needed) to intensify flavours.

3.   Strain the stock and discard the solids except for the meat.

4.   Remove skin and debone the turkey and reserve. Use for any recipe that calls for cooked turkey meat (such as our Turkey Pot Pie or Turkey & Stuffing Turnovers).

5.   Cool the stock completely.

6.   Once cooled, skim off the fat that settles on the top and if desired, save for any poultry recipe that calls for butter. (Turkey fat is full of flavour and lasts fairly long in the refrigerator and can also be frozen.)

7.   Use stock for any recipe that calls for turkey stock like our Turkey Soup with Potato Dumplings or our Turkey Pot Pie. Stock may also be frozen in zip lock bags for later use.

284. TURKEY STOCKBROTH

Ingredients

1.   2 tablespoons coconut oil

2.   1 medium onion, diced

3.   2 cloves garlic, minced

4.   1 pound turkey BONES

5.   1 tablespoon coconut amino

6.   10 cups chicken broth

7.   1/4 teaspoon salt

8.   1/4 teaspoon pepper

9.   4 cups fresh spinach leaves, coarsely chopped

10.   Fresh rosemary, optional

Directions

1.   Heat the coconut oil in a large stockpot over high heat. Add the onion and garlic and sauté for 2 minutes. Add the ground turkey and sauté for an additional 7 minutes.

2.   Add the coconut amines. Stir frequently for 2 minutes.

3.   Add the chicken broth, salt, and pepper. Simmer for about 20 minutes.

4.   Add the spinach and rosemary (if desired) and sauté for 2 minutes.

285. TURKEY BONE BROTH

Ingredients

1 turkey carcass, picked over

turkey neck, if you have it

leftover turkey drippings

1 onion, quartered

2 cloves garlic, mashed and roughly chopped

1 stalk of celery, including leaves and cut into 3 or 4 pieces

large bunch parsley

half a bunch roughly torn sage leaves

several rosemary sprigs

several thyme sprigs

3 bay leaves

5 peppercorns

Directions

Place carcass, skin and giblets (if you kept them) in a large stockpot with other ingredients. Cover with water. Bring to a boil over high heat. Turn burner down to just below medium. Skim any foam or scum that may settle at the top. Simmer for four to five hours. If the bones start to stick out of the water, add just enough boiling water to cover them up.

Pour the stock through a strainer into a large bowl (or two), catching any bones or vegetables. Allow stock to cool before moving to an airtight container and placing in the fridge or freezer. Use as a base for soups or anything that calls for chicken broth. Stock can be stored in the fridge for 2 or 3 days or in the freezer for a few months.

286. FISHY FISH BONE BROTH

Ingredients

1.   5–7 pounds fish carcasses or heads from large non-oily fish such as halibut, cod, sole, rockfish, turbot, or tilapia (see Notes)

2.   2 tablespoons ghee (clarified butter; see page 000)

3.   1–2 carrots, scrubbed and coarsely chopped

4.   2 ribs organic celery, including leafy part, coarsely chopped

5.   2 medium onion, coarsely chopped

6.   Purified water to just cover the bones in the pot

7.   1 bay leaf

8.   1–2 whole cloves

9.   2 teaspoons peppercorns

10.   1 tablespoon bouquet garnish or a small handful of fresh parsley and 4–5 stems fresh thyme

Directions:

1.   Wash the fish and cut off the gills if present.

2.   In a large stockpot, melt the ghee over medium-low to low heat. Add the carrots, celery, and onion and cook, stirring occasionally, for about 20 minutes.

3.   Add the fish and enough water to cover it by 1". Increase the heat to medium and bring the water to a bare simmer. Use a shallow spoon to carefully skim the film off the top of the broth. Add the bay leaf, cloves, peppercorns, and bouquet garnish and reduce the heat to low. Cook at a bare simmer for about 50 minutes, uncovered or with the lid askew. Continue to skim the surface as needed.

4.   When the broth is done, remove the pot from the heat. Using tongs and/or a large slotted spoon, remove all the bones. Pour the broth through a fine mesh strainer and discard the solids.

5.   Let cool on the counter before refrigerating. You can skim off the fat easily after the broth is chilled, if desired. When chilled, the broth should be very gelatinous. The broth will keep for 5 days in the refrigerator and 3 or more months in your freezer.

6.   Notes:

7.   Non-oily fish is necessary because the fish oils in fatty fish such as salmon become rancid in cooking.

8.   The cartilage in fish bones breaks down to gelatine very quickly, so it's best to cook broth on the stove top.

287. BASIC FISH STOCK

Ingredients

1. the bones of 4 whole snapper – spines, heads and tails

2. enough filtered water to cover with a few inches to spare

3. 4 tbsps white wine vinegar

4. 2 white onions, quartered*

5. 2 lemons, quartered*

6. 2 sprigs fresh thyme*

7. 2 cloves garlic*

Directions

1. Put the fish bits, vinegar, onions, lemon, garlic and thyme in a large pot. Cover with the filtered water. Bring to a boil then reduce the heat to a simmer.

2. Simmer for anywhere between six and 24 hours. I usually go about 12-14.

3. Strain the stock, store in sterile glass jars and use within a week or freeze.

288. DIVINE FISH HEAD STOCK

Ingredients

1. *3-4 whole carcasses, including heads, of non-oily fish (sole, turbot, rockfish or snapper (around

2. here I find halibut at Whole Foods))

3. 2 T. butter

4. 2 onions, coarsely chopped

5. 1 carrot, coarsely chopped

6. fresh or dried thyme

7. fresh or dried parsley

8. 1 bay leaf

9. 1/2 c. dry white wine

10. 1/4 c. raw apple cider vinegar

11. 3 qts. Water

Directions:

1. Melt butter in a large stainless steel pot. Sauté vegetables just until they're soft. Add white wine and bring to a boil.

2. Add the fish carcasses (head and body) and cover with water. Add the vinegar and bring it to a boil. Skim off any scum that rises to the top. Now you can go ahead and add the thyme and parsley to the pot.

3. Reduce the heat, cover and simmer for at least 4 hours or as long as 24 hours.

4. Strain the liquid and store in pint-sized jars or containers. Store in fridge or freezer. Be sure to label your stocks as they all look the same.

5. Pick the meat away from the bones (it will just fall off by this time) and refrigerate or freeze it to add to your soup later – or use it as you would can tuna fish.

289. Salmon Head STOCKBROTH

INGREDIENTS

1. 2 salmon heads, or one salmon frame (head, tails, and scraps)

2. 1 large onion, thinly sliced

3. 3 tablespoons butter

4. 8 ounces potatoes, scrubbed and cut into 2 inch cubes

5. 1 large bunch fresh dill

6. 2 bay leaves

7. 1 teaspoon kosher salt, or to taste

To garnish:

8. About 1/3 cup chopped fresh dill

DIRECTIONS

1. Over medium heat, melt the butter in the sauté pan. Add the onions and sauté until softened but not browned, about 7 minutes. Add the salmon parts, the potatoes, bay leaves, salt, and all but a few stalk of the dill. Add enough water to just cover the fish. Bring the water to a steady simmer and cook until fish and potatoes are tender, about 20 minutes.

2. Using a slotted spoon, remove the fish parts from the liquid. When the fish is cool enough to handle, separate the meat and other edible parts (eyeballs, cartilage, etc.) from the skeleton.

3. Add the fish parts back to the soup. Reheat gently at a low simmer, taking care not to break up the fish flesh. Add the chopped fresh dill. Add more salt, if needed, and freshly ground black pepper. Serve immediately. Leftovers may be kept in the refrigerator for up to three days and reheated over a low simmer.

290. TASTY TRINIDAD FISH BROTH

Ingredients

1. 2 pounds firm fish (slices or whole small fish) (Croakers, Snapper/Red Fish)

2. Juice of 1 lime, for washing fish

3. 3 quarts water (12 cups), add more or less depending on the amount of veggies you use

4. 1 large potato, peeled and quartered (about 3/4 pound)

5. 1-3 sweet potatoes, peeled and quartered (about 2 pounds)

6. 2 green bananas(figs), peeled and quartered

7. 1 medium carrot, sliced

8. 6-8 ochre, tops removed

9. 3 small eddoes(yautia), peeled (about 1 pound)

10. 1 large onion, peeled and sliced

11. 1 stalk celery, sliced in 1-inch pieces

1 medium tomato, sliced

12. 1 hot pepper, whole

13. 4 sprigs thyme (If very small use more!)

14. 3 tablespoons organic ketchup, plus more to serve

15. 3 tablespoons lime juice, plus more to serve

16. Salt and black pepper, to taste

Green Seasoning

1. 6-8 large culantro (also called bandania) leaves, minced

2. 6 large cloves garlic

3.   4 large scallions, chopped (about 1 cup)

Directions

1.   Peel, wash and cut veggies, slice tomato (not shown) and onion.

2.   Leave root vegetables immersed in water to prevent them from getting black.

1.   Try to cut veggies evenly. I did add a little cabbage too, but that is optional!

2.   I used two kinds of sweet potatoes. You may also use other kinds of ground provisions, also called root vegetables.

3.   Mince culantro (bandania), garlic and scallions in a food processor or blender.

4.   If using a blender, add 1/2 cup water or enough to get it blending.

5.   Soak fish in water and the juice of a lemon for a few minutes, check for scales, rinse and drain.

6.   Season fish with salt (1 teaspoon), black pepper (1 teaspoon) and half of the green seasoning, reserve the other half. Marinate fish for 1 hour or overnight.

7.   Bring water to boil in a large pot with a cover over high heat. Add onion, potato, sweet potato, green bananas, carrot, eddoes, onion, tomato, celery, thyme, whole hot pepper and the reserved green seasoning to the boiling water.

8.   Bring to a boil again, cover and reduce heat to low and cook until vegetables are fork tender but firm, about 20-40 minutes, depending on the size and amount of vegetables used.

9.   Season to taste with salt (I used low sodium) and freshly ground black pepper (I used 1 tablespoon).

10.   Serve hot in large bowls with extra ketchup, lime juice and sliced hot pepper on the side for everyone to adjust the taste according to their preference.

Don't forget to serve with additional small bowls in which to place the fish bones...Watch out for those bones, eat carefully and enjoy!

291. HOMEMADE FISHY FISH STOCK

1. 3 carcasses (except gills and guts), including heads of non-oily fish such as Snapper, Flounder, or Tilapia

2. 2 tablespoons olive oil

3. 2 carrots, unpeeled and chopped

4. 3 tomatoes, halved

5. ½ cups yellow onions

6. 4 stalks celery, chopped

7. 2 cloves garlic

8. 5 sprigs fresh thyme

9. 3 sprigs parsley

10. ½ cup good white wine

11. Kosher salt

12. 1½ teaspoon freshly ground black pepper

13. 2 quarts water

Directions

1. Warm oil in stockpot. Add carrots, onions, and celery over medium heat for about 15 minutes, or until lightly browned. Add garlic and cook for 2 more minutes.

2. Add fish carcasses, tomatoes, water, white wine, salt, pepper, thyme, and parsley to the pot. Bring to a boil and reduce heat to a simmer for about 3 hours.

3. Remove carcasses with tongs and strain the liquid. Use then or refrigerate and then freeze what you have left over. It will last in the refrigerator for a few days and in the freezer for a year.

292. TRINIDAD FISH BROTH (FISH BROF)

Ingredients:

1. 2 pounds firm fish (slices or whole small fish) (Croaker, Snapper/Red Fish)

2. Juice of 1 lime, for washing fish

3. 3 quarts water (12 cups), add more or less depending on the amount of veggies you use

4. 1 large potato, peeled and quartered (about 3/4 pound)

5. 1-3 sweet potatoes, peeled and quartered (about 2 pounds)

6. 2 green bananas(figs), peeled and quartered

7. 1 medium carrot, sliced

8. 6-8 ochroes, tops removed

9. 3 small eddoes(yautia), peeled (about 1 pound)

10. 1 large onion, peeled and sliced

11. 1 stalk celery, sliced in 1-inch pieces

1 medium tomato, sliced

12. 1 hot pepper, whole

13. 4 sprigs thyme (If very small use more!)

14. 3 tablespoons organic ketchup, plus more to serve

15. 3 tablespoons lime juice, plus more to serve

16. Salt and black pepper, to taste

Green Seasoning

1. 6-8 large culantro (also called bandania) leaves, minced

2. 6 large cloves garlic

3.   4 large scallions, chopped (about 1 cup)

Flour Dumplings

1.   2 cups all purpose flour, preferably organic unbleached

2.   1 teaspoon salt

3.   2 teaspoons sugar

4.   Water for kneading (about 3/4 cup)

Directions;

1.   Peel, wash and cut veggies, slice tomato (not shown) and onion.

2.   Leave root vegetables immersed in water to prevent them from getting black.

3.   Try to cut veggies evenly. I did add a little cabbage too, but that is optional!

4.   I used two kinds of sweet potatoes. You may also use other kinds of ground provisions, also called root vegetables.

5.   Mince culantro (bandania), garlic and scallions in a food processor or blender.

6.   If using a blender, add 1/2 cup water or enough to get it blending.

7.   Soak fish in water and the juice of a lemon for a few minutes, check for scales, rinse and drain.

8.   Season fish with salt (1 teaspoon), black pepper (1 teaspoon) and half of the green seasoning, reserve the other half. Marinate fish for 1 hour or overnight.

9.   Bring water to boil in a large pot with a cover over high heat. Add onion, potato, sweet potato, green bananas, carrot, eddoes, onion, tomato, celery, thyme, whole hot pepper and the reserved green seasoning to the boiling water.

10.   Bring to a boil again, cover and reduce heat to low and cook until vegetables are fork tender but firm, about 20-40 minutes, depending on the size and amount of vegetables used.

11.   Season to taste with salt (I used about 4 teaspoons, maybe more) and freshly ground black pepper (I used 1 tablespoon).

12.   While the vegetables are cooking, make dumplings, if using. [Alternatively, you may use 1-2 cups uncooked pasta.] In a medium bowl, combine flour, salt and sugar. Gradually add water to make a firm dough. Pinch off small pieces and roll between the palm of your hands to shape.

Feel free to make into any shape or size or just "pinch and drop"! Tastes the same!

Desserts

293. Paleo Pumpkin Pie Smoothie

Ingredients

1 frozen banana

2 tbsp pumpkin puree

½ cup unsweetened almond milk

½ tsp vanilla extract

1 tsp honey

1 tbsp hemp hearts

¼ tsp cinnamon

¼ tsp cloves

¼ tsp nutmeg

Instructions

Combine all ingredients in a blender and process until smooth. I find it's easier on the blender if I break the frozen banana into smaller chunks before processing.

Pour into a tall glass and enjoy with your favourite book, your favourite music, or both!

Notes

Calories: 220

Total Fat: 6.4g

Saturated Fat: 0.8g

Carbs: 38.0g

Fiber: 6.1g. Protein: 5.6g

294. Green Kale Smoothie with Mango

Ingredients

2 large leaves of kale

2 frozen bananas (peeled and cut into thirds)

1 frozen mango (diced)

2 tablespoons maca powder

2 tablespoons hemp hearts

3 cups unsweetened almond milk

This recipe makes two large smoothies, can be halved for one serving.

Directions

Add frozen banana chunks and frozen mango chunks into a blender with the almond milk. Blend until smooth. (I freeze my fruit in chunks to make it easier on the blender)

Add in kale, maca powder, and hemp hearts. Blend until smooth.

Serve immediately and enjoy!!

Nutrition Facts (per smoothie)

Calories: 294

Fat: 9.0g

Saturated fat: 0.7g

Sodium: 274mg

Carbs: 51.0g

Fiber: 8.6g

Protein: 7.7g

295. Healthy Fruit Leather

Ingredients

2 apples, finely diced

10 strawberries, diced

1 ruby pink grapefruit, diced

Stevia/rice malt syrup to sweeten if needed

1 tsp cinnamon

Pinch salt

1/4 cup water

Instructions

Place the fruit in saucepan with the water and bring to a boil. Reduce the heat and simmer until the fruit is soft and the liquid has been reduced. Stir through the cinnamon and salt.

Transfer the fruit to a blender and puree until smooth. Taste the mixture and if required add a sweetener. The grapefruit can be quite tart and while suitable for adults children may not appreciate this. If you would like a sweeter roll up than I suggest adding some sweetness to balance out the sourness. If a sweetener is added blend again until combined. You should end up with 2-3 cups worth of pureed fruit.

Heat oven to 120-150°C (250-300F). Line a large baking tray with baking paper (if your baking tray is not very large you may need to use two smaller sized trays). Pour the mixture onto the tray and spread it out thinly by using the back of a spatula. You want it to just cover the baking paper's surface without leaving any gaps (the thinner the better!). Place the baking tray in the oven on the lowest shelf available and bake for 8-12 hours. I left mine overnight baking at about 130°C for 9 hours. Remove the tray from the oven and using a sharp knife cut the fruit leather into strips. Let it cool completely before peeling the fruit leather off the baking paper. Roll up if desired and store in an airtight container for up to a week! Enjoy :)

296. Gummi Orange Slices

Ingredients:

1 T. vanilla extract

½ t. natural orange flavour

Pinch real salt

1 ½ t. liquid stevia (every brand varies in sweetness, so add this 'to taste')

8 T. grass-fed gelatin

1 can coconut milk

1 ½ C. water

Natural orange food coloring to desired colour

orange ice cube tray molds

INSTRUCTIONS:

Heat water and coconut milk over low heat until simmering.

Continue on low heat, slowly adding in each tablespoon of gelatin, whisking the entire time.

Add remaining ingredients and whisk until any clumps of gelatin are gone.

Pour into molds, and pour remaining liquid into 8X8 glass pan.

Put in fridge until solid. Gummis should pop out easily once hardened.

297. Prosciutto-Wrapped Berries

Yields: 12 total strawberries/baby bell peppers

6 strawberries

6 golden baby bell peppers

Honey Basil Ricotta (see below)

1 oz. thinly sliced grass-fed prosciutto, divided into 12 strips

1/4 c. micro greens (about half a small package)

Instructions

Using a sharp pairing knife, cut the tops off the strawberries, pulling the middle completely out and leaving a deep hole. Do the same for the peppers and use your finger to pull any seeds out of the insides.

To assemble: use a butter knife to stuff the berries/peppers with about 1 t. each of the Honey Basil Ricotta (the peppers will hold more ricotta than the berries). Then place a few sprigs of micro greens into the ricotta. Wrap a thin slice of prosciutto around each one and lay down length-wise to hold the prosciutto in place (you could also use toothpicks for this but that's a little too fussy for me).

298. Vanilla Pudding Pops

Ingredients

1 3.4 oz. box vanilla Jell-O instant pudding

2 cups vanilla almond milk, chilled

Instructions

In a medium bowl, combine pudding mix and cold almond milk.

Beat mixture continuously with a whisk for two minutes. Let sit for 5-7 minutes.

Pour mixture into 3 oz. cups

Place in freezer for 30 minutes; Remove and insert popsicle sticks into center.

Place back in freezer for 2-3 hours, or overnight.

299. Vanilla Pumpkin Seed Clusters

Ingredients:

115g (1/2 cup) pumpkin seeds

1 tsp vanilla extract

2 tsp honey

2 tsp coconut sugar

Water (boiled)

Instructions

Preheat oven to 150c.

In a medium bowl, combine the honey, coconut sugar and vanilla. Stir together to create a thick paste then add a small drop of boiled water to thin it out and create a runny syrup.

Pour in the pumpkin seeds and stir them around in the mixture to evenly coat them.

Dollop a generous tsp full of the pumpkin seeds onto a baking sheet, repeat until it's all used up and cook for 15-20 minutes until most of the seeds have browned (but don't let them burn!)

Take out of the oven and leave to cool for a few minutes. Once they've cooled a little (but are still warm) you can press the clusters together to make sure they don't fall apart. They will dry quickly.

Once they're cooled and dried, they're ready to eat! Enjoy on their own or served on top of your cereal.

300. Almond Joy Sunday

Ingredients:

1. 2 cans full fat coconut milk

2. ½ cup honey

3. 1 ½ tablespoons vanilla extract

4. 1 dark baking chocolate bar

5. ¼ cup sliced almonds

6. ½ cup unsweetened coconut flakes

Instructions

1. In a blender, mix together the coconut milk, honey, and vanilla extract. Line a plastic Tupperware with plastic wrap. Pour the mixture into it and freeze it overnight. The next day, take half of the frozen mixture and add it to a food processor. Mix it on high until it resembles frozen yogurt and put it back into a storage container. Repeat this process with the other half of the mixture. Return the blended ice cream to the freeze for 30 minutes before serving.

2. To assemble, melt the chocolate chips in a saucepan over low heat, to prevent burning the chocolate. Serve each Almond Joy Sunday with a scoop of the ice cream. Drizzle the melted chocolate on top, then sprinkle with coconut flakes and sliced almonds. Serve immediately.

301. Spiced Autumn Apples Baked in Brandy

Ingredients

2 apples of your choice (I used gala, but choose your favorite!)

1 cup brandy

1/4 cup walnuts

1/4 cup raisins

1/4 tablespoon nutmeg

1/4 tablespoon cinnamon

1/4 tablespoon ground cloves

Directions

Preheat oven to 350 degrees Fahrenheit.

Slice the very top and very bottom off of each apple. (The top allows for more room to stuff with goodies, the bottom allows the apples to soak up all the nice sauce).

Core both apples to the bottom, but not all the way through.

Mix brandy, spices, walnuts, and raisins in a small bowl.

Pour half of the brandy spice mixture into each apple.

Place on baking sheet and bake 20-25 minutes, or until apples are soft. I like to pour any remaining sauce mixture into the bottom of the pan so the apples can soak up the flavours.

Serve and enjoy! My roommate enjoyed his with a side of vanilla coconut milk ice cream.

Notes

Recipe makes 2 servings

Nutrition Facts Per Serving

Calories: 353

Total Fat: 10.0g

Saturated Fat: 0.6g

Carbs: 32.4g

Fiber: 4.0g; Protein: 4.6g

302. Chocolate Bavarian Cheesecake

Ingredients:
For the base:

15 Easy Chocolate Cookies

¼ cup coconut oil (melted)

OR

2 cups nuts

2. 1 cup dried dates (soaked in water)

For the middle:

2+1/2 cups raw cashews (soaked in water for 6 or more hours)

½ cup honey

¼ cup coconut oil

¼ cup cacao powder

½ cup coconut milk

½ cup orange juice

For the top:

1 can coconut cream (chilled in fridge overnight)

Cacao nibs to decorate

Instructions:

For the base:

Grind the chocolate cookies in a food processor until fine. Add the melted coconut oil and process until mixture sticks together. Add another tablespoon of coconut oil if you need to.

Press the crumbs into the base of a 21cm spring form tin. If you don't have a spring form tin, just line your tin with plastic wrap or baking paper so you can remove it easily.

OR

If you can't be bothered making the cookies (or didn't have any in the freezer like I did), just process 2 cups of nuts in a food processor until finely chopped. (Any combination of nuts works well. I've tried just macadamias and it is beautiful and also a combination of cashews, macadamias, hazelnuts, walnuts and brazil nuts)

When your nuts are finely chopped, drain the soaked dates, getting out as much water as you can. Then add them to the food processor and process until it makes a sticky dough.

Next, scoop the date & nut mixture into your pan. Put small plastic freezer bags onto your hands and use your fingers to spread the mixture evenly into the pan. (No sticky fingers!)

For the filling:

Drain the cashews well. Put all of the filling ingredients into a high speed blender or processor and process until smooth. I have a new Froothie blender that is amazing! I compared it to the Vita Mix and it's cheaper and more powerful. You know I love a bargain. Anyway, I'm really happy with it and it makes amazing cheesecake filling!

You will need to use the tamper if you have one and regularly scrape down the sides to make sure all the ingredients are blended together. Keep processing until it is super smooth. Lots of taste testing needed for this step!

Once the mixture is smooth, scrape it all into your pan, on top of the base mixture. Spread it out with a spatula.

Cover with plastic wrap, then put into the freezer for at least 6 hours to set.

When ready to serve, take it from the freezer and defrost for around 30 minutes to soften slightly before cutting. (15 mins for minis.)

While it's defrosting, beat the cream that rises to the top of the coconut cream after it's been refrigerated. Use electric beaters and add some honey to taste if you like.

Spread or pipe the cream over the top of your cheesecake and decorate with cacao nibs.

303. Raw Brownie Bites

Ingredients

1 1/2 cups walnuts

Pinch of salt

1 cup pitted dates

1 tsp vanilla

1/3 cup unsweetened cocoa powder

Instructions

Add walnuts and salt to a blender or food processor. Mix until the walnuts are finely ground.

Add the dates, vanilla, and cocoa powder to the blender. Mix well until everything is combined. With the blender still running, add a couple drops of water at a time to make the mixture stick together.

Using a spatula, transfer the mixture into a bowl. Using your hands, form small round balls, rolling in your palm. Store in an airtight container in the refrigerator for up to a week.

304. Maple Cinnamon Cheesecakes with Gingerbread Crust

Ingredients

For the crust:

1 heaping cup pecans

6 medjool dates

½ tsp ginger

½ tsp cinnamon

For the cheesecake:

2 cups raw cashews (soaked overnight)

½ cup maple syrup

½ tsp cinnamon

Juice of 1 lemon

⅓ cup coconut oil

½ tsp sea salt

Instructions

For the crust:

Combine all the ingredients in a food processor. You will see the mixture start to get to a crumbly like consistency. Be careful not to over process or you will end up with pecan butter. Once the mixture looks done, you can press a little into the bottom of each muffin cup. I used standard sized pans. Place them in the fridge while you make the cheesecake part.

For the cheesecake:

Make sure your cashews have been soaking overnight. Drain and rinse them. Place them in a food processor with all the other cheesecake ingredients. Mix until everything is smooth.

Spoon a little of the cheesecake mixture into each muffin cup.

Once that is done, place them in the fridge to firm up. It can take up to 12 hours for the cheesecakes to get fully firm.

Notes

Keep these stored in the fridge. You can probably freeze them as well. I have not tried that though.

305. Heavenly Raw Vegan White Chocolate and Raspberry Cheesecake

Ingredients

Base layer:

1 cup almonds

6 medjool dates, pitted

2 tbsp cocoa butter, liquefied

¼ tsp raw ground vanilla beans (or ½ tsp pure vanilla extract)

Cheesecake layer:

1½ cups cashews, pre-soaked (at least a few hours, best overnight) and strained

¼ cup fresh squeezed lemon juice

6 tbsp liquid sweetener of your choice (I used maple syrup)

¼ cup coconut oil, liquefied

⅓ cup cocoa butter, liquefied

1 tsp pure vanilla extract (or ½ tsp more ground raw vanilla bean)

¼ tsp salt

Raspberry topping layer:

1½ – 2 cups fresh or frozen raspberries (I used frozen and slightly thawed out)

3 tbsp liquid sweetener or your choice (I used maple syrup)

⅓ cup cocoa butter, liquefied

Optional:

Reserve a few raspberries for garnish

Instructions

Place all base ingredients into a food processor and process until a medium-fine crumbly mixture is formed. Transfer this mixture into the spring form pan and press down well to create an even flat cake base. Place in the freezer while working on the next step (or for at least 10 minutes).

Place all cheesecake layer ingredients in your blender (a stronger blender like a Vitamix works best), and blend until mixture is completely smooth. Pour it over the crust into the spring form pan. Lightly tap the pan down on the counter to eliminate any air bubbles. Smooth it out as well to create an even surface. Place in the freezer while working on the next step (best if in the freezer for at least 15 – 20 minutes). {Placing cake in the freezer for a bit helps keep the cake layers better separated}

Place all raspberry layer ingredients into your blender and blend until the mixture is smooth. Pour over the cheesecake layer into the spring form pan and return back to the freezer for at least 3-4 hours. Cake can then be served out of the freezer as an icebox cake, or kept refrigerated for a softer and more mousse-like consistency. I kept mine frozen, but allowed it to thaw out for about an hour in the fridge before serving. Decorate with some fresh raspberries prior to serving and enJoy!

306. Samoa Donuts

Ingredients

For the Donuts

2½ cups blanched almond flour (such as Honey Ville)

½ teaspoon baking soda

A scant less than ½ teaspoon salt

6 tablespoons honey

¼ cup coconut oil, softened or liquid

1 tablespoon vanilla

1 teaspoon Lemon juice

3 whole large room temp eggs

Coconut caramel topping

1 can full-fat coconut milk (about 1½ cups), I used guar gum-free Natural Value

½ cup mild flavored honey or maple syrup,

A pinch of sea salt

1 rounded tablespoon ghee or butter (can sub palm shortening or coconut oil)

2 teaspoons vanilla extract

¼ cup finely shredded coconut, plus 2 more tablespoons for garnishing

For the Dipping Chocolate

1 bag Enjoy Life Chocolate chips (melted in a double boiler)

Instructions

Preheat your mini donut making machine OR preheat the oven to 350 degrees if you are using a regular donut pan or making into muffins.

In a large bowl, mix together the almond flour, baking soda and salt.

In another bowl, combine the honey, oil, vanilla, lemon juice and eggs.

Add the oil/honey mixture to the dry ingredients. Mix till just combined.

Add about 2 tablespoons of batter to each mould in the donut machine or scoop the batter into a ziplock bag, twisting the other end to close it. Snip the end off of one of the corners with a scissors. Start with a small cut. You can always make it bigger if you need too. Squeeze batter into moulds.

Close the lid and allow to cook for about 2 minutes. Times will vary with each machine. Open the machine and flip over each donut using the forked 'skewer' that comes with most machines. Close the lid again cook for about one more minute. Remove donuts and let cool on a wire rack. Repeat with the rest of the batter.

If using a regular donut pan, fill each well-greased mould about ¾ full. Smooth the tops if needed and bake for 10-12 minutes. Let cool in the pan for 5 minutes, remove from the pan and cool completely on a wire rack.

Makes 12-15 mini donuts or 6 regular sized ones (depending on how much batter you eat during the prep time.)

For the Coconut Caramel

In a small-medium heavy bottomed sauce pan, bring the coconut milk, honey and salt to a boil over medium high heat, being sure that they are well combined. Reduce to a medium heat, and let the mixture boil down for about 35-40 minutes.

Add the ghee and vanilla, stirring it in till well incorporated. Continue cooking for another 5-15 minutes or as long as needed until it is a deep caramel color. Don't rush the process. Depending on how hot your burner is this process could be faster or slower. Stir often toward the end to keep the bottom from burning too much. A little burning is fine as long as you are stirring it in to the mixture. It will give it a darker flavor.

Remove from heat, transfer to a bowl and let cool for 5 minutes then stir vigorously until it's creamy, shiny and smooth.

While the caramel is cooking, spread the coconut out on an ungreased cookie sheet and toast the coconut in a 325-degree oven. Stir often till golden, about 5-10 minutes. Remove from the oven and let cool.

Mix the toasted coconut into the caramel minus a tablespoon or so for garnishing later. Use coconut caramel while still warm for best spreading results. Caramel can be made ahead of time (w/o the shredded coconut) and reheated in a double boiler.

307. Paleo Cocoa Puffs

Ingredients

¾ Packed Cup of Blanched Almond Flour

1 Cup + 2 Tbsp Tapioca Starch/Flour

½ Cup Cocoa Powder

¼ tsp Salt

⅔ cup Coconut Palm Sugar

2½ tsp. Baking Powder

1 Tbsp Vanilla Extract

⅓ Cup of oil or Melted Butter (dairy or nondairy)

1 Egg + 1 Egg White

Instructions

Preheat Oven to 350 degrees.

Mix together the dry ingredients (Almond Flour, Tapioca Flour, Cocoa Powder, Salt, Palm Sugar, and Baking Powder).

Add in the Vanilla, Oil, and Eggs. Mix really well (don't be afraid to get your hands dirty!)

Line 2 large baking sheets with parchment paper.

Roll teaspoon sized balls of dough (or smaller if you have the patience) in between your palms to create little cocoa puff balls. If you find your hands getting sticky- rinse them off and dry them before continuing and or dust your hands with a little extra tapioca starch.

Use about half the dough to make cocoa puffs for the first baking sheet. Leave a little space between each cocoa puff as they will expand in the oven.

Place the first baking sheet into the oven and bake 18-20 minute. Halfway through baking using a spatula to flip the cocoa puffs over so that the bottoms do not burn.

While the first tray is baking, prepare your second tray of cocoa puffs and follow the same baking instructions.

Let cocoa puffs cool completely before eating. (They will get crispy as they cool).

308. Hummingbird Bread

Ingredients

½ cup tapioca flour/powder

½ cup coconut flour

½ cup coconut sugar

½ teaspoon cinnamon

½ teaspoon baking soda

pinch of salt

2 bananas, mashed

½ cup pineapple, diced

½ cup coconut oil, melted

3 eggs, whisked

1 teaspoon vanilla extract

½ cup pecans, chopped

Instructions

Preheat oven to 350 degrees.

Add tapioca flour, coconut flour, coconut suguar, cinnamon, baking soda, and salt to a large bowl and mix.

Then add the rest of the ingredients, folding in pecans at the end.

Pour mixture into a bread pan (I lined mine with parchment paper for easy removal) and smooth at the top

Bake for 40-45 minutes or until bread is completely cooked through (use the toothpick trick to check). Let cool slightly before serving.

309. Paleo Cookie Butter

Ingredients

For the Cookie Butter

½ cup (128 grams) favorite nut butter, almond, cashew or macadamia

½ cup (128 grams) roasted sunflower butter, such as Sun Butter®

½ cup (128 grams) raw organic coconut butter, such as Artisan®

¼ cup (60 grams) organic ghee (you could also use coconut oil)

4 tablespoons (84 grams) organic raw honey*

1½ tablespoons (20 grams) 100% pure cocoa butter, I use Callebaut®, melted

1½ tablespoons (10.5 grams) organic coconut flour, such as Tropical Traditions®

1 teaspoon (5 grams) unsulphured molasses, such as Brer Rabbit®

1 teaspoon (about 2 grams) pure vanilla extract, such as Nielsen-Massey®

½ to 1 teaspoon ground cinnamon, such as Penzey's® Cinnamon

¼ teaspoon ground allspice

¼ teaspoon freshly grated whole nutmeg

Generous pinch of fine sea salt

Coconut palm sugar or pure stevia extract powder, to taste

*Do not serve raw honey to children under the age of 1 year.

For the Optional Mix-Ins for "Cookie Dough Butter"

Chopped dark chocolate 70% cocoa or more

Gluten free semi-sweet chocolate chips, such as Trader Joe's®

Chopped walnuts or pecans, toasted or not

Unsweetened shredded coconut, toasted or not

Special Equipment

Mini Prep Food Processor

Mason jar with lid, helpful but not necessary

Rubber spatula

Preparation

Place nut butter and Sun Butter into work bowl of prep food processor.

In a small saucepan over medium-low heat, melt and brown the coconut butter and ghee until golden brown, stirring constantly, about 3 minutes for a lighter "blonde" browned coconut butter or 5 minutes for a darker, rich browned coconut butter the color of dark coffee and cream. (The mixture will bubble and foam. Keep stirring.) Remove immediately from heat to prevent overbrowning or burning; stir and allow to cool until still warm (not room temp, but no longer hot). Note: It is important to remove the pan immediately when coconut butter mixture is browned to desired doneness as the residual heat will continue to cook the mixture.

Add browned coconut butter mixture to nut butter and Sun Butter®; process until well combined and smooth scraping down sides of bowl as necessary between pulses. The mixture will be very thin at this point. Do not worry. Add honey, melted cocoa butter, coconut flour, molasses, vanilla extract, spices and salt; process until well combined and smooth. Taste and, if desired, sweeten additionally with coconut palm sugar or pure stevia extract.

Remove work bowl from processor unit. With a rubber spatula, or the plastic spatula that came with your processor unit, scrape and pour mixture into a small to medium bowl. Cover bowl with plastic food wrap and place in refrigerator until thickened, about 1 hour. Stir halfway through chilling time for an even chill. Remove from the fridge and stir to loosen. Transfer to Mason® jar, if desired, or other covered container for storing. Before serving add and stir in favorite mix-ins as desired, about a few tablespoons each. Keep stored in an airtight container, such as a Mason® jar, in refrigerator.

Notes

Tip: This homemade cookie butter softens upon room temperature. If you wish for a thicker cookie butter, either keep it chilled or simply stir in an additional 1 tablespoon of coconut flour (or more to desired thickness).

310. Paleo-friendly Coconut Chocolate Coffee Cake

Ingredients

What you'll need:

(all ingredients are available at Whole Foods or Natural Grocers/health sections; my ordering recommendations listed)

two medium-sized glass bowls for mixing & one square glass baking dish (8"x8")

coconut oil for greasing baking dish

4 eggs

½ cup full-fat coconut milk

¼ cup coconut butter

½ cup brewed coffee or espresso, as strong as you like

¼ cup grade B maple syrup

1 tsp. vanilla extract

½ cup almond flour

½ cup + 1 Tbs coconut flour

½ tsp. baking soda

pinch of sea salt

1 cup dark chocolate chips

½ cup unsweetened coconut flakes

What to do

Preheat the oven to 350° F.

500 Paleo Anti Inflammatory Instant Pot, Bone Broth and Dessert Recipes By Mercedes Del Rey

Combine the first 6 ingredients (eggs, coconut milk, coconut butter, coffee, maple syrup, and vanilla) in a bowl. Mix them together. I always use my favorite kitchen tool, my stick blender, to do the mixing.

In a separate bowl, combine the almond flour, coconut flour, baking soda, and salt. Stir.

Add the liquid, a little at a time, to the dry ingredients, mashing and stirring the mixture until smooth. Then, add half the chocolate chips to the mixture and stir them in.

Pour/push the mixture into the greased baking dish, smoothing it out with a spatula.

Top with coconut flakes, then chocolate chips.

Bake for 35 minutes, then allow it to cool.

311. Earl Grey Lavender Ice Cream

Ingredients

2 cups full-fat coconut milk

1 cup homemade almond milk *

½ cup raw honey

5 large egg yolks **

¼ cup loose leaf earl grey tea

1 tbsp dried culinary grade lavender ***

1 tsp pure vanilla extract

Instructions

Heat coconut and almond milk with the honey over low heat in a saucepan. Make sure it does not boil.

Once milk is hot and honey has been dissolved, remove from heat.

Place the earl grey tea and lavender in a large cotton or paper tea bag and drop it into the milk mixture. Cover saucepan and infuse the milk with tea for 30 minutes (or longer for a much stronger flavor).

Remove tea bag and rewarm the milk over low heat.

At the same time, beat the egg yolks with the vanilla extract and temper it 1 tbsp at a time with the warm milk (until about ¼ cup of milk has been added to the eggs).

Add the rest of the milk to the egg yolk mixture and mix until combined.

Add it back to the pan and heat the mixture over low heat while stirring constantly.

Watch this part carefully to avoid curdling.

Once the mixture has thickened enough to coat the back of a wooden spoon. Remove it from heat and chill for 4-5 hours in the fridge.

Freeze the cooled mixture using an ice cream maker for about 12 minutes. Make sure it does not get too hard.

Place ice cream in a container and freeze for another hour before serving.

This makes a pint of ice cream.

Notes

Homemade almond milk is creamier and has no preservatives compared to the store bought brands.

** Make sure egg yolks are brought to room temperature to avoid curdling.

*** Not all types of dried lavender is edible. Get ones that are used for cooking/baking

312. Blueberry Cream Pie

Ingredients

Crust:

3 cups almonds

½ Teaspoon cinnamon

½ cup honey

2 Tablespoons coconut oil

1 Tablespoon lemon zest

1 Teaspoon almond extract

pinch of sea salt

Filling:

2 Teaspoons kosher plant-based gelatin, dissolved in 2 Tablespoons hot water

⅓ cup freshly squeezed lemon juice

⅓ cup honey

1 can coconut milk, chilled (Native Forest brand is good for this recipe)

4 cups blueberries for serving

Instructions

Place the almonds and cinnamon in a food processor and pulse until your desired texture is reached. I like to leave some bigger pieces for texture. Add the rest of the crust ingredients and pulse until a sticky dough forms. Pat the crust into a pie plate, (use water to keep your hands from sticking to the crust).

For the filling, mix the gelatin and water together. Stir to dissolve and immediately add the lemon juice. If the gelatin gets clumpy, place the mixture over hot water until it melts again. Pour the coconut milk into an electric mixer, add the honey and whip on high until peaks form, about 15 minutes. Add the gelatin mixture to the whipped cream. Pour the filling into the crust. The filling will seem thin, but don't worry it will set up in the refrigerator.

Chill for at least 4 hours until set, and serve with lots of berries!

Notes

Use Grade A maple syrup in place of honey for a completely Vegan version.

313. Jam Ball Donuts

INGREDIENTS

Portions12 portion(s)

125 g Buttermilk or Milk

15 g butter (I used salted)

1 egg

250 g bakers flour

1.5 tsp Yeast

1/4 tsp salt

30 g caster sugar

1/2 Cup raspberry jam

Sugar - For rolling

RECIPE'S PREPARATION

Method

1. Place milk & butter in bowl, and mix on 37 degrees, speed 1 for 2 minutes.

2. Add in egg to milk mixture and mix speed 4, 5 seconds.

3. In this order - Add in Yeast, then flour, then the caster sugar & the salt last. Mix on speed 6 for 6 seconds to combine, then knead for 3 minutes

4. Place dough in a greased bowl and cover and place in a warm place to prove for 1 hour or until dough has doubled in size.

5. Once the dough is proved, knock down onto a floured surface and cut dough in half until you have 2 balls.

6. Roll each ball into a 25cm long log, then cut each log into pieces and roll each piece into a ball and place on piece of baking paper and let prove for a further 15 minutes.

7. While the dough balls are proving, warm up your deep fryer, or oil in a frypan/saucepan (I used solidified oil which is an animal fat that you find in the butter section at the supermarket), to 175 degrees.

8. Drop in 3-4 balls at a time and cook for 5 mins or until nice and brown/golden. Mine turned over on their own in the oil, but you may need to turn them manually

9. When cooked, take out and roll in sugar, then using a piping bag with the long nozzle (Or an old sauce bottle cleaned out and filled with jam), fill the donuts with jam

These taste Just like the donuts you get from the markets and fast food vans etc. Enjoy!

TIP

You can use any flavor jam you like, but raspberry is generally what they use for traditional hot jam donuts

314. Baked Cinnamon Doughnuts

(recipe adapted from Taste, makes 12)

1 cup full cream or reduced-fat milk

15g unsalted butter, melted

400g plain flour

1 1/2 teaspoons instant dried yeast

1/4 cup (50g) caster sugar

1/2 teaspoon ground cinnamon

For cinnamon doughnuts:

35g melted butter

1/2 cup (44g) caster sugar

1 tsp ground cinnamon

Optional strawberry doughnut men decorations:

1 cup icing sugar

1/4 tsp strawberry essence

Pink food coloring

Milk

Brown mini m&ms

Toothpicks (or a safer alternative)

Place milk in a heatproof, microwave-safe jug. Microwave on medium-high (75%) for 30 to 40 seconds or until heated through (do not allow to boil). Stir in melted butter and set aside.

Sift flour into a large mixing bowl. Stir in yeast, sugar and cinnamon. Make a well in the centre. Add milk mixture. Mix to form a soft dough. Turn out onto a lightly floured surface. Knead for 10 minutes or until smooth and elastic (or if you are lucky enough to have a mixer with dough hooks like me, beat using dough hooks on high for 5-7 mins).

Place dough in a lightly oiled bowl. Cover with plastic wrap. Set aside in a warm place for 1 hour or until doubled in size. Line 2 baking trays with baking paper. Using your fist, punch dough down. Turn out onto a lightly floured surface. Knead until smooth. Roll dough out until 2cm thick. Using a 6.5cm cutter, cut 12 rounds from dough. Using a 3cm cutter, cut circles from the centre of each round. Place doughnuts (and doughnut holes), 5cm apart, on prepared tray. Cover with lightly greased plastic wrap. Set aside in a warm place for 30 minutes or until doubled in size.

315. Gluten Free Dairy Free Coconut

Ingredients

3 cans (14 ounces each) coconut milk, 2 of the 3 refrigerated for at least 24 hours*

3/4 cup (150 g) sugar

1 teaspoon (3 g) unflavored powdered gelatin

3 ounces dairy-free chocolate chips (optional)

1 teaspoon pure vanilla extract (optional)

*You must use full-fat coconut milk. Thai Kitchen brand coconut milk and Whole Foods 365 brand coconut milk both work well consistently for this application.

Directions

In a large, heavy-bottom saucepan, place the entire contents of the 1 room-temperature can of coconut milk and the sugar, and mix to combine well. Cook over medium-high heat, stirring frequently to prevent it from splattering, until it is reduced at least by half and thickened (about 10 minutes). You can also cook the mixture over low heat for about 35 minutes, and stir much less frequently. This is now your sweetened condensed coconut milk. Remove from the heat and set aside to allow to cool completely.

Remove the remaining two cans of coconut milk carefully from the refrigerator, without shaking them at all. The solid should have separated from the liquid while it was chilling, and you don't want to reintegrate them. Remove the lids from the cans, scoop out only the solid white coconut (discarding all of the liquid), and place it in a large bowl. With a hand mixer (or in the bowl of a stand mixer fitted with the whisk attachment), whip the coconut on high speed for about 2 minutes, or until light and fluffy and nearly doubled in volume. Place the whipped coconut cream in the refrigerator to chill for about 10 minutes.

Place the gelatin in a small bowl, and mix well with 2 tablespoons of the sweetened condensed coconut milk from the first step. Allow to sit for 5 minutes while the gelatin dissolves. The mixture will swell. Microwave on 70% power for 20 seconds to liquify the gelatin, and then add the mixture to the rest of the cooled sweetened condensed coconut milk.

Remove the coconut whipped cream from the refrigerator and add the sweetened condensed coconut milk mixture and optional vanilla to it. Whip once more until light and creamy, and well-

503

combined (another 1 to 2 minutes). Fold in optional chocolate chips, and scrape the mixture into a 2 quart freezer-safe container. Cover tightly and freeze until firm (about 6 hours). Serve frozen. If it is at all difficult to scoop, allow to sit in the refrigerator for 15 minutes before scooping and serving.

316. Grain Free Steamed Christmas Puddings – GAPS & Paleo Friendly

Ingredients

150g sultanas

80g dried sour cherries or dried unsweetened cranberries, plus extra for garnish

100g currants

30g activated or raw almonds, roughly chopped

200g kombucha or freshly squeezed orange juice

zest of 1 orange

40g blanched almond meal

20g coconut flour

1/4 tsp nutmeg

1/2 tsp mixed spice

1/4 tsp cinnamon

55g tallow or coconut oil

40g apple, peeled & cored

2 eggs

1/4 tsp fine salt

1/4 tsp bicarb soda

Instructions

Weigh dried fruit and almonds into the Thermomix bowl, and add kombucha or orange juice.

Cook 6 mins/80C/reverse/speed soft. Remove to a large bowl and set aside to cool.

Place orange zest into clean, dry Thermomix bowl and chop 20 sec/speed 10.

Add almond meal, coconut flour, spices, salt, soda, apple, eggs and tallow or coconut oil into Thermomix bowl and mix 5 sec/speed 5. Scrape down sides of bowl.

Add soaked fruit and nuts back to bowl and mix 10 sec/reverse/speed 3.

Scoop mixture into silicone cupcake cups or small ramekins and place into the Varoma dish and tray, with lid on. Cups/ramekins should be about 3/4 full.

Place 500g water into Thermomix bowl and place Varoma in position. Cook 25 mins/Varoma/speed 2.

Allow puddings to cool, covered, and store in fridge until needed.

Drizzle with Coconut Vanilla Custard, with a dried cranberry or sour cherry on top for decoration.

Notes

I use my Thermomix to make these puddings - if you don't have a Thermomix, chop by hand, cook fruit gently on stovetop, and mix in remaining ingredients. Steam in a steamer or use traditional Christmas pudding cooking method.

317. Raw Pineapple Coconut Vegan Cheesecake

Crust:

4 dates, soaked until very soft1 cup dried organic, unsweetened coconut

Place soften dates and coconut in food processor and process until well blended. Pat into the bottom of an oiled 7 1/2 inch spring form pan.

Filling:

2 1/2 cups young Thai coconut flesh (about 5 young coconuts)1/4 cup coconut water (from the coconuts)1/3 cup raw agave nectar or liquid sweetener of choice1 cup coconut oil, softened2 cups fresh pineapple chunks, separated

In high-speed blender, pureé the coconut flesh and coconut water together until smooth. Add the agave, coconut oil. You want this to be quite smooth so blend away. Add 1 cup of the pineapple chunks. Blend until incorporated. Pulse the remaining pineapple chunks in the food processor until well chopped. Drain. Stir the pineapple into the coconut mixture, pour over crust and let set up in the refrigerator for 4 hours. Move to freezer and leave until firm.

318. Grain-free Italian Lemon Almond Cake

Ingredients

320 grams (this is about 3 cups + 3 tablespoons) almond flour (not almond meal) or blanched almonds, ground into almond flour

200 grams (1 cup + 3 tablespoons) white chocolate, chopped

2 tablespoons whipping cream or milk (I used 1.5% milk)

180 grams (3/4 cup + 1 tablespoon) unsalted butter, softened

130 grams (about 2/3 cup) granulated sugar or coconut sugar1

zest of 4 lemons, about 2 tablespoons

4 large eggs, separated

1 teaspoon lemon extract

40 grams (about 2 tablespoons) of limoncello or lemon juice

powdered sugar as garnish, optional

Directions

Preheat your oven to 350°F / 176°C and grease a 10" / 26cm pan or line it with parchment paper. If using blanched almonds instead of almond flour, process them in the food processor until they're pretty finely ground. If you grind them too much, they'll release oil and become almond butter.

Combine the white chocolate and milk / cream in a microwave safe bowl.

Heat in 30 second increments and stir after every 30 seconds. Set aside to cool while you prepare the rest. Beat the butter with 100 grams of sugar and beat until fluffy.

Add the lemon zest, egg yolks and lemon extract and beat until well combined. Then add the almond flour / ground almonds and the melted chocolate. Add the limoncello / lemon juice and beat until combined.

In a separate bowl with spotlessly clean beaters, beat the egg whites until soft peaks form. Gradually add the remaining 30 grams of sugar to the egg white mixture. Fold the egg whites into the almond batter until well combined. Spoon the batter into the greased pan and bake for 40 - 45 minutes. If making half the cake, use a 7" / 18cm pan and bake for 30 minutes. The cake will puff up in the oven, but when cooling, it'll fall back down.

Let it cool completely in the pan and then invert the cake onto a plate, and then flip that back into the pan or onto another plate (so that it's not upside down). Sprinkle on some powdered sugar if desired, but only before serving.

Notes

If using coconut sugar, blend in a coffee grinder first so that it's basically like powdered coconut sugar. I'd be worried about how well non-grinded coconut sugar would do with the egg whites. I'm guessing not well. And please note the above comment about how using coconut sugar turns the cake the brown! It's just not possible to make a bright yellow cake with this dark sugar. Also, this recipe originally used 200 grams of sugar. I used 200 grams in the first cake and only 130 in the second and didn't notice much of a difference, but I'm used to not using so much sugar. Feel free to use up to 200 grams.

319. Paleo Antioxidant Berry Shake

Ingredients

1/2 cup coconut milk

1/4 cup cold water

1/2 frozen banana

1/2 cup frozen raspberries

1/2 cup frozen blueberries

1 tbsp chia seeds

Directions

In a large cup (if using an immersion blender) or a blender, combine ingredients and blend until smooth. Add more water if necessary to reach desired consistency. Serve immediately.

Notes

Servings: 1

Difficulty: Easy

320. Gluten Free Tiramisu Roulade Recipe

Ingredients

8 eggs, separated

2/3 cup granulated sugar

2 tablespoons unsweetened cocoa powder (I like the dark kind)

1 tablespoon granulated espresso or instant coffee

For the filling:

16 ounces Mascarpone cheese

6 tablespoons heavy cream

Powdered sugar for dusting

Grated chocolate (optional)

Directions

Preheat oven to 350 degrees. Grease a sheet pan or jelly roll pan that is something close to 15 ½" by 11 ½". Line with parchment paper and grease that too.

Beat egg whites until glossy and soft peaks form. In a separate bowl beat the egg yolks with the granulated sugar until thick and pale yellow in color. Stir in cocoa powder and granulated espresso/instant coffee. Take a big scoop of the egg whites and mix into the yolks, then fold the yolks into the egg whites. Pour into prepared pan and even out with a spatula.

Bake in pre-heated oven for 20 minutes. Remove pan from oven and let cake cool in the pan. When cool, tip the cake onto another piece of parchment paper that has been dusted with powdered sugar.

For filling, mix mascarpone cheese with cream until well mixed and creamy. Smooth the filling over the cooled cake.

Using the parchment paper to help you, roll the roulade up from one of the short ends. Carefully lift it and place on a serving platter. It may crack but that is fine. Dust with additional powdered

511

sugar and grate some chocolate on top if desired. Chill in fridge for at least half an hour but serve the same day as you make it. Slice to serve.

Servings

Makes 12 – 14 gluten free servings.

321. Gluten Free Monster Cookies

INGREDIENTS:

1 cup creamy peanut butter (I use Skippy)

1 large egg

1/2 cup packed brown sugar

1/2 cup granulated sugar

1/2 teaspoon vanilla extract

1/2 teaspoon baking soda

1 teaspoon nonfat milk

1/2 cup gluten-free oats (or substitute regular quick cooking oats)

1/2 cup M&Ms or a combination of M&Ms and raisins

DIRECTIONS:

Preheat oven to 350°F. Line a cookie sheet with a silpat baking mat or parchment paper

Sitr peanut butter, egg, and sugars together until smooth. Stir in vanilla, baking soda, milk, and oats. Stir in M&Ms and/or raisins.

Scoop 2 tablespoon cookie dough balls onto prepared cookie sheet. Use a lightly dampened fork to flatten slightly in a criss cross pattern. (These cookies will not spread much.)

Bake for 8-11 minutes, until they no longer look glossy and are slightly browned on the bottoms. Cool before storing in an airtight container for up to 4 days. Note: these cookies are more crumbly than regular cookies, so be careful when stacking or transporting.

NOTES:

Not all gluten free oats are quick cook oats. To make them quick cook, just give them a few pulses in a food processor or blender to break them up a bit. There are two brands of GF oats that I know of, Bob's Red Mill (rolled oats) and Gluten Free Chex (quick cook).

322. Figgy Apple-Mascarpone Tart, with Green Apple Ice and Cider Caramel

Ingredients:

Shortbread Crust

7 Tablespoons unsalted butter, cut into pieces, at room temperature

¼ cup confectioner's sugar

1 large egg yolk

1¼ cups all-purpose flour

Mascarpone-Fig filling

4 oz of mascarpone cheese, at room temperature*

4 oz of cream cheese, at room temperature*

¼ cup white granulated or lightly packed light brown sugar or a mix of both, depending on your taste

1 large egg

½ - 1 tsp ground cinnamon - again, depending on your taste

½ teaspoon pure vanilla extract

⅓ to ½ cup chopped, dried figs - depending on how 'figgy' you're feeling**

Apple Topping

2 large, 3 medium, or 4 small tart apples (Granny smith, Jonathan, Jonagold etc...OR, whatever looks and smells good at the market)

2 Tablespoon white granulated sugar

¼ teaspoon cinnamon

½ of a lemon

Honey Apricot Glaze

¼ cup apricot preserves

1 Tablespoon honey

1 Tablespoon apple liqueur. such as Calvados

Green Apple Ice

6 Granny Smith apples (or other tart baking apples, or 2 cups apple juice*)

½ cup Simple Syrup (equal parts sugar and water boiled until somewhat thick and clear. In this case, you would combine ½ cup water with ½ cup sugar in a small saucepan, boil until sugar has dissolved)***

4 Tablespoons lemon juice

Cider Caramel

1 cup granulated sugar

¼ cup water

1 teaspoon light corn syrup

½ cup apple cider or unsweetened apple juice

2 Tablespoons unsalted butter

Directions:

For the Shortbread Crust

In a bowl, combine the butter and sugar and blend to make a paste. Add the yolk and blend thoroughly. Add the flour and using your fingers, blend to make a crumbly dough, being careful not to overwork. Pour the crumbles into rectangle 13 x 4 or round 8 or 9-inch spring form pan, then press gently on the bottom and up the sides, until it's uniform, and fills every crevice of the tart pan (or slightly up the sides of a spring form pan). You want to see little pieces of butter in the dough. Let it rest in the refrigerator, covered, at least 2 hours or overnight. Remove from the refrigerator and prick the bottom of the crust with the tines of a fork.

OK, you can do one of two things here...

Place a sheet of parchment or foil in the tart pan (I used a 13 x 4 rectangular tart pan, but a round 8 or 9-inch tart or spring form pan will work just as well) and fill with pie weights or dried beans or rice, and blind bake the crust in a preheated 350-degree oven for 10 minutes. Remove the pie weights and foil and bake for another 5 minutes or until somewhat firm and very lightly golden brown. This is the method I used for the apple tart you see. I find the crust gets too dark in certain areas upon baking again, so next time I'm going to use the number 2 method below.

Do NOT prick the crust prior to letting it rest in the fridge. When ready to bake, brush the chilled shortbread crust with some beaten egg white and let dry for a few minutes. NOW prick the bottom and sides of the crust. Fill with the mascarpone-fig mixture, smoothing it out so it's even. Cover and chill for about 1-2 hours until it firms up (this makes it easier to keep the apple slices from slightly sinking when you pile them on top, although, if aesthetics isn't a big deal to you, skip the refrigeration/firming of the cheese mixture.).

For the Mascarpone-Fig filling

Combine the mascarpone, cream cheese and sugar and mix until smooth. Add the egg, vanilla, and cinnamon, and mix until uniform. I feel that hand mixing this is better, as you get a feel for the smooth, lump free consistency you're seeking. However, using electric beaters or a stand mixer is perfectly fine, just don't over-mix! Mascarpone doesn't react well to over-mixing.

Fold in the chopped, dried figs and pour into the partially baked and cooled crust, or egg white brushed raw crust. Let set in the fridge, covered, for 1 to 2 hours.

For the Apple Topping

Preheat oven to 425F. Combine the cinnamon and sugar in a small bowl.

Peel and core the apples. Slice in half or into quarters, then slice each half or quarter into ¼-inch thick slices. If you want the 'fanned' look. Hold apple slices together on top of the filling, then fan out (spread, sliding in one direction). Continue until you've covered the top completely, filling in any gaps with leftover slices or pieces of slices. You can spread them over the top any way you like...from concentric circles if using a round tart pan, to fanned out rows.or just pile them on, whichever suits your fancy. Squeeze some lemon juice over the apples (making sure to keep the seeds from sneaking in), then sprinkle the cinnamon sugar mixture evenly over the top.

Place the tart on a baking sheet, to catch any drips, and bake at 425F for 10 minutes, then turn the oven down to 400F, and bake for another 25 to 35 minutes, until the apples are soft and can be pierced easily with a knife. If the crust looks like it's browning too fast, cover the exposed area as best you can, with some aluminum foil. Remove from oven, and let cool on a wire rack. If using the egg white-raw crust method, bake at 425F for 15 minutes, then turn it down to 400F, and bake for 30-40 minutes more, checking on it periodically.

For the Honey Apricot Glaze

In a small saucepan over medium high heat, bring all the ingredients to a boil. Let boil for about 1 to 2 minutes, until slightly thickened. Brush glaze over the cooled apples.

For the Green Apple Ice

Quarter apples and juice them through a fruit juicer with peels on (this helps keep the color of the ice a nice bright green).

Add simple syrup and lemon juice to taste. Pour into a shallow pan or a glass baking dish and place in the freezer. After 30-40 minutes, scrape the pan to break up the frozen bits and create slush. Do this again after another 30-40 minutes, then put the pan in the freezer until you're ready to serve. (You can also do this in an ice cream maker following the manufacturer's directions.)

For the Cider Caramel

In a small saucepan, combine ¼ cup water, sugar, and corn syrup, and bring to a simmer over medium heat, stirring until the sugar dissolves. Increase heat to high and boil the mixture, swirling the pan occasionally until the mixture turns a medium amber color.

Remove the from heat and carefully whisk in the apple cider or juice, and butter from a distance (as the caramel may splatter). Whisk the mixture over low heat until smooth. Pass through a fine mesh sieve, and reserve until ready to use, or refrigerate for up to two days.

To Serve

Place a wedge or two (depending on how small or large you slice the tart, or if you'd like to make it a dessert for two), on a plate. Add a quenelle or scoop of the green apple ice next to the wedges, or as I did, in a small, clear or pretty bowl since it melts pretty fast, especially if it's a muggy day/night. Drizzle the cider caramel around the plate.

notes:

*All cream cheese or all mascarpone can be substituted for the combination of both.

** Dates would also be great in this, especially Medjools or Honeyballs (Bahri dates). In fact, that's what I'll be trying next time. Raisins can also be substituted, golden or dark.

*** The original Green Apple Ice recipe calls for ¾ cup of simple syrup, but I felt that was a tad too sweet, and the ice didn't need that much. If you prefer it sweeter, use ¾ cup. If using store-bought apple juice, reduce to ¼ cup sugar plus ¼ cup water for syrup.

UPDATE. 2014: Add the coconut cream from a cold can of coconut milk, or just ½ cup coconut milk to the Green Apple Ice mixture, prior to freezing, if you want it creamier.

Also, you can freeze the apple mixture overnight into a solid block, then scrape it to make it a Green Apple Granita, if desired.

333. Cheeky Cherry Crisp

Ingredients:

3 cups cherries, pitted and sliced

2 tsp almond extract

1/3 cup unsweetened coconut milk

A few drops stevia to taste

For the topping:

1/4 cup hemp seeds

1/4 cup almond flour

1/4 cup coconut flour

2 Tbl coconut oil

1 Tbl water

1 tsp cinnamon

pinch of low sodium salt

Instructions:

In a medium bowl, combine the cherries, almond extract, coconut milk and sweetener if using. Make sure there are no pits!

In another bowl combine all of the topping ingredients and mix well until crumbly.

Pour the cherry filling into one large, 4 medium, or 8 small greased ramekins or oven proof dishes.

Top with the crumble mixture and bake for 20 minutes in a preheated 375 degree (F) oven. Remove from the oven and let cool before serving. Yum!

334. Stunning Key Lime Pie

Ingredients:

Filling:

6 avocados

3-4 drops stevia

1 cup coconut oil

2/3 cup lime juice

Crust :

1 1/2 cups almond flour/meal

2 TBSP almond butter

3-4 drops stevia

1/4 cup unsweetened coconut, shredded

1/4 cup coconut flour

Instructions:

Place all crust ingredients in food processor and pulse until grainy. It should stick together when you press on it, but not form a ball by itself. If it does, add more almond flour.

Dump blended ingredients into spring form pan and press down to form crust.

Wipe out food processor and place all filling ingredients within. Blend for several minutes (4-5) until completely smooth.

Pour over crust and smooth out.

Place pie in freezer for 1-2 hours. Serve chilled.

335. Mouthwatering Dark Chocolate Cherry Scones

Ingredents:

3 cups blanched almond flour

1½ teaspoons baking soda

½ teaspoon fine low sodium salt

4 tablespoons olive oil

2 large pastured eggs

2 tablespoons apple cider vinegar

3-4 drops stevia

1 teaspoon vanilla extract

3 ounces of 80+% cacao dark chocolate, cut into bite-size chunks

⅓ cup dried cherries

Instructions:

Preheat the oven to 350°F with the rack in the middle position, and line a baking sheet with parchment paper. In a large bowl, combine the almond flour, baking soda, and fine low sodium salt.

Use your hands or a pastry cutter to work the pieces of cold butter into the dry ingredients until a crumbly mixture is produced.

In a separate bowl, thoroughly whisk together the eggs, apple cider vinegar, stevia, and vanilla extract.

Make a well in the middle of the dry ingredients, and pour the egg mixture into it.

Gently mix with a spatula until a wet, chunky dough forms, and then throw in the chocolate chunks and cherries.

Combine the ingredients with your hands, and form two small balls of dough.

On a sheet of parchment paper or a nonstick surface, gently flatten the balls with your hands. The rounds of dough should be about ¾-inch thick. (If the dough's a little too sticky to handle, refrigerate it for a half hour to firm it up before proceeding.)

Using a pastry cutter or a sharp knife, cut each round of dough into 4 equal-sized wedges, and arrange all 8 pieces on the parchment-lined baking sheet.

Bake for 20 to 25 minutes, rotating the tray halfway through. The scones are ready when they're golden brown, and an inserted toothpick comes out clean. Transfer the scones onto a wire rack to cool before serving.

336. Delectable Cocoa-Nut Apples

Ingredients:

1 ½ cups coconut flakes

2 tablespoons cacao powder

1 tablespoon cacao nibs

1 ½ teaspoons cinnamon

1/8 teaspoon nutmeg

3-4 drops stevia

1 organic green apple

2 tablespoons heated coconut oil

A half tablespoon of water if consistency is too dry

Instructions:

In a medium sized mixing bowl add coconut flakes, cacao powder, cacao nibs, cinnamon, nutmeg and coconut oil. Stir well, for 2-3 minutes, Clean and dry the apple. Thinly slice the apple starting from the outside and working your way toward the center. Repeat on the other side. Then lay the apple flat on one of the cut sides and chop thin slices of the remaining sides of the apple core

Transfer the sliced apple to a serving tray.

Pour the cocoa-nut mixture on top of each apple.

Now you can serve them right away or let them sit for an hour or longer to let the coconut flake mixture soften, totally up to you.

337. Fruity Fruit Salad

Ingredients:

4 cups chopped watermelon

1lb strawberries, chopped

6oz raspberries

6oz blueberries

1/4 cup packed mint, chopped (NOT 1/4 cup chopped mint)

1/4 cup fresh lime juice (about 3 limes)

3-4 drops stevia

Instructions:

Add watermelon, strawberries, raspberries, blueberries, and mint in a large bowl. Stir together lime juice and stevia in a small bowl then pour over fruit and berries.

Gently toss with a spatula then let sit in the refrigerator for at least 15 minutes before serving to allow the natural juices in the fruit to start coming out.

338. Delicious Almond Butter Banana

Ingredients:

1 Medium-Sized Banana

1 Tbl Almond Butter

½ tsp Cinnamon

Instructions:

Preheat your oven to 375 degrees.

Using a butter knife, cut about ½" deep down the length of your banana.

With the back of a spoon, widen the cut to make room for the almond butter.

Spoon the almond butter throughout the opening in the banana.

Sprinkle with cinnamon.

Wrap completely in aluminum foil.

Bake for 15 minutes at 375 degrees.

Remove from oven and let cool for 1-2 minutes (or until it's cool enough to handle).

Unwrap and either eat directly from the foil or move to a plate.

339. Outstanding Hazelnut Banana

Ingredients:

1 banana, sliced

1 tablespoon hazelnut butter

Cinnamon

Olive oil or coconut oil

Instructions:

Lightly drizzle oil in a skillet over medium heat.

Arrange banana slices in pan and cook for 1-2 minutes on each side.

Remove pan from heat and place bits of hazelnut butter over banana.

Allow to cool and sprinkle with cinnamon.

340. Cookies with Dark Chocolate

Ingredients:

2.5 cups unsweetened dark chocolate, in 1 oz chunks

3 large eggs

1/3 C coconut oil

3/4 drops stevia

1 T vanilla

3/4-1 C almond flour(sunflower seed flour for nut-free)

1/4 C organic cocoa powder

1/4 teaspoon low sodium salt

1/4 teaspoon baking powder

coarse low sodium sea salt or pink low sodium salt for sprinkling

Instructions:

Melt chocolate together into a smooth consistency (double boiler or microwave in blasts of 30-60 seconds), stirring constantly and making sure that one does not over cook or seize before they both come together.

Sift dry ingredients and set aside. Combine wet ingredients, except chocolate, by whisking until combined.

Temper in melted chocolate by adding in about 1/4 C and whisking. Then add another 1/4 C of the warm chocolate and whisk again. Then add the remaining melted chocolate to the remaining wet batter.

Slowly add in the dry ingredients, stirring on low until just incorporated together - final batter will be smooth and plyable.

If you used 3/4 C flour you'll want to set your dough aside to chill for a little while, only 10 minutes or so. This will allow the chocolate to cool a bit and make the dough more plyable. If you used 1 C flour, the dough should be firm enough to shape into balls right away.

Form tablespoon sized balls, sprinkle with low sodium salt then press semi-flat onto a parchment-lined baking sheet. Bake at 350 degrees for 9 minutes, or until the center of the cookie begins to firm - will further harden as it rests.

341. Lemon Almond Delight

Ingredients:

6 Tbl coconut oil

2 cups almond flour

3-4 drops stevia

1 tsp freshly grated lemon zest

Instructions:

Melt the butter in the microwave or a small saucepan. Add the almond flour, stevia, and lemon zest, stirring until fully combined.

To make a tart or pie crust:

No need to pre-chill, just press dough into tart or pie tins. Bake in a preheated oven at 350 degrees (F) for 15 mins until firm and golden brown.

To make the cookies:

Form dough (it will be crumbly, this is normal) into a cylinder and wrap tightly with plastic wrap to compress. Chill in freezer for 30 minutes or until firm, or in the refrigerator for 2 hours. With a sharp knife, slice into 1/2 inch thick cookies (if they crumble apart your dough isn't cold enough). Bake in a preheated oven @ 350 degrees (F) on a greased or parchment lined cookie sheet for 15 minutes, or until firm and golden brown. Allow to cool before removing.

342. Ginger Vanilla Extravaganza

Ingredients:

3-4 drops stevia

3 Tbsp Organic Coconut Oil

2.5 cup Blanched Almond Flour

1/2 tsp low sodium Salt

1/2 tsp Baking Soda

1/2 tsp ground Cloves

1/2 tsp ground Cinnamon

1/2 tsp ground Nutmeg

1/2 tsp ground Ginger

More stevia to taste – administer the drops slowly

Instructions:

Preheat oven to 350 degrees.

In a large mixing bowl, combine blanched almond flour, low sodium salt, baking soda, cloves, cinnamon, nutmeg, ginger, and stevia. Stir ingredients with a wooden spoon to combine.

In a small sauce pan, bring molasses to a boil over medium heat.

Add coconut oil to the sauce pan, and stir until combined with the molasses.

Remove sauce pan from heat and pour into the dry ingredients.

Mix batter with a wooden spoon until you have formed a dark golden cookie dough, and all the dry ingredients are combined with the molasses and coconut oil.

Place a sheet of parchment paper onto a flat cooking surface, and dust parchment with arrowroot flour.

Form dough into a ball, and place on the parchment paper. Lightly press dough down to flatten, and sprinkle with a small amount of arrowroot flour. Place another sheet of parchment paper on top of the dough, and roll into a thin sheet with a rolling pin (about 1/4 inch thick).

Sprinkle almond flour on a small plate, and place cookie cutters into the arrowroot to coat the bottom for cutting. This will keep the cookie dough from sticking to the batter for an easy release after cutting.

Once you have made cuts throughout the entire sheet of cookie dough, carefully peel away the excess dough, and lightly transfer the cut out cookies to a parchment lined baking sheet. Form dough into another ball, and roll out again to repeat until all the dough is used.

Bake gingerbread people at 350 degrees for 10 minutes. Remove from oven and cool on a cookie rack before frosting.

343. Cute Cupcakes Recipe

Ingredients:

2/3 Cup coconut flour

1/4 Cup almond flour

1/2 tsp cinnamon

1 tsp baking powder

1/2 tsp low sodium salt

6 eggs

2 egg whites

304 drops stevia

1 Tbsp vanilla

1/2 Cup coconut milk (canned)

Buttercream Frosting Recipe

1 1/4 Cup Grass-fed Butter softened (20 T. or 2 ¼ sticks)

3-4 drops stevia

1/2 tsp cinnamon

2 1/2 Tbsp coconut flour

5 Tbsp coconut cream (the thick coconut cream skimmed off the top of canned coconut milk)

1/4 tsp cinnamon

Instructions:

Preheat the oven to 350 degrees.

Line 2 muffin tins with a total of 16 cupcake liners.

Place the coconut flour, almond flour, cinnamon, baking powder, and low sodium salt in a small bowl and mix together with a whisk.

In another bowl, combine the eggs, egg whites, stevia, vanilla, and coconut milk, beating together well with a whisk.

Add the dry ingredients to the wet ingredients, whisking until well combined.

Add the melted butter to the batter and mix in well.

Let the batter sit for 5 minutes to allow the coconut flour time to absorb the liquids.

Divide batter evenly between cupcake liners and bake for 20-22 minutes, or until tops of cake are firm to the touch and spring back.

Remove and cool completely on a wire rack.

Buttercream Frosting Instructions

Place the butter, stevia, cinnamon, and coconut flour in a bowl and beat with a mixer until well combined.

Beat in the coconut cream, 1 t. at a time, until fully incorporated.

Mixture should be thick and glossy.

Scoop into a piping back and pipe on top of cooled cupcakes.

Mix more stevia and ¼ t. cinnamon together and sprinkle desired amount on top of cupcakes.

344. Strawberry Chessecake Delight

Ingredients:

1 cup almonds course ground

1 heaping cup soaked raw cashews (soaked overnight or at least 4 hours)

1/2 cup peeled and diced zucchini

1/4 cup coconut oil, melted

2 tablespoons canned coconut milk, full fat, room temperature

4-5 drops stevia

1/2 tablespoon vanilla extract

1/8 teaspoon low sodium salt

juice of one and a half lemons, separated

1 cup fresh organic strawberries, hulled and diced

Instructions:

Divide the cup of almond crumbs into the bottom of 4 (8-ounce) wide mouth mason jars and set them aside.

In a high-powered blender, process the raw cashews until they are blended. Add the zucchini, coconut oil, coconut milk, stevia, vanilla extract, low sodium salt, and the juice of one lemon. For the lemon juice go by taste as not to overdo it with lemon flavor. I started by juicing half of the lemon, mixing and tasting, and adding the rest. Add lemon juice as needed to your preference. Then blend again until a super smooth and creamy batter is formed.

Pour the cheesecake batter evenly into the 4 (8-ounce) wide mouth mason jars leaving some room for the strawberry sauce. Place them in the freezer and allow them to set for at least an hour or longer. While the cheesecake is setting go ahead and make your strawberry sauce.

In a heavy bottomed sauce pot over medium-high heat, add the juice of half a lemon, the strawberries, and honey. Mash the strawberries together until they are combined with the rest of the ingredients. Let the mixture boil and reduce, stirring intermittently, for about 10-12 minutes or so. Once the mixture has reduced and thickened remove from heat and set aside.

When your cheesecake is ready, remove mason jars from the freezer, let thaw for about 15 minutes before serving. Top with strawberry sauce. Garnish with fresh strawberry slices and a sprinkle of almond crumbs. Enjoy!

345. Creative Cardamom Cupcakes

Ingredients:

1/2 cup coconut flour

6 eggs, at room temperature (that's important)

3-4 drops. stevia

6 Tbs. coconut oil or butter

2 Tbs. coconut milk, room temp. (this one doesn't have any icky additives or BPA)

1 tsp. vanilla extract

1/2 tsp. ground cardamom

1/4 tsp. baking soda

1/2 tsp. apple cider vinegar

Instructions:

Preheat the oven to 350 degrees and prepare a muffin tin with 8 liners (I like unbleached parchment paper baking cups).

Combine the coconut flour and eggs until smooth. Add the remaining ingredients and stir well.

Divide evenly between the muffin tins. Bake until golden and a toothpick comes out clean, about 20 minutes.

Cool completely and frost with the lemon mousse.

Makes 8 cupcakes. Feel free to double the recipe if you want more cupcakes! These last in an airtight container for a few days at room temperature. They also freeze really well!

346. Apple, almond & blackberry Bonanza

Ingredients:

Filling:
3 sweet apples

100 g blackberries, frozen are fine

3-4 drops stevia

1 knob of coconut oil

1/2 tsp cinnamon

1/4 tsp cardamom

1/8 tsp cloves/all spice

1/8 tsp ground ginger

Batter:
3/4 cup ground almonds (100 g)

2 Tbsp stevia

1/2 tsp ground vanilla

1/2 tsp baking powder

a pinch of low sodium salt

1 Tbsp melted coconut oil or butter

1 egg, whisked

Around 1/5 cup full fat coconut milk(50 ml)

Instructions:

Preheat oven to 200 °C/ 400 °F. Cut apples on bite-sized chunks. You need to use an oven proof skillet* about 20 cm i diameter. Melt coconut oil and stevia on high heat and add the apples and spices. Sauté for 5 min until the apples are caramelized and slightly tender.

Meanwhile make the batter. Mix almond flour with vanilla, stevia, baking powder and low sodium salt. Stir in the egg, coconut oil and coconut milk.

Place the blackberries among the apples in the skillet. Pour the batter on top if the fruit until it covers the surface. It is okay if there is small cracks where the fruit can release some moist.

Bake in the oven for 15-20 min. depending on your oven. The cake should be golden brown on the entire surface and the batter just set.

Serve the cake while it is still a little warm with a dollop of yoghurt, whipped cream or splash of coconut milk – and maybe a few fresh black berries on top.. Enjoy.

347. Almond Happiness Bars

Ingredients:

First Layer:

3/4 cup raw almond butter (I make my own from this recipe: Almond Butter)

1/4 cup coconut oil, melted

1/3 cup cacao powder

3-4 drops stevia

1/4 teaspoon vanilla bean paste

pinch low sodium salt

Second Layer:

2 cups of dried, unsweetened, raw coconut

2/3 cup coconut butter, softened

3-4 drops stevia

1-2 teaspoons organic almond flavoring (not raw)

Third Layer:

1/3 cup almonds, coarsely chopped

Ganache:

1/2 cup cacao powder

3-4 drops stevia

1/4 cup coconut oil, melted

Instructions:

First Layer:

Whisk all ingredients together and pour into oiled, parchment lined 8 x 8-inch glass pan. Set in refrigerator aside making topping. The bottom layer should be set up (but not completely hard) before adding the next layer.

Second Layer:

Place coconut in medium bowl.

Whisk coconut butter (not the same as coconut oil), agave and almond flavor. Pour over coconut and mix well.

Pat over first layer, top with chopped almonds and ganache.

Refrigerate to set.

Ganache:

Whisk all ingredients together.

348. Sexy Coconut Crack Bars

Ingredients:

1 cup unsweetened shredded coconut (80g)

1/4 cup water and 2-3 drops stevia

2 tbsp virgin coconut oil (For all substitutions in this recipe, see nutrition link below)

1/2 tsp pure vanilla extract

1/8 tsp low sodium salt

Instructions:

Combine all ingredients in a food processor....and fridge for an hour before trying to cut. (Or freeze for 15 minutes.) Can be stored in the fridge or freezer, for at least a few weeks.

349. Lemonny Lemon Delights

Ingredients:

Crust:

1 cup almond flour

1/4 cup almond butter

Stevia to taste

1 tbsp coconut butter

1 tsp vanilla

1/2 tsp baking powder

1/4 tsp low sodium salt

Filling:

3 eggs

A few drops Stevia to taste

1/4 cup lemon juice

2 1/2 tbsp coconut flour

1 tbsp lemon zest, finely grated

Pinch of low sodium salt

Instructions:

Preheat oven to 350.

Coat 9×9 baking dish with coconut oil or butter.

Combine all crust ingredients in food processor until a "crumble" forms.

Press crust evenly into the bottom of pan.

Using a fork, prick a few holes into crust.

Bake for 10 minutes.

While crust is baking, combine all filling ingredients in a food processor until well incorporated.

When done, remove crust from oven and pour filling evenly over top.

Continue to bake for 15-20 minutes, or until filling is set, but still has a little jiggle.

Cool completely on wire rack. (You can also chill in the fridge if desired, to further set the filling).

350. Macadamia Pineapple Bonanza

Ingredients:

Crust:

½ cup almond flour

4 tablespoons raw cacao powder

⅓ cup macadamia nuts

½ teaspoon vanilla extract

Stevia to taste

1½ teaspoons coconut oil, melted

Filling:

2 eggs

1 cup fresh pineapple, chopped

1⅓ cup shredded coconut, unsweetened

1 tablespoon fresh lime juice

1 tablespoon vanilla extract

Stevia to taste

½ cup almond flour

pinch of low sodium salt

Instructions:

Crust:

In a large bowl, mix the almond flour and cacao powder.

Chop the macadamia nuts in a food processor and add it to the bowl.

Add vanilla extract and coconut oil to the dry mixture and using your hands, mix to combine ingredients.

Spread the mixture evenly on the bottom of an 8x8-inch pan lined with parchment paper. Be sure to use one large piece of paper covering the entire pan that overlaps on all four sides.

Filing:

In a large bowl beat the 2 eggs

Mix in the pineapple, 1 cup of shredded coconut (reserve the remaining ⅓ cup for the top), lime juice, vanilla and stevia.

Gently mix in the almond flour and low sodium salt with rubber spatula.

Pour mixture over the crust and sprinkle top with remaining shredded coconut.

Bake at 350°F for approximately 20 minutes or until the top starts to brown and the pineapple/coconut layer is firm.

Set pan on a wire rack and allow it to cool before cutting into squares. Store in the refrigerator.

351. Banana Shake

Ingredients

1 frozen banana, sliced

1/2 cup ice cubes

1/2 cup strong coffee**

2 tablespoons cocoa powder

1 tablespoon coconut butter (optional)

small splash of vanilla extract (optional)

Instructions:

Place all ingredients in a blender and process until smooth.

Makes approximately 1 serving

352. Lemon Cookies

Ingredients:

2 cups blanched almond flour

1/4 cup coconut flour

1/2 cup granulated sugar

1 teaspoon baking powder

1/8 teaspoon salt

1/2 cup unsalted butter, melted and cooled slightly

1 large egg, room temperature

1 tablespoon lemon zest (from 1 lemon)

1 teaspoon lemon extract

1/3 cup lemon curd*

powdered sugar, optional

Directions:

In a medium mixing bowl, stir together the almond flour, coconut flour, sugar, baking powder and salt. Set aside.

In another medium mixing bowl, stir together the melted butter, egg, lemon zest, and lemon extract.

Add the dry mixture to the wet and stir just until combined. The dough will feel quite wet. Let it sit for 10 minutes to allow the coconut flour to absorb the liquid while the oven preheats.

Preheat the oven to 350 degrees F and line a cookie sheet with a piece of parchment paper.

Roll the dough into 1" balls and place 2" apart on the prepared cookie sheet. The dough will feel quite greasy.

Bake the cookies for 6 minutes and remove from the oven.

Using the rounded part of a 1/2 teaspoon measuring spoon, make an indentation about 3/4 of the way down into each cookie.

Fill each indentation with 1/2 teaspoon of lemon curd. Be sure not to overfill them.

Return the pan to the oven and bake for another 5-7 minutes or until the cookies feel like they have a firm outer layer. The cookies shouldn't brown around the edges - just on the bottom.

Let the cookies, which will be very soft at this point, cool for 5 minutes on the baking sheet and then remove to a wire rack to cool completely. The parchment paper may be a little greasy, but the cookies will not be.

10. Refrigerate in an airtight container for up to 4 days. Dust with powdered sugar before serving, if desired.

Notes:

I've never seen lemon curd containing gluten but if you eat gluten-free, please check the ingredients label on your jar to ensure that your lemon curd doesn't have gluten.

353. Macadamia Pineapple Bonanza

Ingredients:

Crust:

½ cup almond flour

4 tablespoons raw cacao powder

⅓ cup macadamia nuts

½ teaspoon vanilla extract

Stevia to taste

1½ teaspoons coconut oil, melted

Filling:

2 eggs

1 cup fresh pineapple, chopped

1⅓ cup shredded coconut, unsweetened

1 tablespoon fresh lime juice

1 tablespoon vanilla extract

Stevia to taste

½ cup almond flour

A pinch of low sodium salt

Instructions:

Crust:

In a large bowl, mix the almond flour and cacao powder.

Chop the macadamia nuts in a food processor and add it to the bowl.

Add vanilla extract and coconut oil to the dry mixture and using your hands, mix to combine ingredients.

Spread the mixture evenly on the bottom of an 8x8-inch pan lined with parchment paper. Be sure to use one large piece of paper covering the entire pan that overlaps on all four sides.

Filing:

In a large bowl beat the 2 eggs

Mix in the pineapple, 1 cup of shredded coconut (reserve the remaining ⅓ cup for the top), lime juice, vanilla and stevia.

Gently mix in the almond flour and low sodium salt with rubber spatula.

Pour mixture over the crust and sprinkle top with remaining shredded coconut.

Bake at 350°F for approximately 20 minutes or until the top starts to brown and the pineapple/coconut layer is firm.

Set pan on a wire rack and allow it to cool before cutting into squares. Store in the refrigerator

354. Pumpkin crepes

Ingredients

Apple Butter:

apples - 5 lb, peeled and sliced

cinnamon - to taste

Crepes:

egg yolk - 1

egg whites - 4

pure pumpkin puree - 1/3 cup

canned full-fat coconut milk - 1/3 cup

coconut flour - 3-4 tablespoons

arrowroot starch - 1/4 cup

pure vanilla extract - 1 teaspoon

ground allspice - 1/4 teaspoon

pure maple syrup - 3 tablespoons

Instructions

Preheat oven to 425 degrees Fahrenheit.

Combine the apples and cinnamon to taste on 2 9 inch by 13 inch baking dishes.

Roast for 1-2 hours, stirring every 15 minutes, or until the apples have lost quite a bit of moisture.

Puree until smooth, adding water if necessary.

Preheat a nonstick skillet to 350 degrees Fahrenheit. Whisk together all crepe ingredients in a large bowl until smooth.

Lightly grease the skillet with coconut oil and add 4-5 tablespoons of batter, spreading it around with the back of a spoon.

Cook until the batter looks dry. Flip and cook until golden. Repeat with remaining batter.

Serve crepes with apple butter.

355. Choco Zucchini Cookies

Ingredients

2 cups shredded zucchini (squeezed)

½ cups pitted dates (7 pieces)

2 tbsp. unsweetened cocoa powder

1 egg

1 tsp baking powder

1/8 tsp salt

1 tsp instant coffee

1 tbsp. vanilla extract

1 tsp flax oil

¼ cup dark chocolate chips

Flourless Chocolate Zucchini Cookies

PRINT

Instructions

Preheat oven at 350 degree Fahrenheit. Prepare a cookie sheet with a liner and grease it.

In a food processor combine all the ingredients (except chocolate chips) and grind smooth.

Pour the batter into the mixing bowl and mix in chocolate chips.

With the help of a round spoon or ice cream scoop spoon the batter into 12 round shapes.

Put the sheet on the middle rack of the oven and bake for 30 minutes.

Take it out and let it cool completely. Put the cookies in the refrigerator for 15 minutes to stiffen.

356. Choco - Coconut Berry Ice

Ingredients:

Follow recipe of berry ice cream and almond delight for the ice cream only

4 ounces sugar free dark chocolate - 75% cacao content

¼ cup coconut milk

2 cups fresh berries (I used raspberries)

Instructions:

Make the Homemade Coconut Ice Cream,

While the ice cream is freezing in the machine, break the chocolate into pieces and place in a small saucepan.

Add the coconut milk and melt the two together, stirring over low heat.

When the chocolate mixture is completely smooth, pour the chocolate over the ice cream and stir to create 'ripples'. If your ice cream if thoroughly frozen, soften in the fridge for 20 minutes before stirring in the chocolate.

Serve immediately with the fresh berries, or freeze for an additional 3-4 hours for a firmer texture.

357. Best Banana Nut Bread

Ingredients:

3 bananas, mashed, or 1 cup

3 eggs

1/2 cup almond butter

1/4 cup coconut oil, melted

1 tsp vanilla extract

1/2 cup almond flour

1/2 cup coconut flour

2 tsp cinnamon

1 tsp baking soda

1/4 tsp low sodium salt

1/2 cup chopped walnuts

1-2 drops stevia

Instructions:

Preheat the oven to 350 degrees F. Line a loaf pan with parchment paper. In a large bowl, add the mashed bananas, eggs, almond butter, coconut oil, and vanilla. Use a hand blender to combine.

In a separate bowl, mix together the almond flour, coconut flour, cinnamon, baking soda, and low sodium salt. Blend the dry ingredients into the wet mixture, scraping down the sides with a spatula. Fold in the walnuts.

Pour the batter into the loaf pan in an even layer. Bake for 50-60 minutes, until a toothpick inserted into the center comes out clean. Place the bread on a cooling rack and allow to cool before slicing.

358. Perfect Paleo Loaf

Makes 1 traditional loaf

Ingredients:

1/2 cup + 2 tbsp coconut flour, sifted

2 tbsp finely ground golden flaxseed

1 tsp baking soda

6 eggs, separated

4 tbsp coconut oil, melted

1/2 cup coconut milk

1 tsp apple cider vinegar or lemon juice

Low sodium salt (to taste)

Instruction:

1. Preheat your oven to 375 degrees F. Line a loaf pan with a sheet of parchment paper on it, brush some butter on the remaining uncovered sides.

2. In a large mixing bowl, sift together all dry ingredients; make sure all lumps are smoothed out.

3. Separate eggs, adding the yolks to the flour mixture and set aside the whites to a medium mixing bowl.

4. Add the melted coconut oil, coconut milk, and apple cider vinegar/lemon juice to the flour, mixing thoroughly. Expect the mixture to be dene and dry.

5. Whip egg whites with hand mixer until stiff peaks begin to form.

6. Fold egg whites into batter.

7. Spoon bread batter into a greased loaf pan. Smooth out the top with a spatula so that bread will bake evenly.

8. Bake for 35-40 minutes, covering bread with foil the last 5-10 minutes of baking.

9. Allow bread to cool for 5-10 minutes before transferring the bread to a cooling rack.

10. Slice and serve. Store any remaining bread in the refrigerator for up to 4 days.

Tips

It is very important to sift the coconut flour to remove any lumps, as it is a very dense flour.

Golden flaxseed as it adds a nice color to the bread making it look like a "multi-grain."

Whipping the egg whites allows the bread to be more fluffy and "slice-able."

This bread is not sweet. Many bread recipes have added honey or sweeteners, but if you want it to be a bit sweet, you can add a few drops of stevia.

359. Carrot Coconut Surprise

Ingredients

1/4 cup coconut flour

2 smallish-medium-sized carrots, about 2.5 oz/70 gr each

1/4 cup almond milk

2 eggs

Low sodium salt and pepper, to taste

Instructions

1. Preheat your oven to 400 degrees and line a baking sheet with parchment paper.

2. Put the carrots and coconut in your food processor and blend for about 30-60 seconds, until the mixture looks like orange crumbs. Add everything else into the food processor and blend for about a minute or until the mixture is smooth.

3. Divide the mixture into 8 parts and form into rounds on the baking sheet. If necessary, slightly dampen your hands to flatten the rounds and prevent the dough from sticking to your hands. The rounds should be a bit thicker than 1/4 inch - not too thin, or they won't hold together.

4. Bake for about 15-17 minutes until slightly browned on the bottom and dry on the top. Let cool for a few minutes before removing from the pan.

**These biscuits are best to eat within an hour after baking, so I won't recommend to bake plenty. Bake just enough.

360. Relishing Raisin Bread

Ingredients:

6 room temp eggs *see tip below

1/3 cup melted coconut oil

1/3 tsp stevia

1/2 cup coconut milk

1/2 tsp vanilla extract

1/2 cup coconut flour

1 tsp cream of tartar

1/2 tsp baking soda

Low sodium salt (to taste)

For the Swirl:

2 tbsp water

1/2 tbsp cinnamon

1tsp stevia

A pinch of low sodium salt (to taste)

1/4 cup raisins

Directions:

1. Pre-heat your oven to 325 degrees. Cover the bottom of an 8×4 loaf pan with parchment paper and grease the sides (and bottom if you do not have parchment paper) with palm shortening (or other baking fat you chose).

2. Separate the eggs – this will allow you to whip up your egg whites and ensure a good light texture. Place your egg whites in a medium, clean bowl, and set it aside. Place your egg yolks in a large mixing bowl.

559

3. Add the rest of the wet ingredients to your yolks. Cream until smooth.

4. Add your dry ingredients, mix until well-combined.

5. Get your cinnamon swirl ready – simply mix together the first 4 swirl ingredients in a small bowl – Keep your raisins separate.

6. With a hand mixer or KitchenAid mixer – using clean beaters – on a medium speed whip up your egg whites until soft peaks begin to form when you remove the beaters. Fold the egg whites into the batter until just combined.

7. Add about 1/3 of the batter to your loaf pan – drizzle 1/2 of your swirl, and then quickly with a knife lightly zig-zag the swirl on top of the batter. Sprinkle with half of your raisins

8. Add another third of the batter and drizzle the rest of the swirl.

9. Top with rest of batter.

10. Place in oven to cook for 47-50 minutes – until the top is bouncy or until when a toothpick is inserted in the top it comes out clean.

11. Remove and let cool for 5-10 minutes. Flip out to complete cooling. Can be tightly wrapped and stored on counter for 5-7 days, or placed in fridge for 10-14 days.

361. Luscious Lemon Delight

Ingredients:

6 eggs

1/4 cup coconut oil, melted

zest from 2 lemons

1/3 cup lemon juice

1 cup milk (almond or coconut)

2/3 cup coconut flour (do not substitute another flour)

1 heaping teaspoon baking soda

Pinch of low sodium salt (to taste)

Lemon Glaze:

2 Tbsp coconut oil

1tbsp water

1 tsp stevia

2 Tbsp almond milk

zest and juice from 1 lemon

1/2 tsp pure vanilla extract

Directions:

1.   Preheat oven to 350 F.

2.   Combine all bread ingredients in a mixing bowl and mix well. Pour into a greased pan and bake for 32-45 minutes or until golden on top and the middle is cooked through. Remove from oven and let cool.

3.   While the lemon loaf is baking, mix all glaze ingredients together in a small pot over low heat until it starts to simmer. Remove from heat and let sit to cool until the lemon loaf is finished cooking and cooling. Pour the glaze all over the top of the loaf. Refrigerate the loaf at least 30 minutes – 1 hour until both the glaze and the loaf firms up a bit.

4.   Enjoy! You can store leftovers in the refrigerator for up to 3 days.

362. Sexy Sweet Potato

Ingredients

300 grams cooked sweet potato flesh*

1/2 cup coconut flour

3 eggs

3 tablespoons of coconut milk

1 teaspoon baking soda

Juice of half a lemon

A pinch of low sodium salt

*I roast a purple skin / white flesh sweet potato and keep the flesh for this recipe, I personally think the skins are delicious ad eat them as they are. You can use whatever sweet potato you like.

Instructions

1. Preheat your oven to 180 Degrees Celsius or 350 Degrees Fahrenheit.

2. Grease and line a mini loaf tin (mine is 6" x 2.5") with baking paper hanging over the sides for easy removal.

3. Put the ingredients into your food processor or blender and pulse until well combined. Spoon the mixture into the prepared tin, smooth over the top with a spoon. Bake for 40 minutes. Cover the loaf with foil and bake for a further 20 minutes. Remove from the oven and allow the bread to cool before slicing. Enjoy.

363. Cheeky Coconut Loaf

Ingredients

1/2 cup coconut flour, sifted

3 eggs

zest of one lemon

1/2 cup desiccated coconut

1 cup coconut yoghurt

1 teaspoon ground cardamom

¼ cup almond milk

2 tsp stevia

A pinch of low sodium salt

1/2 teaspoon concentrated natural vanilla extract

1 teaspoon baking soda

Instructions

1. Preheat your oven to 175 degrees Celsius or 350 degrees Fahrenheit

2. Grease a mini loaf tin (mine is 16cm x 6cm)

3. Combine the flour, zest, coconut, baking soda and cardamom. Add the eggs, mix together. Add the yoghurt, milk and stevia, combine. Add the salt and vanilla, combine. Spoon the mixture into your prepared pan. Bake for 35 minutes. Cover with foil and bake for another 10 minutes. Remove from the oven and allow it to cool slightly before flipping onto a cooling tray. Leave to cool for a few minutes before cutting into thick slices.

4. This is great toasted and served with butter. Enjoy.

364. Heavenly Herb Flatbread

Ingredients:

1/2 cup Coconut Flour

3 eggs

1 cup coconut milk or almond milk

1/2 tsp low sodium salt

1/2 tsp dried oregano

1/2 tsp dried basil

1/2 tsp garlic powder

drizzle of coconut oil

Instructions

1. Preheat oven to 375 degrees.

2. Mix together the coconut flour, salt, herbs, & garlic powder in a bowl.

3. Whisk the eggs and coconut milk in a separate bowl.

4. Pour the wet ingredients into the coconut flour mixture.

5. Stir until no lumps are left. Let the batter sit for at least 5 minutes (so the coconut flour absorbs all the liquid). It should resemble a thick paste.

6. Prepare your pan. Drizzle some coconut oil on the bottom of pan (10 x 15 " rimmed pan) and then place the parchment paper (oil first helps the corners stick). I also drizzled some coconut oil on top of the paper and spread it out with a pastry brush.

7. Pour out all the mixture into the pan. Tap the pan until the upper part is flat. (this will help your bread to cook evenly)

8. Cook for 30- 40 minutes or until the toothpick comes out clean.

9. Allow the bread to cool before transferring it to your container or serving plate.

365. Naked Chocolate Cake

Ingredients

1/2 cup (2 3/4 oz) Naked Chocolate or a good quality cocoa

1/2 cup (2 3/4 oz) coconut flour

2 1/2 teaspoons gluten free baking powder

1/2 teaspoon ground cinnamon

Pinch of low sodium salt

6 free-range eggs

1/2 cup (4 1/2 fl oz) coconut oil

3/4 cup coconut milk

1 teaspoon stevia

1 teaspoon vanilla paste

Instructions:

Preheat oven to 160°C (320°F)

1. Combine the cocoa, coconut flour, baking powder, cinnamon and salt into a mixing bowl.

2. Add the eggs, stevia, vanilla, coconut milk and coconut oil.

3. Mix well until smooth and combined – a whisk works well for this.

4. Pour into a 20 cm (9 inch) baking tin lined with baking paper.

5. Bake the cake for 55 – 60 minutes or until cooked through. Best to test after 45 to make sure as oven temps may vary.

6. Remove from the oven and cool.

7. Spread with ganache or healthy chocolate mousse and enjoy.

366. Blueberry Sponge Roll Surprise

Ingredients

6 eggs, separated

1/3 cup almond milk

1/2 cup coconut flour

1/2 teaspoon baking soda

1/4 teaspoon vanilla powder

1 tsp stevia

For filling:

1 can coconut cream (chilled in fridge overnight)

¼ cup blueberry

A few drops of stevia

Instructions:

1. Heat oven to 170 degrees Celsius (338F)

2. Line a 24 x 30cm (base measurement) Swiss roll pan with baking paper.

3. Beat egg whites with electric beaters until they form soft peaks.

4. In a separate bowl, beat egg yolks and honey until pale yellow. (1-2 mins)

5. Add coconut flour, vanilla powder and baking soda to yolks, add milk and stevia and beat until well combined.

6. Using a metal spoon, mix 1/3 of the egg white mixture into the egg & flour mixture.

7. Gently fold in the remaining egg whites.

8. Spread into lined pan and bake for 12-15 mins until golden brown.

9. When cake comes out of the oven, lift it from the pan using the baking paper.

10. Leaving the cake on the paper, start from the short end and roll the cake into a log.

11. Place in fridge to cool with seam side down.

12. While cake is cooling, use electric beaters to beat the coconut cream that has separated to the top of the can and put a few drops of stevia on it. (About 1 cup) After doing the cream, slice blueberries into small pieces.

13. After cake has cooled, unroll and spread the coconut cream and put sliced blueberries at the top of the cake.

14. Using the paper as a guide, re-roll again from the short side.

15. Sprinkle top with coconut flour if you like.

16. Serve straight away, or store in the fridge.

367. Lemon Mousse Mouthwatering Cupcakes

Ingredients

1/2 cup coconut flour

6 eggs, at room temperature (that's important)

6 Tbs. milk

2 tsp stevia

6 Tbs. coconut oil

2 Tbs. coconut milk at room temperature

1 tsp. vanilla extract

1/2 tsp. ground cardamom

1/4 tsp. baking soda

1/2 tsp. apple cider vinegar

Instructions

1.   Preheat the oven to 350 degrees and prepare a muffin tin with 8 liners (I like unbleached parchment paper baking cups).

2.   Combine the coconut flour and eggs until smooth. Add the remaining ingredients and stir well.

3.   Divide evenly between the muffin tins. Bake until golden and a toothpick comes out clean, about 20 minutes.

4.   Cool completely and frost with the lemon mousse.

5.   Makes 8 cupcakes. Feel free to double the recipe if you want more cupcakes!

368. Lemon Mousse Frosting

Ingredients

3/4 cup stevia-sweetened lemon curd (recipe below)

1 cup coconut milk

1 Tbs. light coconut milk

1 tsp stevia

Pinch of salt to taste

Instructions

1.   First, make the stevia-sweetened lemon curd, by simply whisking the whole eggs, yolks and 1tsp stevia in a saucepan until smooth, then place pan over a low heat. Add the coconut oil, juice and zest and whisk continuously until thickened. Strain through a sieve. Lemon curd keeps, covered, in the fridge for 2 weeks. Chill until thickened and cold before using it.

2.   In a small saucepan, whisk together the coconut milk and gelatin. Let it sit for 10 minutes. Then turn the heat on medium and whisk until the gelatin dissolves. Pour into a bowl and refrigerate until set, about 4 hours.

3.   In a food processor, blend together the set coconut milk and the lemon curd until smooth. Add stevia to taste and a small pinch of salt.

369. Chocolate Raspberry Cake Delight

Ingredients

For the cake

1/2 cup (120g) of Coconut Oil

1/4 cup (30g) of Coconut Flour

1/3 cup (45g) of Arrowroot Starch

1/4 cup (35g) of Unsweetened Cocoa Powder

1 teaspoon of Baking Soda

1/4 cup almond milk

1/4 cup of Strong Hot Coffee

1 tbsp Stevia

4 large Eggs

1 teaspoon of Vanilla Extract

For the raspberry sauce

10 ounces of Raspberries

1 teaspoon of Lemon Juice

1/4 cup almond milk

1 tsp Stevia

1/2 teaspoon of Gelatin

For the chocolate ganache

3 ounces of Chocolate Chips

1/3 cup of Full Fat Coconut Milk

Instructions

1. FOR THE CAKE: Whip together the coconut oil and stevia in a large mixer until combined, about 3 minutes on high speed.

2. Sift together the coconut flour, arrowroot flour, cocoa powder, and baking soda in a separate bowl. Whisk together the eggs, milk, stevia, coffee, and extract in a large glass.

3. Add about a third of the dry ingredients and a third of the liquid ingredients to the mixing bowl and mix until combined. Repeat adding the ingredients in batches until all mixed and uniform.

4. Evenly portion the cake batter into muffin tin cups. Bake at 350F for 25-28 minutes, until an inserted toothpick comes out clean.

5. Remove from the oven and let the cakes cool for about 10 minutes. Gently remove the cakes from the tin cups using a rubber spatula and set on a cooling rack upside down.

FOR THE RASPBERRY SAUCE: Reserve a few raspberries for garnish.

Gently heat the raspberries, lemon juice, and milk and stevia for about 5 minutes. Remove from heat when the mixture looks uniform. Sprinkle the gelatin on the jam and mix until dissolved.

FOR THE CHOCOLATE GANACHE

Heat the coconut milk to a very low boil. Add to the half of the chocolate chips and mix until fully combined. Then add the rest and mix until uniform. Let cool to a thick yet pourable consistency before use.

ASSEMBLY: Scoop out a portion of cupcake from the center, careful not to puncture it completely. Fill the hole with about a tablespoon of the raspberry sauce. Pour about 2 tablespoons worth directly on top of the raspberry center.

* *Use a frosting spatula or the back of a spoon to spread the chocolate in a circular motion toward the cupcake edges. Let the chocolate goodness fall to the sides. Top with a raspberry and enjoy!

370. Strawberry Dashing Doughnuts

Ingredients:

4 large eggs, room temperature

3 tablespoons coconut oil, melted

¾ cup coconut milk, warm

1 tsp Stevia

1 teaspoon apple cider vinegar

1 teaspoon pure vanilla extract

½ cup coconut flour

¼ cup strawberries, grind

½ teaspoon baking soda

¼ teaspoon low sodium salt

Topping

1 ounce raw cacao butter, melted

2 tablespoons coconut butter

1 teaspoon stevia

¼ cup strawberries, grind

Instructions:

1.   Preheat a doughnut maker. If using a doughnut pan, preheat the oven to 350F and grease the pan liberally with butter.

2.   Using a stand mixer or electric hand mixer, beat the eggs with the coconut oil on medium-high speed until creamy.

3.   Add the milk, stevia, vinegar, and vanilla and beat again until combined.

4.   Using a fine mesh sieve or sifter, sift the remaining dry ingredients into the bowl. Beat on high until smooth.

5.   Scoop the batter into a large Ziploc bag, seal the top, and snip one of the bottom corners.

6.   Pipe the batter into the doughnut mold, filling it completely.

7.   Cook until the doughnut machine indicator light goes off. If you are using an oven, bake for 17 minutes. Remove the doughnuts and cool on a wire rack. Trim if necessary.

Make the glaze

1.   Mix the cacao butter, coconut butter, and stevia in a shallow bowl. Place in the freezer for 5 minutes to thicken.

2.   Once the donuts are completely cooled, sprinkle ground strawberries on top.

3.   Place in the refrigerator for 20 minutes to allow the glaze to set.

371. Perfect Plantain Cake Surprise

Ingredients

4 eggs, separated

2 tsp cream of tartar

1/2 cup extra virgin coconut oil

1/4 cup almond milk

2 tsp Stevia

1 cup ripe plantain, mashed (equals one plantain)

4 tsp vanilla extract

1/2 cup coconut flour, sifted

1/2 tsp baking soda

1/4 tsp low sodium salt

Instructions

1. Preheat oven to 350 degrees F. In a bowl combine egg whites and cream of tartar.

2. Whip the egg whites until stiff peaks form.

3. In a separate bowl cream together coconut oil, stevia and milk. Do that for a few minutes.

4. Add the egg yolks. Mix until smooth. Add mashed plantain and vanilla until mixed.

5. Add the sifted coconut flour, baking soda and salt to the egg yolk mixture. Mix until smooth. Slowly add the egg yolk mixture to the whipped egg whites.

6. Line an 8 x 1.5 inch cake tin with parchment paper and grease the sides.

7. Bake for 35 minutes until the top is firm to the touch and a toothpick can be inserted and comes out dry.

372. Lemon Blueberry Cake Delight

Ingredients

½ cup coconut flour, sifted

3 eggs, beaten

⅓ cup unsweetened coconut milk or almond milk

2 tbsp lemon juice, (use lemon squeezer to get all the juice)

1 tbsp lemon zest

2 ½ tbsp. coconut oil, melted

½ tbsp liquid stevia

1 tsp lemon extract (organic GF kind).

½ tsp baking soda + 1 tsp apple cider vinegar, mixed in separate pinch bowl (should be very fizzy)

½ cup blueberries *optional.

Lemon Ice Glaze:

2 tbsp coconut oil, melted

1½ tbsp coconut butter, melted

1 ½ tbsp unsweetened coconut milk

1½ tbsp lemon juice

½ tsp lemon extract (organic GF kind)

2 tsp lemon zest

1/3 tsp liquid stevia (as sweetener)

Instructions

1. Preheat oven to 350 F, and grease or oil a 9" round cake pan.

2.   In a large mixing bowl combine: all the first 8 cake ingredients. Stir together thoroughly; break up any coconut flour lumps. Add in baking soda and vinegar mixture and stir.

3.   Gently add and mix in the blueberries.

4.   Spoon cake batter into prepared pan and spread around evenly.

5.   Bake in 350 F oven for 30 minutes or until center is firm.

6.   Remove cake from oven and let cool for 10 minutes while you make the lemon ice glaze.

7.   Heat a small sauce pan over low heat and melt: coconut oil, and coconut butter. Stir the mixture as it melts and break up any coconut butter lumps.

8.   Once melted, remove from heat and add all the rest of the lemon ice glaze ingredients. Stir the glaze thoroughly until well mixed and set aside to cool.

9.   Use a metal or wooden skewer, or large toothpick to poke holes all over the cake. Be sure to poke all the way down to the bottom of cake.

10.   Spoon or pour lemon ice glaze all over the top of cake, making sure to cover well. Use the back of a spoon to spread around evenly.

11.   Let cake cool and glaze set awhile. It should only take 5 minutes or so for glaze to solidify a bit.

12.   Slice and serve. Unused portions should be stored in the fridge.

373. Delicious Coconut Flour Cake with Strawberry Surprise

Ingredients

1 dozen eggs

2 cups coconut milk (I used homemade)

¼ cup milk

2 teaspoons Stevia

2 teaspoons vanilla extract

2 cups coconut flour

1/2 teaspoon baking soda

1/4 teaspoon low sodium salt

coconut oil for greasing the pan

Instruction

1. Preheat oven to 350F.

2. Whisk together the eggs, coconut milk, milk, stevia and vanilla extract. Mix until smooth.

3. Add coconut flour, baking soda and salt to the egg mixture and whisk until a smooth batter forms.

4. Grease 2 – 9 inch round cake pans with coconut oil.

5. Divide up the batter evenly between the 2 cake tins. Use a rubber spatula to smooth it out.

6. Bake for 40 minutes, or until a toothpick inserted into the center of the cake comes out clean.

7. Allow the cake to cool.

8. Fill the center with cooked strawberries (recipe below). You can also use the strawberry filling to decorate the cake.

Strawberry Filling

Ingredients

2 cups organic strawberries, stems removed and sliced

1. Place the strawberries in a saucepan over medium heat.

2. After a few minutes, the strawberries will release their juices.

3. Allow them to cook uncovered, occasionally stirring and smashing them.

4. Keep cooking them until the strawberries are soft, smashed and the sauce has reduced. About 30 minutes.

374. Titillating Berry Trifle

Ingredients:

1/2 cup plus 2 tsp coconut flour, sifted

1/4 tsp low sodium salt

1/4 tsp baking soda

5 whole eggs (2 of them separated)

1/2 cup coconut oil, softened

1/2 cup almond milk

2 tsp stevia

1 tablespoon vanilla extract

2 teaspoons lemon juice

1 1/2-2 cups washed & diced strawberries (cut large if using a traditional Trifle bowl)

1 1/2-2 cups washed blueberries

1 1/2-2 cups washed raspberries

3-4 cans full-fat coconut milk, cream only

Instruction:

1. Preheat oven to 350 degrees.

2. Sift the dry ingredients together and set aside.

3. Separate 2 of the eggs, setting the whites aside and putting the 2 yolks in a medium sized bowl. Crack open the rest of the eggs, adding them to the bowl with egg yolks.

4. Using a mixer or hand whisk, beat the coconut oil (liquid or solid, doesn't matter), milk, vanilla and lemon juice until they are well combined.

5. On low/medium-speed, mix the dry ingredients into the wet ingredients. Continue to mix till the batter is smooth and has no lumps.

6. Add the eggs (not including the 2 egg whites) in three phases to the batter. Allow each addition to be incorporated completely before adding the next.

7. In a small bowl, beat the egg whites till thick soft peaks form. Fold into the batter.

8. Pour the batter into a greased 8 inch square brownie pan or 7X10 small casserole dish lined with parchment paper, allow a few inches of flaps to hang over the two long sides of the pan. This will help later with removing the cake ensure that the sides of the cake won't stick to the pan. Alternatively, you could make cup cakes with the batter and cube those up for the trifle. Baking times will vary depending on the depth of the cake pan. I find that a 1 or 2 inch high cake produces the best texture instead of a thicker cake. However, I have made this in a standard size bread pan as well, and it turns out very nice.

9. Bake for 30-45 min. or until a toothpick in the center comes out clean.

10. Allow the cake to cool for 5-10 minutes, run a sharp knife along the edges and carefully remove from the pan. Cool completely.

For the coconut whipped cream:

1. Chill 2-3 three cans of full-fat coconut milk (a few hours or overnight).

2. Open the cans and scoop the thick cream in to a medium bowl. Try to keep as much coconut liquid out of the cream as possible. Discard the liquid or freeze it into ice cube trays to use in smoothies.

3. With a hand/stand mixer, beat the cream on high for a minute or so. Add ½ tsp. stevia as sweetener if desired. Continue beating until well combined.

Assembling the Trifle:

Assembly is super easy. Just add some cake to the bottom of your dish, then whipped cream, strawberries/raspberries, whipped cream, more cake, blueberries, more whipped cream, then more fruit if desired or cake crumbles. Really just layer it however you like!

This recipe should make enough for 4 individual 12 oz trifles or you can make two cakes, add extra fruit and more coconut cream (2-3 more cans) for one, 2-quart trifle or glass bowl.

375. Gingerbread Cream Delight

Ingredients

For the Gingerbread Cake

½ cup (80g) of packed Coconut Flour

½ cup (64g) of Arrowroot Flour

1 teaspoon of Baking Powder

½ teaspoon of Baking Soda

½ teaspoon of low sodium Salt

1½ teaspoon of Ginger Powder

1½ teaspoon of Cinnamon

¼ teaspoon of Nutmeg

Pinch of Cloves

½ cup of almond milk

1 teaspoon of Vanilla Extract

4 Eggs, room temperature

½ cup (100g) of Coconut Oil (softened solid)

2 tsp Stevia

For the Cream Cheese Frosting

8 oz Cream Cheese, room temperature

4 oz of Coconut oil at room temperature

2 tbsp Stevia

¼ cup of Arrowroot Flour

Instructions

For the Gingerbread Cake

1. Preheat oven to 350F and grease an 8"x4" loaf pan.

2. Sift together the coconut flour, arrowroot flour, baking powder, baking soda, salt, and spices in a bowl to form the dry mixture.

3. Combine the milk and vanilla extract in another bowl to form the liquid mixture.

4. Separate the eggs whites from the egg yolks.

5. Beat the egg whites at high speed in a mixer bowl with a whisk attachment until a meringue forms. Remove the whites from the mixer bowl and set aside.

6. Add the coconut oil and coconut sugar to the mixing bowl and beat on medium high for about a minute until uniform.

7. Add the egg yolks one at a time to the mixing bowl and beat on medium until combined. Scrape the sides if necessary.

8. Add half of the dry mixture to the mixing bowl and beat until combined.

9. Add half of the liquid mixture to the mixing bowl and beat.

10. Repeat the previous two steps until all mixed.

11. Portion a heaping of the egg whites and add to the mixing bowl and mix.

12. Fold in the rest of the egg whites until uniform.

13. Pour batter into the loaf pan and bake, centered rack, at 350F for 35-40 minutes.

For the Frosting

1. Whip the coconut oil and cream cheese until smooth.

2. Add the arrowroot flour and stevia.

3. Whip on low until the flour is absorbed into the butter, then whip on high for a few minutes until light and fluffy.

376. Mouthwatering Coconut Custard Cake

Ingredients:

4 eggs

2 ½ cups almond milk

1/2 cup coconut flour

1 tsp pure vanilla extract

2 tsp baking powder

2 tsp stevia

1/4 cup coconut, melted

1 1/2 cups unsweetened, coconut flakes

1/2 cup chocolate chips or broken chocolate bar

Instruction

1. Pre-heat oven to 350F.

2. In a large bowl of a stand mixer (or whisk by hand) eggs, milk, coconut flour, stevia, vanilla, coconut oil, and baking powder until smooth.

3. Stir in coconut flakes and chocolate.

4. Pour into an 8" cake pan and bake for 45 - 50 minutes or until a toothpick inserted into middle comes out clean.

5. Allow to cool before slicing in pan, and serving.

6. Sprinkle with cinnamon just before serving.

377. Cranberry Orange Upside Down Revolution

Fruit:

unbleached parchment paper

2 cups fresh cranberries

1 tablespoon coconut oil (at room temperature)

1 teaspoon stevia

1 tablespoon arrowroot powder

Dry Ingredients:

6 tablespoons coconut flour

6 tablespoons arrowroot powder

2 teaspoons baking powder

1/4 teaspoon low sodium salt

Wet Ingredients:

4 large pastured eggs

4 tablespoons melted coconut oil

4 tablespoons almond milk

2 tablespoons freshly squeezed orange juice

A zest of 1 organic orange

1 teaspoon vanilla

Instruction

1. Preheat oven to 350 degrees F. Place a 9-inch cake pan onto a sheet of parchment paper and draw a line around the bottom with a pencil. Cut out the circle and place it onto the bottom of the cake pan. Grease the sides of the pan with coconut oil.

2. In a small bowl mix together the coconut oil, milk, and arrowroot powder. Spread it onto the parchment paper in the cake pan (I use an offset spatula to do this). Arrange the cranberries on top of the mixture.

3. Whisk together the dry ingredients. In a separate bowl, whisk together the wet ingredients. Pour the wet into the dry and quickly whisk together until combined. Pour batter over fruit and spread evenly with the back of a spoon or spatula.

4. Bake for 30 to 35 minutes. Let pan cool on a wire rack for 15 to 20 minutes then carefully flip out onto a plate; peel off parchment paper. Let cool and then serve. Enjoy!

378. Baked Vanilla Cardamom Delights

Ingredients:

1/2 cup coconut flour

1/8 teaspoon baking soda

3/4 teaspoon baking powder

1/4 cup Stevia liquid drops

1/4-1/2 teaspoon cardamom (we did 1/2 because we love cardamom)

2 egg, room temperature

2 tablespoons coconut oil, liquid (or oil of choice)

1/2 cup warm water

Instructions:

1. In a bowl place all dry ingredients into bowl and whisk together. Set aside.

2. Next grab your stevia, coconut oil and egg and whisk together in mixing bowl. Once that is all mixed together add in your dry ingredients. Begin to stir the donut batter.

3. End with adding in your warm water to the batter and stir till smooth and combined.

4. Pre-heat your mini donut maker. Once your green light turns off it is ready. Begin to scoop your donut batter into each mini donut ring. We used a cookie scooper to help with the scooping.

5. Once all rings are filled close the donut maker and let bake for 2-3 minutes. Check and see if they feel done. If so remove carefully with a knife. Repeat process till all our donut batter has been baked.

6. Remove donuts from pan with a knife. Serve and enjoy.

379. Pumpkin Cream Cookies

Ingredients

For the donuts

6 dried medjool dates, pitted

½ cup pumpkin puree

¼ cup coconut oil, melted

4 eggs

3 tablespoons coconut flour

½ tablespoon cinnamon

¼ teaspoon nutmeg

⅛ teaspoon ground cloves

⅛ teaspoon ground ginger

½ teaspoon baking powder

A pinch of low sodium salt

For the cream

1 (14 ounce) can of coconut cream OR coconut milk refrigerated overnight*

1 tablespoon stevia

¼ teaspoon cinnamon

For the chocolate

1 cup Enjoy Life Chocolate Chips, melted

3 tablespoons coconut milk

Instructions

1. Place dried dates in a food processor and pulse to break down.

2. Add pumpkin puree, melted coconut oil, and eggs to the food processor and puree until smooth.

3. Add coconut flour, cinnamon, nutmeg, ground cloves, ginger, baking powder, and a pinch of salt and puree once more.

*To make the donuts easy to pour and keep them a round shape, place donut puree into a plastic bag or pastry bag, cut the end off of the plastic bag so you can squeeze to mixture in a circle in the donut maker. If you are using a donut pan for the oven, preheat oven to 350 degrees.

4. Heat up a mini donut maker, grease the donut maker or pan, and use the bag to squeeze about 2 tablespoons of the mixture into each donut round.

5. In a mini donut maker, cook for 5-7 minutes. Times will vary with the different donut maker. If you are using a donut pan, cook for 20-25 minutes.

6. Remove donuts once cooked through and let rest and cool on a wire rack.

7. Once cooled, place in refrigerator for about 10 minutes. (The donuts will be easier to work with once they are a bit harder).

8. While the donuts cool, in a bowl, remove the coconut cream that sits on top of the coconut water (keep the coconut water for later) and whip together the coconut cream with a fork or whisk. Then add maple syrup and cinnamon and mix well. Place cream in a piping bag or plastic bag and then cut off the end.

9. In a bowl, melt chocolate chips and coconut milk that was left behind from the coconut cream via a double boiler or in a microwave.

10. Cut the donuts in half, carefully. On the bottom donut, pipe on the cream around the donut then place the top donut half on top of the cream. Then finish the donuts off by dipping them halfway into the melted chocolate.

11. Place donuts on a parchment lined baking sheet and into the freezer to harden the chocolate.

12. Once chocolate has hardened, eat up! Makes 8 mini donuts.

380. Delicious Lady Fingers

Ingredients

4 Pastured Eggs, separated

1/4 cup almond milk

1/4 tsp Baking Soda

1/2 tsp Pure Vanilla Extract

1/3 cup Coconut Flour, sifted

1 tsp freshly ground Coffee

Instructions

1. Preheat oven to back at 400 degrees.

2. Beat egg whites until stiff in a standing kitchen mixer, or with a hand mixer.

3. In a medium sized mixing bowl, combine egg yolks, baking soda, vanilla extract, and milk. Whisk until combined.

4. Sift in the coconut flour, and continue to whisk until smooth.

5. Fold in the egg whites, followed by the coffee grounds.

6. On a parchment lined baking sheet pipe out 3 inch long cookies with a round piping tube.

7. Bake at 400 degrees for 13 minutes, or until cookies are golden brown.

8. Allow to cool and enjoy.

381. Cheeky Coconut Chocolate Cookies

Ingredients

1/2 cup Virgin Coconut Oil, melted

1/4 tsp stevia

1/2 tablespoon vanilla extract

4 eggs

1/8 teaspoon low sodium salt

1 cup coconut flour

1/2 cup shredded coconut

3/4 cup chocolate chips

Instruction

1. Preheat oven to 375 degrees F.

2. Mix together coconut oil, sugar, vanilla, eggs, and salt together. Blend thoroughly. Add flour, coconut and chocolate chips; mix thoroughly.

3. Form into small cookies on a parchment lined pan and bake in preheated oven for about 15 minutes, or until lightly browned.

382. Scrumptious Peanut Butter Parcels

Ingredients:

½ cup sifted coconut flour

1 cup natural peanut butter

½ cup peanuts, coarsely chopped (optional)

1 tsp Stevia Drops

4 eggs

½ teaspoon vanilla

½ teaspoon low sodium salt

Directions:

1. Mix together peanut butter, sugar, eggs, vanilla and salt. Stir in peanuts and coconut flour. Batter will be runny.

2. Drop by the spoonful 2 inches apart on greased cookie sheet. Bake at 375 Degrees F for about 14 minutes.

3. Cool slightly and remove from cookie sheet.

**Makes about 3 dozen cookies.

383. Chocolaty Pumpkin Muffins

Ingredients

⅓ cup pumpkin puree

⅓ cup almond milk

¼ cup coconut oil, melted

3 eggs, whisked

1 teaspoon vanilla extract

¼ cup coconut flour

½ teaspoon cinnamon

¼ teaspoon nutmeg

⅛ teaspoon ground cloves

⅛ teaspoon powdered ginger

½ teaspoon baking soda

½ teaspoon baking powder

pinch of low sodium salt

½ cup Enjoy Life Mini Chocolate Chips

1 tsp stevia

Instructions

1. Preheat oven to 350 degrees.

2. Mix together wet ingredients in a bowl: pumpkin puree, milk, coconut oil, eggs, and vanilla extract.

3. In another bowl, whisk together coconut flour, cinnamon, nutmeg, ground cloves, powdered ginger, baking soda, baking powder, and salt.

4. Pour dry ingredients into wet ingredients and mix well.

5. Fold in chocolate chips.

6. Use an ice cream scoop to scoop batter into 5 silicone baking cups.

7. Bake for 35-40 minutes

384. Succulent Shortbread Cookies

Ingredients:

3/4 cup + 1/2 cup extra coconut flour

1/4 cup arrowroot starch

1/2 cup coconut oil or butter, melted

1/8 tsp low sodium salt

5 tablespoons milk

1 tsp stevia

1/4 cup dark chocolate chips

Instruction

1. Preheat oven to 350 degrees.

2. Combine all ingredients except chocolate and 1/2 c extra coconut flour in a mixing bowl. Mush up with a fork and add additional coconut flour until the mixture is crumbly.

3. Dust a clean, smooth surface with coconut flour. Press the crumbly mixture out with your fingers to make it smooth and somewhat flat. Dust with coconut flour.

4. Roll the dough to about 1/8-1/4 inch thickness using a rolling pin. Cut shapes out of the dough. Roll the scraps up into a ball and flatten to cut more shapes out.

5. Bake on a lightly greased cookie sheet for 15 minutes. Allow the cookies to cool.

6. Microwave the chocolate chips for 10 second intervals, stirring between intervals, until they are melted. Drizzle cookies with the chocolate. If the chocolate is not very runny, add a tiny amount of coconut oil and stir.

7. Allow the cookies to cool in the fridge or freezer for a few minutes until the chocolate is set.

385. Tasty Coconut Pancakes

Ingredients:

1/4 cup coconut flour

1/8 tsp baking soda

Pinch of low sodium salt

1/3 - 1/4 cup coconut milk

2 tbsp organic, cold-pressed coconut oil

3 eggs

1 tsp stevia

1/2 tsp vanilla extract

Coconut oil for cooking

Instruction

1. Thoroughly mix the eggs, coconut oil, and stevia together.

2. Add the coconut milk and vanilla extract.

3. Throw in the coconut flour, baking soda, and salt. Mix, but remember, not too much!

4. Place a little coconut oil in your skillet and then using a measuring cup, add a little batter to the pan. I recommend figuring out how many pancakes you'd like to make beforehand so that you can use an appropriately sized cup or ladle. This recipe should yield around 8 or so pancakes.

5. Remember that you aren't likely to see many bubbles forming on the top, so carefully check the underside of your pancake before flipping.

6. For best results, serve your pancakes with Blueberry sauce

386. Blueberry Sauce

Ingredients

2 cups fresh or frozen blueberries (no need to thaw before use if frozen)

1/4 cup water

2 tsp. arrowroot powder

1 Tbs. water

Instruction

1. Place the berries and 1/4 cup water (or juice) in a small saucepan over medium heat. Cook for 5-10 minutes, until bubbling. Slightly smash some of the blueberries with the back of a fork.

2. In a small bowl, stir together the arrowroot powder and 1 Tbs. of water. Remove the saucepan of berries from the heat. While stirring constantly, add the arrowroot mixture into the blueberry mixture. Let cool until no longer hot and serve. The sauce with become even thicker when chilled.

**You can store the sauce in the fridge for a few days.

387. Fluffy Coconut Flour Waffles

Ingredients

8 free-range organic eggs

1/2 cup melted butter or ghee (organic and preferably grass-fed)

1/2 cup coconut flour

1/4 teaspoon low sodium salt

1/4 teaspoon baking soda

1/4 cup canned coconut milk

1 tsp stevia drops

Instructions:

1. Take out your waffle maker.

2. In a large bowl add the eggs and beat with an electric hand mixer for 30 seconds until the eggs are well beaten.

3. Add the melted butter or ghee slowly into the eggs while you are still mixing.

4. Add the coconut flour, pink salt, baking soda and coconut milk.

5. Mix with the hand mixer for 45 second on low until the batter becomes thicker.

6. Heat up your waffle maker and make the waffles according to your maker's specifications..

7. Serve with butter or ghee, mashed strawberries (recipe here) or fresh maple syrup

388. Sexy Savory Pannukakku

Ingredients

1/4 cup coconut oil

1/4 cup coconut flour

1/4 cup arrowroot powder

1/4 teaspoon low sodium salt

1 cup light coconut milk (canned)

8 eggs

2 teaspoons pure vanilla extract

1 tsp stevia

Instructions

1. Preheat the oven to 400 degrees. Place the butter in a 9 by 13 inch baking pan and place it in the oven to let it melt.

2. In a medium mixing bowl, stir together the coconut flour, arrowroot, and salt. Whisk in the coconut milk until there are no lumps of starch. Whisk in the eggs, vanilla, and stevia.

3. Remove the hot pan from the oven and pour the batter onto the hot butter (pour slowly to avoid splatters of hot butter). Return the pan to the hot oven and bake for 15-20 minutes, or until the edges has puffed up and the center is set. Serve right away, topped with warmed berries, if desired.

389. Fudgy Coconut Flour Brownies

Ingredients

1/2 cup minus 1 Tbs. coconut

1/2 cup cocoa powder

1/2 cup plus 2 Tbs. coconut oil, melted

3 eggs, at room temperature

1/2 cup almond milk

2 Tsp stevia

1 tsp. vanilla extract, optional

Instructions

1. Preheat the oven to 300 and grease a glass baking dish (8x8 or 9x9).

2. Mix together all ingredients. You can do this by hand or with an electric mixer or high-powered blender.

3. Pour into the baking dish and bake for 30-35 minutes, until a toothpick inserted into the center comes out clean. Cool for 30 minutes before cutting or removing from the pan.

4. These store well at room temperature or in the fridge for a few days. Make sure you keep them in an airtight container.

390. Delectable Pumpkin Bars

Ingredients:

15 oz. pumpkin puree (about 1 1/2 cups)

3/4 cup coconut flour

3/4 cup almond milk

1 1/2 teaspoons ground cinnamon

3/4 teaspoon ground ginger

1/4 teaspoon ground cloves

3/4 teaspoon baking soda

1/4 teaspoon low sodium salt

2 large eggs

Instruction

1. Preheat the oven to 350F and grease a 9"x9" baking dish well with coconut oil. Combine all of the ingredients in a large mixing bowl, and stir well until no clumps remain. Transfer the batter to the greased baking dish, and use a spatula to smooth the top.

2. Bake at 350F for 40-45 minutes, or until the edges are golden and the center is firm.

3. Allow to cool completely, then cut into squares and serve. Store in in the fridge for up to a week. (They're delicious straight out of the fridge, too!)

391. Mouthwatering Lemon Bars

Ingredients:

Crust:

2 cups Sifted Coconut Flour

½ teaspoon low sodium Salt

½ cup almond milk

1tsp stevia

16 tablespoons Room Temperature Virgin Coconut Oil {= 1 cup}

Filling:

1 ½ cup Fresh Lemon Juice

1 cup almond milk

½ cup coconut oil

1 tsp stevia

2 tablespoons Lemon Zest

8 Eggs

Instructions:

Crust:

1. Preheat oven to 350 F.

2. Line a 9×13 inch baking dish with parchment paper.

3. Whisk the coconut flour with salt.

4. Thoroughly stir in the milk and coconut oil until it's evenly mixed and crumbly.

5. Add the room-temperature coconut oil and stir until it's evenly combined.

6. Pat the dough down into the bottom of the baking dish for an even thickness.

7. Bake at 350 for approximately 17 minutes or until it starts to brown.

8. Remove from the oven and let cool on the counter while you prepare the filling.

FILLING:

1. Mix stevia with the lemon juice.

2. Working quickly, whisk in the eggs.

3. Whisk in the lemon zest.

4. Pour the filling into the now cooled crust.

5. Bake at 350 for 25 – 30 minutes or until it's stiffened.

6. Let it cool on the counter for 30 minutes than the refrigerator for 3 hours or overnight.

7. Cut into squares and serve chilled.

392. Yummy Pumpkin Bars

Ingredients

1/2 cup coconut manna

1/2 cup coconut oil

1/4 heaping cup coconut flour

1 1/2 cup cooked winter squash (butternut or pumpkin)

A pinch of low sodium salt

2 tsp. cinnamon

1 tsp. ginger

1/4 cup almond milk

1 tsp stevia

Instructions

1. On the stove, gently melt coconut oil and manna until melted.

2. In food processor, add squash, spices, coconut flour, salt, milk and stevia. Pour melted coconut oil and manna on top and blend for 30 seconds being sure all the big pieces of squash are blended.

3. Line a square 8x8 brownie pan with parchment paper. Scoop the bar filling into the pan and use a spatula to smooth it out. Bake for 25 min at 350 degrees. Remove from oven, let cool, cover and put in fridge until completely chilled; about 3 hours.

393. Delicious Coconut Biscuits

Ingredients

4 large eggs, yolks and whites divided

1/2 cup coconut flour

1/4 teaspoon baking soda

1/2 teaspoon cream of tartar

1/2 teaspoon low sodium salt

4 tablespoons coconut oil, room temperature

1 tsp stevia

Instructions

1. Preheat oven to 400 degrees.

2. In a medium bowl, whisk the egg whites until frothy and at least doubled in size. Mix in the yolks until no streaks remain then add stevia.

3. In a separate bowl, combine the flour, baking soda, cream of tartar and salt.

4. Using a fork or pastry cutter, mix the butter into the dry ingredients until you have pea-sized bits of butter.

5. Fold the flour mixture into the egg mixture, incorporating well (the batter will be rather wet, but the coconut flour will start to absorb some of the liquid. Do not add more coconut flour!).

6. Using a 1/4 cup measuring cup, scoop the batter onto a parchment lined baking sheet.

7. Bake for 15-20 minutes or until golden brown and a toothpick inserted into the biscuit comes out clean.

394. Beautiful Butternut Pitta Surprise

Ingredients

1 Tbs. coconut flour

1 1/2 tsp. grass fed gelatin

3 Tbs. well-cooked and mashed butternut squash (or sweet potato)

1 Tbs. coconut oil

1 egg

Low sodium salt (to taste)

**(You can double the recipe if desired)

Instructions

1. Prepare all the ingredients and have them at room temperature.

2. Preheat the oven to 400 and line a baking sheet with parchment paper. Stir together the coconut flour and gelatin.

3. Stir together the squash and the coconut oil until smooth. Stir in the coconut flour/gelatin mixture until combined, and then stir in the egg and salt.

4. Spoon into rounds on the baking sheet. Make sure that you spoon out the same sizes. It's up to you but I prefer a bit thicker.

5. Bake for about 12 minutes, and then carefully peel them off the parchment paper and flip. Bake for another 5 minutes (or longer), until they are dry to the touch and pliable. (They will take longer to cook if they are thicker and they will cook faster if they are thinner.)

6. Let cool completely, then enjoy within an hour or so of baking for the best texture.

395. Onion Herb Coconut Biscuits

Ingredients

6 Tbsp. coconut flour

6 Tbsp. coconut oil, melted

2 eggs

1/4 cup very finely minced onion

2 garlic cloves, finely minced

2 Tbs. GAPS/SCD yogurt or additive free coconut milk

1 Tbs. fresh chopped herbs (parsley, dill, thyme... whatever you have) OR 3/4 tsp. dried herbs

1/4 tsp. baking soda

1/2 tsp. apple cider vinegar

Instructions

1. Preheat the oven to 350. Line two baking sheets with parchment paper.

2. Mix together the coconut flour, oil, eggs, onion, garlic, yogurt/coconut milk, and herbs Let sit for 5 minutes; the batter will thicken slightly.

3. Mix in the baking soda and vinegar. Drop a spoonful of batter onto the baking sheets. Use the back of a spoon to spread the batter into circles about 1/2" thick. The batter will not spread very much when baking.

4. Bake for 12-15 minutes, until moist but cooked through. Cool at least 10 minutes before serving, or they will be too crumbly.

396. Oniony Delishy Biscuits

Ingredients

1/3 cut coconut flour

¼ cup coconut flour, melted

4 eggs

1/4 tsp low sodium salt

1/4 tsp cream of tartar

1/8 tsp baking soda

1 cup shredded onion

Instruction

1. Preheat oven to 400 degrees

2. Put flour, salt, cream of tartar and baking soda in a small bowl

3. Put eggs and coconut oil in a mixing bowl, and whisk until smooth

4. Add flour mixture, and whisk until no lumps remain

5. Stir in the onion

6. Drop by spoonful onto lightly oiled baking sheet

7. Bake 8-10 minutes until lightly browned

8. Remove from baking sheet

397. Crisp Coconut Flour Tortillas

Ingredients

1/2 cup coconut flour

1/2 teaspoon grain free baking powder

1/4 teaspoon low sodium salt

1 1/2 cup egg whites (or 16 egg whites)*

3/4 cup almond milk

Instruction

1. Mix all of the ingredients in a non-reactive bowl.

2. Let it sit for 10 minutes so the coconut flour can soak up some of the moisture, and then whisk again. The batter should be runnier than that of pancakes, about the same as a crepe batter.

3. Heat a non-stick skillet over medium high heat and spray with oil or melt enough butter to coat the bottom and sides of pan.

4. Pour 1/4 cup of the batter into the pan, swirling the pan while you pour to ensure the bottom is coated and the tortilla is thin.

5. Once the bottom looks set (about 1 minute), carefully release the sides of the tortilla with a rubber spatula and turn over. Alternatively, you could use a frittata pan, or turn the tortilla into another hot and greased pan or greased griddle. This may help the tortilla to stay in one piece. If your first couple breaks, don't fret and don't throw them away. Add a little more coconut flour and try again, but keep the broken ones to use as filling if you're making enchiladas.

6. Spray the pan again, and repeat above steps until all the batter is used. Layer the tortillas on a plate and set aside until you're read to fill them and bake.

398. Easy Delish Pizza Crust Recipe

Ingredients

1 cup tapioca flour (starch) (plus more for rolling out dough)

1/3 cup + 2-3 tablespoons coconut flour, separated

1 teaspoon low sodium salt

1/2 cup olive oil

1/2 cup warm water

1 large egg, whisked

Instructions

1. Preheat oven to 450 degrees F

2. Combine the tapioca flour (you can substitute arrowroot flour/starch), salt and 1/3 cup coconut flour in a medium bowl.

3. Pour in oil and warm water and stir. Your mixture will look something like this.

4. Add the whisked egg and continue mixing until well combined.

5. Add two to three more tablespoons of coconut flour – one tablespoon at a time – until the mixture is soft but somewhat sticky dough.

6. Turn out the dough onto a surface sprinkled with tapioca flour and knead it gently until it is in a manageable ball that does not stick to your hands.

7. Place the pizza dough ball onto a sheet of parchment paper. Use a tapioca floured rolling pin to carefully roll out the dough until it is fairly thin. You may end up using another few tablespoons of tapioca at this point. You will need it to keep the dough from being too sticky. But don't overwork the dough or add TOO much more tapioca or your dough will be too dense.

8. Place the rolled out dough (on its parchment paper) into the preheated oven onto a hot pizza stone or sheet pan. I used a pizza stone that was left in the oven while it was heating up. You may have different results if you put it on a sheet pan or with the paper directly on the oven rack.

9. Bake for 12-15 minutes depending on how "done" the crust should be before putting on toppings. Here's what it looked like after 12 minutes on the pizza stone.

399. Coconut Pretty Pizza Crust

Ingredients

1 egg

1 tablespoon cream of buckwheat

1 tablespoon coconut flour

1/8 teaspoon baking soda

Instructions

Preheat oven to 425.

1. Mix all ingredients in a bowl until well combined.

2. Line a cookie tray with parchment paper and spread the cheese mixture on the paper as thinly as possible, using the back of a spoon or fork.

3. Reduce heat to 400 and bake on the top rack for about 15 minutes, or until the crust is starting to look golden in places. Remove from the oven and add desired toppings.

4. You can store this in the fridge for up to 3 days.

400. Creamy Appetizing Croissant

Ingredients

3 eggs, separated.

¼ tsp cream of tartar, where to buy this

2 tbsp organic coconut cream, softened.

2 tbsp coconut oil, melted

2 tbsp coconut flour

15 drops liquid stevia

½ tsp baking soda + ¼ tsp cream of tartar, mix together in separate pinch bowl.

⅛ tsp low sodium salt

Kitchen Tools:

2 large mixing bowls

1 donut pan, or bagel pan

1 electric hand mixer or stand mixer

1 pinch bowl (small bowl)

Instructions

1. Preheat oven to 300 F, and grease or oil a bagel or donut pan (even if it's a non- stick type).

2. Separate egg whites from yolks, and place whites in one mixing bowl, and yolks in another mixing bowl.

3. Add cream of tartar to egg whites and whip with stand mixer or hand mixer until stiff peaks form. Set aside.

4. Beat egg yolks in separate mixing bowl and add: creamed coconut, melted coconut oil, coconut flour, stevia, baking soda and cream of tartar mixture, and sea salt. Beat egg yolk mixture until thoroughly combined.

613

5. Gently fold egg yolk mixture into egg white mixture until combined (careful not to stir or beat (should still be a whipped meringue texture).

6. Spoon mixture into bagel pan, and spread around, with the back of a spoon, in the pan forms. Wipe off excess that gets on the bagel hole with a damp paper towel.

7. Bake for 20 to 25 minutes or until tops and edges are slightly browning. Should check at 20 minutes, as all oven temperatures can vary.

8. Remove and cool. Use a butter knife in between the pan and the croissant, and slide around to loosen from pan.

Store unused portions in a covered container or zipper bag, put it in the fridge. Bagels can be reheated.

401. Delicious Gnocchi Balls

Ingredients

3 eggs, beaten

4 tbsp coconut flour

1 tsp garlic powder

1/4 tsp low sodium salt

Instructions

1. Mix the coconut flour and beaten eggs well.

2. Add the garlic powder and salt and mix well into dough.

3. Place the dough on a sheet of cling film and roll into a long sausage shape.

4. Wrap up with the cling film and place in the refrigerator. Chill the dough for a minimum of 30 minutes.

5. Bring a saucepan of water to the boil.

6. Remove the Gnocchi dough from the refrigerator and cut into small bite sized pieces.

7. Place the pieces into the boiling water, reduce the heat to medium and cook for 4-5 minutes. Remove with a slotted spoon. Repeat until all gnocchi are cooked.

8. Top with the sauce of your choice.

*Makes about 8-10 gnocchi.

402. Crispy Coconut Crackers

Ingredients

4 ounces shredded coconut

4 tablespoons butter (2 ounces or 1/2 stick), softened

1/4 cup tapioca flour

1 tablespoon coconut flour

1/2 teaspoon baking soda

1/4 teaspoon powdered mustard

1/4 teaspoon powdered onion

Instructions:

1. Preheat your oven to 350F. Line a baking sheet with parchment paper or a silicone mat.

2. Combine all ingredients in a food processor. Buzz until a ball of dough has formed.

3. Use your hands to shape dough into 1-inch balls. Place balls on the baking sheet, leaving about 3 inches of space between each.

4. Bake until the edges are slightly browned, about 10 minutes.

403. Tempting Custard Pie

Ingredients

4 eggs 2 cups coconut milk

1/4 cup expeller-pressed coconut oil (softened works best)

1/2 cup almond milk

1 tsp stevia

1/2 cup coconut flour

1/2 teaspoon baking powder

1/2 teaspoon low sodium salt

1 tablespoon vanilla (or 2 vanilla beans scraped)

1 cup shredded dried coconut

Instructions

1. Preheat oven to 325 degrees ºF.

2. Place all ingredients into a blender and blend for about 10 seconds (or until thoroughly mixed)

3. Pour into a pie dish greased with coconut oil.

4. Bake for 55 minutes in preheated oven. Serve warm (or cold the next day for breakfast!)

* For the freshest coconut milk make homemade coconut milk.

404. Nutritious Paleo Tortillas

Ingredients

1/4 cup coconut flour (40 g)

1/4 teaspoon baking powder

8 egg whites (240 g or 1 cup)

1/2 cup water

A pinch of low sodium salt

coconut oil (as needed, for greasing the press or pan)

Instructions

1. In a bowl mix all ingredients. Set aside for five minutes. The batter takes about that long to hydrate and thicken.

*If necessary grease your tortilla press or pan with coconut oil.

Make the tortillas:

1. In a preheated electric tortilla press: Pour about a little less than 1/4 cup of batter onto the tortilla press. Quickly smooth out using a heat resistant spoon, and press the top of the press down to distribute the rest of the batter. Cook until the indicator on the press goes off.

2. In a pan over medium heat: Pour a little less than 1/4 cup of batter onto the pan. Quickly smooth out using a heat resistant spoon. Cook for 1 to 2 minutes or until the edges of the tortilla start to turn golden brown. Then flip and cook for an additional minute or two.

3. Transfer tortillas to a plate and cover with a paper towel to keep warm.

4. Serve with desired toppings and do your best to keep away from within hungry doggy mouths.

405. Luscious Chocolate-Caramel Brownies

Ingredients

1/4 cup coconut flour

1 1/4 cup cacao powder

4 eggs

1 teaspoon low sodium salt

1 teaspoon baking soda

1/2 cup almond milk

1 ½ tsp stevia

1 tablespoon vanilla extract

1/3 cup coconut oil

1/3 cup dark chocolate chips

1 homemade caramel recipe

Instructions:

1. Preheat oven to 350 degrees Fahrenheit.

2. Mix dry ingredients in one bowl and wet ingredients in a second bowl.

3. Combine both mixtures and stir until all ingredients are incorporated together.

4. Pour the mixture into a greased 8x8 pan.

5. Top with chocolate chips and/or nuts if desired, and bake for 25–30 minutes.

6. Let cool and then drizzle with caramel sauce.

406. Grain-Free Raw Brownie Bites

Ingredients

1 1/2 cups walnuts

Pinch of salt

1 cup pitted dates

1 tsp vanilla

1/3 cup unsweetened cocoa powder

Instructions

Add walnuts and salt to a blender or food processor. Mix until the walnuts are finely ground.

Add the dates, vanilla, and cocoa powder to the blender. Mix well until everything is combined. With the blender still running, add a couple drops of water at a time to make the mixture stick together.

Using a spatula, transfer the mixture into a bowl. Using your hands, form small round balls, rolling in your palm. Store in an airtight container in the refrigerator for up to a week.

407. Fudgy Pumpkin Blondies

Ingredients

2 cups blanched almond flour

½ cup flaxseed meal

2 teaspoons ground cinnamon (optional)

½ cup raw coconut palm sugar

½ teaspoon salt

1 egg

1 cup pumpkin puree

1 tablespoon vanilla extract

⅓ cup (or more) chocolate chunks

Instructions

mix together the almond flour, flaxseed meal, cinnamon, coconut palm sugar, chocolate chunks and salt

in a separate bowl, whisk the egg, pumpkin and vanilla extract

using a rubber spatula, gently mix dry and wet ingredients to form a batter being careful not to over mix or the batter will get oily and dense

spoon the batter onto a 9-inch pan lined with parchment paper

bake at 350°F until a toothpick inserted into the centre comes out clean, approximately 25 minutes

408. Spinach Brownies Revisited

Ingredients:

1 ¼ cups frozen chopped spinach (measured frozen)

1 cup pureed green plantain (1 large plantain or 1 1/2 medium plantains)

6 oz semisweet chocolate (substitute bittersweet for a less sweet brownie)

½ cup extra virgin coconut oil

½ cup palm shortening (or substitute butter)

6 eggs

1 Tbsp honey

1 Tbsp molasses

½ cup cocoa powder

1 Tbsp vanilla (or substitute espresso)

¼ tsp baking soda

½ tsp salt

½ tsp cream of tartar

pinch cinnamon

Instructions:

Preheat oven to 325F. Line a 9"x13" baking pan with wax paper or use a silicone baking pan.

Melt coconut oil and chocolate together over low heat on the stove top or medium power in the microwave. Add vanilla and stir to incorporate. Let cool.

Mix cocoa powder, baking soda, cream of tartar, salt and cinnamon.

Blend spinach, plantain, egg, honey and molasses together in a food processor or blender, until completely smooth (2-4 minutes).

Add palm shortening to food processor and process until full incorporated.

Add melted chocolate mixture to egg mixture slowly and processing/blending constantly.

Mix in dry ingredients and process/stir to fully incorporate.

Pour batter into prepared baking pan and spread out with a spatula. Bake for 40 minutes. Cool completely in pan. Cut into squares. Enjoy!

409. Celebratory Chocolate Hazelnut Cupcakes

Ingredients:

2 large (or 3 medium) zucchini, grated (about 3 cups grated)

4 eggs

2 cups Hazelnuts

5 drops stevia liquid (May need a few more – please taste test)

1/4 cup coconut oil (room temperature)

1/3 cup Tapioca Flour (this is the same thing as Tapioca Starch)

1 cup cocoa powder

1 Tsp Vanilla Extract

1 tsp Baking Soda

½ tsp low sodium Salt

Instructions

Preheat oven to 350F. Line a muffin pan with paper liners, use Silicone Muffin Cups. or bake in a silicone muffin pan.

Grind hazelnuts in a Food Processor or Magic Bullet until they are super fine and almost turning into hazelnut butter.

Finely grate zucchini (you could even process in a food processor).

Combine ground hazelnuts, grated zucchini and the rest of the ingredients together in a bowl. The batter is quite runny. That's okay–that's why these cupcakes are so fudgy.

As an alternative you can combine all ingredients in a food processor or blender and process/blend until smooth.

Pour mixture into prepared muffin pan and bake for 30 minutes.

Let cool completely before icing or serving. Enjoy!

410. Bursting Banana Cupcakes (nut-free) with Whipped White Chocolate Sesame Frosting

Ingredients (frosting):

3 oz cocoa butter

1 Madagascar vanilla bean

5 drops stevia liquid (May need a few more – please taste test)

1/4 cup tahini (aka sesame seed butter)

1 tsp arrowroot powder

1/4 `room temperature coconut oil

Instructions

Melt cocoa butter (you can do this in a double boiler or in the microwave). Add stevia to melted cocoa butter and whisk until cane juice has dissolved.

Cut the vanilla bean lengthwise and scrape out the vanilla seeds with a sharp knife (save the pod for making vanilla ice cream or some other dish where you simmer the vanilla pod in coconut milk). Add to cocoa butter.

Add the remaining ingredients and whisk together until fully combined.

Allow to cool to room temperature (because of the high melting point of cocoa butter, this takes a long long time—if you want to speed it up, put it in the fridge and whisk aggressively every 5 minutes while it cools). Whisk every so often (maybe every half hour) just to make sure it doesn't separate or clump up.

Whip aggressively by hand (or you could use a hand mixer or blender) and generously frost your cupcakes!

Ingredients (cupcakes):

3 large (or 4 medium) overripe bananas

3 eggs

3 Tbsp extra virgin coconut oil

5 drops stevia liquid (May need a few more – please taste test)

1 tsp vanilla

1/3 cup coconut flour

1/3 cup arrowroot powder

1 tsp baking soda

1/8 tsp low sodium salt

Instructions

Preheat oven to 350F.

Grease a muffin pan or put paper liners. I actually use a silicone muffin pan just because it's so easy and ends up saving me tons of time!

Combine all of the ingredients in a blender or food processor (yes, it really is that easy). Blend or process about 1-2 minutes until you have a thick and smooth batter.

Pour batter into prepared muffin pan. You can make your cupcakes a bit bigger by dividing into 10 muffin cups or a bit smaller by dividing into 12 muffin cups.

Bake for 40 minutes (45 if you only make 10). Remove from oven and let cool completely before frosting. Enjoy!

411. Lovely Lemon Cupcakes with Lemon Frosting (2 Variations)(Nut-Free

Ingredients (Lemon Caramel Frosting):

5 drops stevia liquid (May need a few more – please taste test)

2/3 cup fresh Lemon Juice

¼ tsp Baking Soda

½ room temperature coconut oil

Instructions

1.   Heat stevia and lemon juice in a medium-sized saucepot over low heat. Reduce to 1 cup volume, being very careful not to let it burn (this will take 10-15 minutes).

2.   Remove from heat and immediately stir in baking soda. It will froth and expand. Stir vigorously for 15-20 seconds, then pour into a bowl and let cool to room temperature.

3.   Mix in coconut oil until completely combined.

4.   Store in an airtight container at room temperature for several days or store in the fridge for longer-term storage (warm up to room temperature before frosting cupcakes).

Ingredients (Lemon Coconut Butter Frosting):

½ cup Coconut Cream Concentrate (a.k.a. Coconut Butter or Creamed Coconut)

¼ cup fresh Lemon Juice

5 drops stevia liquid (May need a few more – please taste test)

1.   If you are opening a new bottle or box of coconut cream concentrate and the oil has separated out, heat the jar (or remove the contents of the box to a glass jar) by placing it a pot or bowl and surrounding with hot water. Let it sit until it's warmed enough to stir thoroughly. Let cool to room temperature.

2.   Mix coconut cream concentrate, lemon juice and stevia until thoroughly combined.

3.   Store in an airtight container at room temperature for several days or store in the fridge for longer-term storage (warm up to room temperature before frosting cupcakes).

627

Ingredients (Lemon Cupcakes):

½ cup Coconut Flour

¼ cup Tapioca Flour

½ tsp Baking Soda

6 Eggs

5 drops stevia liquid (May need a few more – please taste test)

¼ cup fresh Lemon Juice (roughly juice of two lemons)

2 Tbsp finely grated Lemon Zest (roughly zest from two lemons)

Instructions

1. Preheat oven to 350F. Line a muffin tin with paper muffin cup liners.

2. Blend all ingredients together in a a until a smooth batter forms. Let the batter rest for 2-3 minutes to thicken.

3. Pour batter into prepared muffin tin. Each cup should be filled approximately ¾ full (or slightly more).

4. Bake for 22-23 minutes, until starting to turn golden brown along the edges (should pass a toothpick test).

5. Carefully remove cupcakes from pan and cool on a wire rack. Let cupcakes cool completely before frosting.

6. Spread a generous amount of frosting (which ever you chose) on each cupcake. Candied lemon zest and edible flowers make great decorations for these cupcakes.

7. Enjoy!

412. Sexy Red Velvet Chocolate Cupcakes With Coconut-Cherry Glaze

Ingredients

¼ cup beets, peeled and finely grated

1¼ cup blanched almond flour

½ teaspoon baking soda

2 tablespoons raw cacao powder

¼ cup coconut oil, melted

7 tablespoons coconut milk, full fat

1 teaspoon vanilla extract

1 teaspoon apple cider vinegar

2 tablespoons raw stevia (add more if you like it sweeter)

1 egg

¼ cup chocolate chips

Coconut-cherry Glaze:

1 can (13.5 ounces) coconut milk, full fat

1 teaspoon vanilla extract

6 fresh cherries, pitted

Instructions

Preheat the oven to 350°F and line a muffin tin with baking cups.

Mix together the blanched almond flour, baking soda and raw cacao powder.

In a separate bowl, whisk together the coconut oil, coconut milk, vanilla extract, apple cider vinegar, stevia, egg and grated beets.

Using a rubber spatula, gently mix the wet and dry ingredients together.

Fold chocolate chips into the batter.

Spoon batter into prepared muffin tin, filling each to the top.

Bake until a toothpick inserted into the center comes out clean, about 30-35 minutes.

Set pan on a wire rack to cool, then top with the coconut glaze and a fresh cherry.

Coconut Glaze:

Place a can of full fat coconut milk in the fridge overnight.

Scoop the coconut cream that forms on top of the can into a bowl, being careful not to mix with the water in the bottom of the can.

Add the vanilla extract and using a handheld or stand electrical mixer, whip the coconut cream until fluffy.

413. Party Pink Velvet Cupcakes with Vanilla Frosting

Ingredients

Cupcakes

1/2 cup coconut oil, melted

5 drops stevia liquid (May need a few more – please taste test)

3 eggs

1 teaspoon vanilla extract

3/4 cup tapioca flour

1/2 cup coconut flour

1 teaspoon baking powder

2 tablespoons beet powder (works without it)

pinch of low sodium salt

Frosting

1/2 cup room temperature coconut oil

5 drops stevia liquid (May need a few more – please taste test)

1 teaspoon vanilla extract

2 tablespoons tapioca flour or arrowroot powder

2 teaspoons coconut flour

1 tablespoon chilled coconut milk fat (thick stuff from top of can)

Instructions

Cupcakes

Preheat oven to 350 degrees Fahrenheit

In a stand mixer or large bowl, mix together coconut oil, stevia, eggs and vanilla extract with a mixer or whisk

In a separate bowl, whisk tapioca flour, coconut flour, baking powder, beet powder and salt together

Slowly mix the dry mixture in with the wet mixture, adding ¼ cup at a time until well mixed

Scoop your batter into muffin liners in a muffin pan. Fill each well 2/3 of the way and you should get 10 cupcakes

Place in oven and bake for 18-20 minutes or until cooked through. Use a toothpick to poke through a muffin to make sure the toothpick comes out clean

Frosting

Combine the coconut oil shortening, stevia, vanilla, tapioca flour and coconut flour in the bowl of a stand mixer with a whisk attachment or a large mixing bowl

Using the stand mixer or a hand mixer, beat until smooth

Add your chilled coconut milk and beat until well combined. Do not over mix or your frosting might separate

Once your cupcakes are completely cool, use immediately by placing in a piping bag or ziploc bag with a corner cut off to frost your cupcakes

414. Perfect Paleo Bananacado Fudge Cupcakes

Ingredients

2 1/2 c. almond butter

1 1/4 c. stevia (or you can lower this to 3/4 c. and add an additional banana)

2 lg ripe bananas

3 medium avocados

3 eggs, beaten

3/4 c. cocoa powder

1 tbsp. vanilla

1 tsp baking soda

2 tsp baking powder

Instructions

In a large bowl, mix the almond butter and stevia.

In a blender or mixer, beat the eggs, banana, vanilla, cocoa powder and avocado to form a mousse-like consistency.

Add baking soda and baking powder.

Fold into the almond butter to make batter.

Pour into mini-cupcake tin (use the paper, it really makes a difference)

Bake at 350 for 15-18 minutes depending on size and desired consistency.

415. Chocolate Cupcakes with Coconut Cream Filling

Ingredients

Cupcakes

1/4 cup coconut flour

1/4 cup organic cocoa powder

4 large eggs (at room temperature)

1/4 cup coconut oil

5 drops stevia liquid (May need a few more – please taste test)

1/4 tsp baking soda

1 tsp lemon juice

Pinch of low sodium salt

Cream Filling (Optional)

Cream from 1 13.5 oz can of full fat coconut milk (refrigerate the can overnight and scoop out the cream that rises to the top)

5 drops stevia liquid (May need a few more – please taste test)

1 tsp vanilla extract

Chocolate Frosting

3 very ripe avocados

1/2 cup organic cocoa powder

5 drops stevia liquid (May need a few more – please taste test)

2 Tbsp grass fed butter or coconut oil, melted

Instructions

Preheat oven to 350 F

Combine the coconut flour, cocoa powder, sweetener, baking soda, and low sodium salt.

In a separate bowl, combine the eggs, coconut oil, and lemon juice.

Add the dry ingredients to the wet and mix to combine.

Line a muffin tin with 7 cupcake liners.

Fill cupcake liners evenly with the batter and bake for 18 - 20 minutes or until cooked through.

Allow to cool before filling with cream and topping with the icing.

Once cool, cut a small whole in the middle of each cupcake, reserving the lid/top of the hole that was cut out.

Fill with cream (directions below) and place the lid/top back on the cupcake to cover the hole.

Pipe chocolate frosting (directions below) onto each cupcake and serve.

For the cream filling

Combine the coconut cream, sweetener, and vanilla and mix until smooth. Pipe the cream into the hole cut out of the cupcake.

For the chocolate frosting

Place the meat of the avocados in a mixer and mix until completely smooth.

Add the cocoa powder and sweetener and mix until thoroughly incorporated.

Add the butter and mix to combine.

416. Delish Apple Pie Cupcakes with Cinnamon Frosting

Ingredients:

WET INGREDIENTS

5 Eggs, room temperature

1/2 cup applesauce (you can make your own or use a sugar-free pre-made brand)

5 drops stevia liquid (May need a few more – please taste test)

1/3 cup coconut oil, melted

DRY **INGREDIENTS**

1/4 cup finely ground blanch almond flour

1/2 cup coconut flour

1/2 tsp. low sodium salt

1/2 tsp. baking powder

FROSTING INGREDIENTS:

1 cup coconut oil

3 drops stevia liquid

2 tsp. cinnamon

Dash low sodium salt

Instructions

1. Preheat oven to 350F. Line muffin pan with baking cups.

2. Combine all wet ingredients in a medium sized mixing bowl. Beat on medium with a hand mixer for about 30 seconds.

3. Combine all dry ingredients in another medium sized bowl. Mix together with a fork to break apart any clumps.

4. Add the dry ingredients to the wet ingredients and beat for about 20 seconds. Make sure all ingredients are combined.

5. Fill each lined muffin tin about 3/4 of the way full. Bake for 25-30 minutes or until a toothpick comes out clean in the center.

6. Take the cupcakes out of the oven and set aside to cool completely. All the way cooled! But feel free to sneak one to nibble on while the rest cool off.

7. Once the cupcakes have cooled, make the frosting! Combine all of the ingredients into a medium mixing bowl and beat on medium speed for about 30 seconds until well combines. Ice those cupcakes and get to eating!

417. Paleo Sticky Date Pudding Cupcakes

Ingredients

For the muffins

Coconut Butter grease the muffin tray with

10 tbsp water

12 dates

1 ½ ripe banana, peeled and roughly chopped

2 ½ -3 tbsp coconut flour

1 tbsp vanilla extract or essence or 1 fresh vanilla bean, seeds scraped out

2 eggs

5 drops stevia liquid (May need a few more – please taste test)

½ tsp baking powder

For the sticky date ganache

5-6 dates, chopped

½ of orange, juice only

3 tbsp almond milk (coconut milk or water can also be used)

1 tsp vanilla extract or essence

2 drops stevia

Fresh raspberries or strawberries for garnish

Instructions

Preheat oven to 185°C (365 °F).

Grease muffin tins with the butter and set aside.

Heat the dates and water in a small saucepan over low heat until the dates break down and thicken. Use a fork to mash them together and set aside.

Place the coconut flour, egg, banana, vanilla extract and baking powder in a blender or food processor and mix well until well combined and aerated.

Add the dates to the banana mixture and combine. Evenly distribute into the ramekins. Cook in the oven for about 20-22 minutes.

While the muffins are in the oven, place the sticky date ganache ingredients in a small saucepan over a low heat and cook for about 3-4 minutes or until the dates break down. Mash with a fork and whisk until thickened. Set aside.

Allow the muffins to rest for 5 minutes before removing them to a serving plate. Scoop a dollop of sticky date ganache paste on top and garnish with a few raspberries.

418. Pumpkin Coco Cupcakes with creamy cinnamon filling

Makes 12 cupcakes

Cupcake:

1 cup pumpkin puree

3 eggs

5 drops stevia liquid (May need a few more – please taste test)

1 Tbs raw apple cider vinegar

2 Tbs melted butter or coconut oil

1 tsp vanilla extract

1 ½ cups almond flour

2 Tbs coconut flour

2 tsp cinnamon

½ tsp cardamom powder

1/2 tsp ginger powder

¼ tsp each nutmeg, allspice and cloves

¾ tsp sea low sodium salt

¾ tsp baking soda

2 oz unsweetened baking chocolate (can also use chocolate chips)

Instructions

Preheat oven to 350 F. Line a cupcake pan with liners.

In a medium bowl, whisk together the pumpkin puree, eggs, stevia, butter and vanilla extract. Mix until smooth. Add in the flours, spices, low sodium salt and baking soda and stir until well combined. Add the vinegar.

Using a sharp knife, cut the baking chocolate into small chunks. Fold into the cupcake batter to evenly distribute.

Portion out into lined cupcake tins, until they are almost completely full of batter; these will not rise very much, so no need to worry too much about them getting too big.

Bake for 25 minutes. Check with a toothpick to make sure they are done; if the toothpick comes out clean, they are ready. If not, add 5 more minutes to the baking time.

Let cool completely before frosting.

Frosting:

8 oz. Full fat organic creamed coconut

¼ cup coconut butter, softened

5 drops stevia liquid (May need a few more – please taste test)

1 tsp vanilla extract

1 ½ Tbs cinnamon

Using a strong fork, cream together the cream and butter until smooth. Stir in the stevia, vanilla and cinnamon, and stir well until creamy and well combined.

Use a piping bag or simply a knife to top the cooled cupcakes with the buttercream frosting.

419. Bursting Banana Choco Cupcakes

Ingredients:

2 cups almond meal

1/2 cup almond butter

2 ripe bananas

1/4 cup cocoa powder, unsweetened of course

1/2 cup coconut palm sugar

1/2 cup chocolate chips (I like Enjoy Life brand)

2 eggs

1 tsp pure organic vanilla extract

1 tsp low sodium salt

1/2 tsp baking soda

1 tsp apple cider vinegar

paper muffin liners

Instructions

1. Instead of mixing wet and dry ingredients separate from each other, I just built it all in one bowl. Any opportunity I get to save myself from having more dishes to do, you bet I will take!

2. Preheat the oven to 350 degrees. Mash the bananas, mix in the almond butter and coconut palm sugar, add the vanilla extract, salt, eggs, baking soda and vinegar. Make it chocolaty and dump in the cocoa powder. Mix that in good and start adding the almond meal a cup at a time to make sure it all incorporates well. When a nice batter forms, make it even chocolatier and dump in the half cup of chocolate chips.

3. Line a muffin pan with the paper liners, fill each cup with batter. You'll get a dozen.

4. Bake for 20 minutes and let cool before eating. The tops get a brownie-like crust, the cake is moist and light.

420. Jam and 'Cream' Cupcakes

cupcakes

1/2 cup coconut flour, sifted

1/4 cup arrowroot (tapioca flour), sifted

4 eggs

5 drops stevia liquid (May need a few more – please taste test)

3 tablespoons coconut oil

1 cup full fat coconut cream

1/2 teaspoon concentrated natural vanilla extract

pinch of low sodium salt

1 teaspoon baking powder

sugar free strawberry jam*

1 punnet of strawberries (250 grams or approximately 1 heaped cup of chopped strawberries)

2 tablespoons chia seeds

2 drops stevia

Place the ingredients into blender or food processor and blend until smooth and well combined. Pour / spoon the mixture into a container and place in the fridge to thicken.

'cream'*

1 cup raw macadamias

1/2 teaspoon concentrated natural vanilla extract

pinch of low sodium salt

Instructions

1. Place the ingredients into your blender or food processor and blend at high speed until you have a lovely, smooth macadamia butter. I leave this at room temperature as I find it easier to work with when assembling the cupcakes. After that I store the remaining butter in the fridge.

2. Preheat your oven to 175 degrees Celsius or 350 degrees Fahrenheit.

3. Line nine holes of a standard muffin tray with cupcake cases.

4. In a medium sized bowl beat together your stevia and coconut oil. Add in the eggs, coconut cream and vanilla. 5. Add the flours and when smooth and well combined gently add the salt and baking powder.

6. Spoon the mixture evenly into your nine cases.

7. Bake for 25 minutes.

8. Allow to cool slightly before moving from the tray to a cooling rack.

9. Leave the cakes to cool completely before using a small, sharp knife to remove the tops of the cupcakes and create a small indent in the cake. Fill the cake with a teaspoon of jam and a teaspoon of 'cream' (macadamia butter).

10. Gently place the cupcake 'lid' back on top.

11. Eat and enjoy!!!

421. Delicious Yellow Cupcake Recipe

Ingredients

Cake

½ cup of sifted Organic coconut flour

5 large eggs

⅓ cup of butter or ghee or coconut oil

1 teaspoon vanilla

5 drops stevia liquid (May need a few more – please taste test)

1 cup of applesauce

1 teaspoon baking powder

1 teaspoon baking soda

Instructions:

Combine the coconut flour, baking powder and baking soda in a bowl and blend.

Add in all the liquid ingredients; mix well with a spoon.

Pour into the cupcake tins and bake at 350 degrees for 20 minutes.

Frost and enjoy!

422. Perfect Pear & Nutmeg Cupcakes

Ingredients

2 ripe pears, peeled, de-cored and chopped into small pieces

1 tsp nutmeg

1 tbsp water

1/4 cup coconut flour

2 large eggs

1/4 cup coconut oil or melted butter

5 drops stevia liquid (May need a few more – please taste test)

1/4 tsp baking powder

Instructions

Add the pear, water, 5 drops stevia and 1/2 tsp of nutmeg to a saucepan. Let the mixture simmer over a medium heat until the pears soften (about 15 mins). Either mash with a hand-masher or transfer to a blender and puree. Set aside to cool.

Sieve the coconut flour, the remaining tsp of nutmeg and baking powder into a mixing bowl. In a separate bowl, beat the eggs, coconut oil/butter and stevia together.

If the pear puree is cool, stir it into the eggs.

Gradually add the wet ingredients to the dry and stir until it forms a semi-runny batter.

Spoon into a muffin tray (it should make 6 muffins). Bake at 375 for 12-15 mins.

423. Vanilla Paleo Cupcakes

Ingredients:

Apple Cakes:

4 tablespoons (or ¼ cup) of Grass-Fed/Clarified Butter or Extra Virgin Coconut Oil

½ cup Unsweetened Applesauce

4 Eggs

1 teaspoon Vanilla Extract

5 drops stevia liquid (May need a few more – please taste test)

¾ cup Almond Flour

2 teaspoons Cinnamon

½ teaspoon Baking Powder

1/8 teaspoon low sodium Salt

Cinnamon Frosting:

1 cup room temperature coconut oil

5 drops stevia liquid (May need a few more – please taste test)

1 teaspoon Vanilla Extract

4 tablespoons (or ¼ cup) Arrowroot

2 teaspoons Coconut Flour

2 teaspoons Cinnamon

2 tablespoons Chilled Coconut Milk Cream

Topping:

½ Apple Thinly Sliced

Cinnamon for Dusting

Instructions

Apple Cakes:

Preheat oven to 350 degrees F. Line mini cupcake pan with 24 paper liners.

Melt the butter then whisk in with the applesauce, eggs, vanilla, and stevia.

Add the almond flour, cinnamon, baking powder, and salt to the wet ingredients and mix until evenly combined.

Evenly distribute into the 24 mini cupcake liners {about 1 tablespoon of batter each} and bake at 350 F for 18 – 19 minutes. The cakes are done when a toothpick can be poked in and come out without any batter on the stick.

Let the cool completely.

Cinnamon Frosting:

Whisk the shortening, stevia, vanilla, arrowroot, coconut flour, and cinnamon together until smooth.

Add the chilled coconut milk cream and whisk again until smooth.

Use immediately. Either spoon the frosting into a gallon plastic bag or a pastry bag.

Gently frost each cupcake with your desired amount of frosting.

Store the rest of the frosting in the refrigerator. Let it come to room temperature before you use as frosting again.

Topping:

Top each cupcake with a thin slice of fresh green apple and dust with ground cinnamon.

If you don't enjoy the cupcakes immediately, store them in an airtight container in the refrigerator.

424. Xmas Chocolate Chip Cupcakes

Ingredients

1/2 c Coconut Flour

5 Eggs

2 Egg Whites

1/2 c Cashew Butter (or coconut oil for nut free)

1/2 t low sodium Salt

1/2 t Baking Soda

1/2 t Gluten Free Baking Powder

5 drops stevia liquid (May need a few more – please taste test)

3/4 c Egg Nog

1/4 t Vanilla

1/2 t Nutmeg

1 c Chocolate Chips

Vanilla Frosting

1 c coconut oil

2 T Canned Coconut Milk

1 t Vanilla

Instructions

Whisk together the dry ingredients.

Beat the eggs, whites, egg nog, butter, vanilla, and stevia. By 1/2 cup-fulls, add the dry mixture and whisk until smooth. Fold in the chocolate chips.

Preheat the oven to 350 degrees. Fill lined muffin tins 1/2 full with batter. Bake for 25-30 minutes, or until a toothpick.

If you want to do a loaf instead, bake in a loaf pan, same temp, for 50-55 mins.

For the frosting, beat all the ingredients till light and fluffy!

425. Boston Cream Pie Cupcake Bonanza

Vanilla Cream

Ingredients:

2 organic cage-free egg yolks

5 drops stevia liquid (May need a few more – please taste test)

2 tablespoons coconut palm sugar

2 tablespoons plus 1/2 teaspoon arrowroot starch/flour

pinch of pink low of sodium salt

1 cup canned coconut cream/milk, full fat, room temperature

1/2 teaspoon vanilla

Cupcakes

Ingredients:

1 & 1/2 cups fine blanched almond flour

1 & 1/2 teaspoons baking powder

1/2 teaspoon pink low sodium salt

1/2 cup canned coconut cream/milk, full fat, room temperature

6 tablespoons unsalted grass-fed butter, plus more for greasing

3 organic cage-free eggs

1 cup coconut palm sugar

1 teaspoon vanilla

Chocolate Ganache

Ingredients:

1 cup Enjoy Life Mini Chocolate Chips

1/4 cup canned coconut cream/milk, full fat, room temperature

4 tablespoons unsalted grass-fed butter

1 teaspoon vanilla

Directions:

1. Start by making the Vanilla Cream. In a small bowl whisk egg yolks together until smooth, set aside. In a medium saucepan combine stevia, coconut palm sugar, arrowroot, and salt and stir over medium heat. Add milk in a slow steady stream. Stir and let cook until the mixture begins to boil and thicken, about 5 minutes.

2. Pour 1/3 of the milk mixture into the yolks and stir together with a whisk until combined. Then pour back into the saucepan with the rest of the milk mixture and cook over medium heat, stirring often, until thick, about 3 minutes. Now stir in the vanilla.

3. Use a fine sieve to pour the vanilla mixture through into a small bowl. Cover it with plastic wrap and press the wrap down directly on to the surface of the cream. Refrigerate until very cold, an hour at least. While you wait prepare your cupcakes and chocolate ganache.

4. Preheat oven to 350. Grease a mini cupcake pan very liberally with butter. In a large bowl combine almond flour, baking powder and salt, use a fork to stir together. Warm coconut cream/milk and butter in a saucepan over low heat.

5. In a separate large bowl, whisk together eggs and coconut palm sugar. Then fold in the dry mixture.

6. Bring the coconut cream/milk and butter mixture to a boil. Add this mixture to the batter and whisk until smooth. Now stir in the vanilla. Pour batter into a Ziploc bag, cut a small hole in the corner. Transfer batter to prepared pan, filling to the top. Bake for 10-12 minutes or until a toothpick comes out clean. While you are waiting for the cupcakes to cool, go ahead and make your chocolate ganache.

7. Using the double boiler method melt together the chocolate, coconut cream/milk and butter. Once melted and combined stir in the vanilla. Transfer ganache to a Ziploc bag once it's cool enough, and cut a small hole in the corner tip.

8. Once your cupcakes are cool, remove two from the pan at a time. Squeeze a layer of vanilla cream over the top of one cupcake and then flip the other one upside down and use it to sandwich the two together. Then pour your chocolate ganache over the top and enjoy!

Notes:

You may have noticed above it says Coconut Cream or Coconut Milk. Coconut Cream can be found at health food stores like Sprouts or Whole Foods next to the regular coconut milk. I prefer it because it's a little thicker than normal coconut milk, so if you can find it use it, if not coconut milk will work just fine.

426. Vanilla Bean Cupcakes with Mocha Buttercream

Ingredients

(makes 5-6 cupcakes):

For the cupcakes

1/4 cup coconut flour, sifted

1/4 teaspoon low sodium salt

1/8 teaspoon baking soda

Seeds scraped from half a vanilla bean

1/2 teaspoon vanilla extract

3 large eggs

1/4 cup coconut oil

5 drops stevia liquid (May need a few more – please taste test)

Instructions

Preheat the oven to 350 and line a muffin tin with paper liners. Whisk together the coconut flour, salt, and baking soda in a medium bowl. Add the vanilla bean seeds, and mix together with your fingers, pinching the mixture to evenly distribute the vanilla seeds. In a small bowl, whisk together the vanilla extract, eggs, coconut oil, and stevia. Add the wet ingredients to the dry and whisk well, or beat with a hand mixer, until very smooth. Pour the batter into the cupcake cups and bake for 15-20 minutes, or until a toothpick comes out clean.

For the frosting:

8 tablespoons 1 stick) unsalted butter, at room temperature

5 drops stevia liquid (May need a few more – please taste test)

1 tablespoon cocoa

Tiny pinch of low sodium salt

1/4 teaspoon vanilla extract

1/4 teaspoon finely ground coffee

Coffee beans for garnish

Using a hand mixer, beat the butter until very smooth. Add the remaining ingredients and beat until incorporated. If your frosting does not seem stiff enough, refrigerate for a little while, then beat again. Once the cupcakes are completely cool, pipe or spread on the frosting (I used a Wilton 1M tip). Top with a coffee bean if desired.

427. Meaty Meatloaf Cupcakes

Ingredients

1.5-2 pounds of ground beef (grass-fed if possible)

3 eggs

¼ cup almond flour (or enough to thicken- this will depend partially on the fat content of the meat and the texture of the almond flour)

1 teaspoon dried basil

1 teaspoon garlic powder

1 medium onion

2 tablespoons worcestershire sauce

Salt and pepper to taste

5-6 sweet potatoes

¼ cup butter or coconut oil

1 teaspoon low sodium Salt

Instructions

Preheat the oven to 375 degrees

Finely dice the onion or puree in a blender or food processor.

In a large bowl, combine the meat, eggs, flour, basil, garlic powder, pureed onion, Worcestershire sauce, and salt and pepper and mix by hand until incorporated.

Grease a muffin tin with coconut oil or butter and evenly divide the mixture into the muffin tins to make 2-3 meat "muffins" per person. If you don't have a muffin tin, you can just press the mixture into the bottom of an 8x8 or 9x13 baking dish.

Put into oven on middle rack, and put a baking sheet with a rim under it, in case the oil from the meat happens to spill over (should only happen with fattier meats if at all)

For sweet potatoes: if they are small enough, you can put them into the oven at the same time, if not you can peel, cube and boil them until soft.

When meat is almost done, make sure sweet potatoes are cooked by whichever method you prefer, and drain the water if you boiled them.

Mix with butter and salt or pepper if desired and mash by hand or with an immersion blender.

Remove meat "muffins" from the oven when they are cooked through and remove from tin. Top each with a dollop of the mashed sweet potatoes to make it look like a cupcake.

428. Gushing Guava Cupcakes with Whipped Guava Frosting

Ingredients

For the Cake

¾ cup (120g) of Coconut Flour

¾ cup (96g) of Tapioca Flour

¾ cup of Light Olive Oil

6 Tablespoons (85g) of Granulated Sugar or Coconut Sugar

5 drops stevia liquid (May need a few more – please taste test)

½ cup of Concentrated Guava Puree ('applesauce thick')

6 Eggs

1 teaspoon of Lime Juice

1½ teaspoon of Cream of Tartar

¾ teaspoon of Baking Soda

½ teaspoon of low sodium Salt

For the Whipped Guava Frosting

¾ cup of room temperature coconut oil

6 Tablespoons of Concentrated Guava Puree ('applesauce thick')

5 drops stevia liquid (May need a few more – please taste test)

½ cup of Arrowroot Starch, sifted

1 teaspoon of Lime

Pinch of low sodium Salt

Instructions

For the Cake

You may have to boil the guava puree until applesauce thick. I used Goya brand and let it boil for about 10 minutes.

Preheat oven to 350F. We will drop the temperature to 325F to bake. Line the muffin tin with cupcake liners.

Separate the eggs into egg yolks and egg whites.

Combine the egg whites and cream of tartar and beat with a whisk attachment on high speed. Place the whites in a bowl and set aside, or store in the refrigerator while preparing the rest of the ingredients.

Combine the olive oil, egg yolks, stevia, lime juice, and guava puree in the mixing bowl and beat on high speed for about 30 seconds.

Sift together the coconut flour, tapioca flour, baking soda, sugar, and salt to make the dry flour mixture.

Add half of the dry flour mixture to the wet mixture and whip until the flours absorb and the batter becomes fluffy. Scrape the sides with a spatula to incorporate.

Add the rest of the dry flour mixture and beat on high speed with the whisk until combined and fluffy.

Scoop in a heaping of the egg white meringue and hand mix into the batter. Gently fold in the rest of the meringue until combined.

Portion the batter into each cake pan and place tin in the oven centered.

Reduce the temperature to 325F and for 25-30 minutes until an inserted toothpick comes out clean. This method will give a nice dome to the cupcakes and prevent over browning of the stevia.

Let cool to room temperature or colder before frosting.

For the Frosting

Chill the beaters and mixing bowl in the freezer for about 15 minutes.

Combine the raw stevia and guava puree in a cup until it forms a thicker syrup.

Whip the coconut shortening and optionally the cream cheese.

Add the arrowroot starch and salt and whip.

While mixing on medium speed, pour the guava mixture slowly. Whip until pink and pretty.

Add more stevia to taste if you like.

Dollop onto a cooled cupcake and enjoy!

429. Blushing Blueberry Muffin Recipe

Ingredients

2 1/2 cups almond flour

1 Tablespoon coconut flour

1/4 teaspoon low sodium salt

1/2 teaspoon baking soda

1 Tablespoon vanilla

1/4 cup coconut oil

5 drops stevia liquid (May need a few more – please taste test)

1/4 cup coconut milk*

2 eggs

1 cup fresh or frozen blueberries

2-3 Tablespoons cinnamon

Instructions

Preheat oven to 350. Line a 12 count muffin tin and lightly oil with coconut oil.

In a mixing bowl combine almond flour, coconut flour, salt, and baking soda and stir to combine.

Pour in coconut oil, eggs, stevia, coconut milk, and vanilla; mix well.

Fold in blueberries and add cinnamon.

Distribute into muffin tin. Sprinkle with additional cinnamon.

Bake for 22-25 minutes. Allow to cool and enjoy!

Notes

*Coconut milk can come in different textures depending on the brand you use. If you use a thicker brand like THAI, then use 1/8 cup of coconut milk and 4 Tablespoons of water. If your coconut milk is thinner, stick to the 1/4 cup of coconut milk.

430. Healthy Carrot Ginger Muffins

Ingredients:

2 cups blanched almond flour

½ teaspoon low sodium salt

1 teaspoon baking soda

½ tsp allspice

½ tsp powdered ginger

a pinch of clove

½ cup shredded coconut shreds , unsweetened

3 eggs, preferably pastured

½ cup coconut oil, melted

5 drops stevia liquid (May need a few more – please taste test)

1-2 Tbs grated fresh ginger

1 cup grated carrot

3/4 cup raisins, soaked in water for 15 minutes and drained

Instructions:

In a large bowl, combine almond flour, salt, baking soda, spices, and coconut shreds

In a smaller bowl whisk together eggs, oil, and syrup. Add fresh ginger, grated carrot, and raisins.

Stir wet ingredients into dry

Spoon batter into paper- lined muffin tins

Bake at 350° for 18-20 minutes for mini muffins OR 24-26 minutes for regular muffins.

Cool and serve.

431. Pecan Muffins

(makes 12)

Ingredients

1/3 cup coconut flour

1/4 cup butter, melted

3 large eggs

1/3 cup chopped pecans

1/4 tsp baking powder

stevia drops to taste

Instructions

Whisk together the butter, eggs and molasses.

Sieve the coconut flour and baking powder into a large mixing bowl.

Gradually add the wet ingredients to the dry, stirring until it forms a thick, runny Fold in the pecans.

Spoon about a tbsp into small (I used 4cm) muffin cups. It should stretch to 12. Bake at 350 for 10-12 minutes.

432. Temptingly Perfect Plantain Drop

Ingredients

3 tablespoons coconut oil

2 brown plantains (they must be brown)

1 tsp stevia

¼ cup coconut oil, melted

3 eggs

1 tablespoon canned coconut milk

3 tablespoons coconut flour

1-2 teaspoons cinnamon (I used 2 because I love cinnamon)

1 teaspoon baking powder

A pinch of low sodium salt

Instructions

1. Preheat oven to 350 degrees.

2. Cut the ends off of the plantains, then use your knife to cut them in half lengthwise and then peel the skin off, cutting off any excess skin that sticks to the plantains. The browner the plantains are, the sweeter they will be and the easier the skin is to take off.

3. Now place a large skillet over medium-high heat, add 3 tablespoons of coconut oil to heat up, then add the halved plantains to the skillet. Cook on both sides for about 3-4 minutes until browned, making sure not to burn them.

4. Once the plantains are done cooking, add them to the food processor and puree until they begin to clump together.

5. Then add the stevia, coconut oil, eggs, and coconut milk and puree until smooth. No clumps should be present at this point.

6. Now add coconut flour, cinnamon, baking powder, and salt to the food processor and puree one more time to combine everything well.

7. Now line a baking sheet with parchment paper and grab an ice cream scoop to help form perfect sized biscuits.

8. Scoop the batter out and plop each biscuit on the baking sheet about 1 inch away from each other. My batter made 8 biscuits.

9. Place in oven and bake for 20-25 minutes until slightly brown and completely cooked through.

10. Let cool. These babies are hot and need to settle afterwards.

433. Sweety Potato Muffins

Ingredients

1/2 c Coconut Flour

6 Eggs

2 t Vanilla

1 t low sodium Salt

1 t Baking Soda

2 t Cinnamon

1/2 c Ground Flax

2 Sweet Potatoes or Yams, baked and mashed (discard skins)

1 c Raisins or Chocolate Chips (optional)

Instructions:

Whisk together all the dry ingredients. Beat the eggs and add dry mix by spoonfuls until well blended. Add the mashed sweet potatoes.

Spoon batter into lined muffin cups. Bake at 350 degrees for 30-35 minutes.

Enjoy!

434. Zesty Zucchini Muffins

Ingredients

3/4 C applesauce

5 drops stevia liquid (May need a few more – please taste test)

1/4 C coconut oil, melted

3 eggs

1 Tbsp vanilla

2 C almond flour

1 1/2 tsp baking soda

1 C zucchini, shredded

3/4 C raisin

Instructions

With electric or stand mixer, beat applesauce, stevia and oil

Add eggs and vanilla and mix until combined

Slowly mix in almond flour and soda, then beat until batter forms

Fold in zucchini and raisins

Bake at 350 degrees for 25 minutes, makes 15 muffins

435. Cozy Coconut Flour Muffins

Ingredients

1/2 cup coconut flour

6 eggs, at room temperature (that's important)

¼ cup almond milk

2 tsp stevia

6 Tbs. coconut oil

2 Tbsp coconut milk at room temperature

2 tsp. vanilla extract

1/4 tsp. baking soda

1 tsp. apple cider vinegar

Instructions

Preheat the oven to 350 degrees and prepare a muffin tin with 8 liners (I like unbleached parchment paper baking cups).

Combine the coconut flour and eggs until smooth. Add the remaining ingredients and stir well.

Divide evenly between the muffin tins. Bake until golden and a toothpick comes out clean, about 20 minutes.

Cool completely.

**Makes 8 cupcakes. Feel free to double the recipe if you want more cupcakes! These last in an airtight container for a few days at room temperature. They also freeze really well!

436. Lemon Mousse Mouthwatering Cupcakes

Ingredients

1/2 cup coconut flour

6 eggs, at room temperature (that's important)

6 Tbs. milk

2 tsp stevia

6 Tbs. coconut oil

2 Tbs. coconut milk at room temperature

1 tsp. vanilla extract

1/2 tsp. ground cardamom

1/4 tsp. baking soda

1/2 tsp. apple cider vinegar

Instructions

Preheat the oven to 350 degrees and prepare a muffin tin with 8 liners (I like unbleached parchment paper baking cups).

Combine the coconut flour and eggs until smooth. Add the remaining ingredients and stir well.

Divide evenly between the muffin tins. Bake until golden and a toothpick comes out clean, about 20 minutes.

Cool completely and frost with the lemon mousse.

Makes 8 cupcakes. Feel free to double the recipe if you want more cupcakes!

437. Sexy Savory Muffins

Ingredients

½ cup coconut flour

1 tsp baking soda

½-1 tsp low sodium salt

¼ cup coconut oil

½ cup + 2 tbsp coconut milk

4 pastured eggs

1 tsp apple cider vinegar

1 tsp garlic powder

½ tsp each of rosemary, thyme, sage

Instructions

1. Pre-heat the oven to 350°. Melt the coconut oil and combine with remaining muffin ingredients in a food procssor or bowl, mix well.

2. Place batter in a muffine tin lined with muffin liners. The muffins will raise a small amount, so you can fill the muffin liner about ¾ full–almost to the top. Bake for about 20-30 minutes or until a toothpick inserted comes out clean and the tops are slightly browned.

3. Let it cool and slice in small squares.

438. Molten Lava Chocolate Cupcake

Ingredients:

4 oz Semi-Sweet or Bittersweet chocolate

½ tsp Vanilla Extract

1/8 tsp Salt

5 drops stevia liquid (May need a few more – please taste test)

1 tsp Coconut Flour

2 tsp Cacao Powder

2 eggs

4 Tbsp extra virgin coconut oil (plus a little more for greasing the ramekins)

Instructions:

1.   Preheat oven to 375F. Grease four 6oz ramekins with coconut oil.

2.   In a 4 cup measuring cup or medium microwave-safe bowl, melt chocolate and coconut oil in the microwave on low power. Stir until smooth and let cool.

3.   In a small bowl, beat eggs, vanilla, salt and sugar with a hand mixer until light and frothy, about five minutes (this can seem like an eternity with a hand mixer, but hang in there because it's worth it!).

4.   Pour egg mixture over chocolate. Sift cocoa and coconut flour over the top. Then gently fold all the ingredients together.

5.   Pour batter into prepared ramekins (they should be filled to within ½" of the top). Place the ramekins on a baking sheet and place in the oven (you can chill the ramekins for a few hours if you want to make them ahead of time, just make sure you bring them back to room temperature before baking). Bake for 11-12 minutes.

6.   Remove from oven and serve immediately. Enjoy!

439. Party Carrot Cupcakes

Ingredients

Wet

3 eggs

6 tablespoon non-dairy milk

6 tablespoon extra virgin coconut oil, melted

6 tablespoon carrot juice

5½ tablespoon egg whites

30 drops liquid stevia*see note

¾ teaspoon pure vanilla extract

Dry

6 tablespoon coconut flour

1 teaspoon baking powder

¼ teaspoon low sodium salt

pinch ground cinnamon

Instructions

Preheat oven to 350F and line 12 muffin tins with medium-sized paper liners.

Place eggs and egg white in blender and beat well, about 30 seconds. My magic bullet worked great for this!

Pour in carrot juice, milk, coconut oil, stevia and vanilla. Blend quickly to mix.

Drop in dry ingredients and mix for about 10 seconds. The batter should be slightly thicker than pancake batter.

Pour into prepared muffin tins and bake for 25-30 minutes or until inserted toothpick comes out clean. Mine took 26 minutes.Remove from pan and allow to cool on cooling rack for at least 1 hour before applying buttercream.

440. Cinnamon Chocolate Chip Muffins

Ingredients

Muffins

6 large eggs

5 drops stevia liquid (May need a few more – please taste test)

1 teaspoon vanilla extract

8 tablespoons (1 stick) unsalted butter, melted

3/4 cup coconut flour

1 tablespoon ground cinnamon

2 teaspoons baking powder

1 teaspoon baking soda

small pinch low sodium salt

Instructions

Muffins

Preheat oven to 375 Fahrenheit and adjust rack to middle position

Line with muffin liners

Whisk eggs, stevia, vanilla, butter, and applesauce in a large mixing bowl or use a stand mixer

Sift coconut flour, cinnamon, baking powder, baking soda, and salt over a medium bowl

Add dry ingredients to wet ingredients and until well blended

Fold in chocolate chips ensuring an even distribution throughout your batter

Spoon batter into muffin cups and bake for 16-18 minutes, or until a toothpick in the center comes out clean

Remove the muffins from the oven and let cool

Once cool you can head below and make the frosting to go with them

Notes

*You cannot let Coconut flour sit long, as soon as you mix this batter, ensure you put it right into the oven *If you want chocolate muffins, you can add between 1/4 - 1/2 cup of cocoa powder to your taste liking *You can store these in an airtight container for 3 days *You can substitute the butter with Coconut Oil but I haven't tested it and 8 tablespoons would probably be too oily. If you do test it, start with half and please let me know how it worked.

441. Strawberry Shortcake Cupcakes

Ingredients:

2½ cups blanched almond flour

¾ teaspoon baking soda

¼ teaspoon low sodium salt

5 drops stevia liquid (May need a few more – please taste test)

⅓ cup coconut oil, melted

4 large eggs, room temperature

1 tablespoon lemon juice

2 teaspoons vanilla extract

½ teaspoon lemon zest

½ cup finely chopped strawberries

Frosting

2 egg whites, room temperature

5 drops stevia liquid (May need a few more – please taste test)

¼ teaspoon lemon juice or vinegar

1½ tablespoons strawberry preserves (freshly pureed strawberries will work too)

Instructions:

Preheat the oven to 325 degrees F.

Line a standard muffin tin with baking cups.

Combine the stevia, coconut oil, eggs, lemon juice, vanilla, and lemon zest in the jar of a blender. Puree on medium speed for 20 seconds or until frothy and smooth.

Add the dry ingredients and blend on high for 30-45 seconds. The batter should be very smooth and contain no lumps. If needed, scrape down the sides with a spatula and blend again for a few seconds until all of the dry mixture is incorporated.

Gently fold the chopped strawberries in by hand. Divide the batter evenly into the muffin tin, filling about ¾ of the way full.

Bake for 16-18 minutes, until a toothpick can be inserted into the middle and comes out clean.

Let the cupcakes cool completely on the counter before frosting.

Frosting

Once the cupcakes have cooled, make your Italian meringue.

Bring your stevia to a boil in a saucepan over medium-high heat.

Meanwhile, beat the egg whites and lemon juice until frothy and you can just begin to see trail marks from your beaters. When you lift out the beaters, you should see soft peaks.

With the beaters or mixer running, slowly pour in the boiling stevia in a steady stream. Continue beating for 6-8 minutes, until the meringue is cool to the touch.

Gently fold in the strawberry preserves. Put the frosting into a piping bag for a pretty design, or spread onto cupcakes with a knife.

Tips

For easier separation, separate the whites from the yolks when they are cold.

Meringue will not stiffen if you use a dirty bowl (usually because of leftover oil) or let any of the yolk get in with the whites

Over beating will cause the meringue to fall. Stop once you can lift the beaters out and see stiff peaks.

The frosting needs to be piped immediately and is best served immediately as well. Once it's on the cupcakes though, it will hold up in the refrigerator for 24 hours.

442. Thin Mint Mini Cupcakes

Ingredients

For the Cupcakes

1/4 cup coconut flour

1/4 cup organic cocoa powder

4 large eggs (at room temperature)

1/4 cup coconut oil

5 drops stevia liquid (May need a few more – please taste test)

1/4 tsp baking soda

1 tsp lemon juice

Pinch of low sodium salt

1/4 tsp mint extract

6 Tbsp chopped dark chocolate or dairy free chocolate chips (for Paleo)

For the frosting:

2/3 cup powdered sweetener or coconut sugar, powdered for Paleo

2 ripe avocado

1/2 cup coconut milk

1/4 tsp mint extract

Instructions

Preheat oven to 350 F

Combine the coconut flour, cocoa powder, sweetener (if granular), baking soda, and low sodium salt.

In a separate bowl, combine the eggs, coconut oil, and lemon juice (and stevia if using).

Add the dry ingredients to the wet and mix to combine.

Line a mini muffin tin with 24 cupcake liners.

Fill cupcake liners evenly with the batter and bake for 13-15 minutes or until cooked through.

Allow to cool before topping with the icing.

Pipe on the frosting (directions below) onto each cupcake and serve.

For the frosting

Place the meat of the avocados in a blender and mix until completely smooth.

Add the sweetener, coconut milk, and mint extract. Mix until thoroughly incorporated.

Notes

Total Carb Count: 3.1 g (for 1 mini cupcake plus the carbs for the sweetener used)

Net Carb Count: 1.2 g net carbs (for 1 mini cupcake plus the carbs for the sweetener used)

*Note carb counts are estimated based on the products I used. Check nutrition labels for accurate carb counts and gluten information.

443. Lemon-Coconut Petit Fours

Ingredients

For the Cake

1/2 cup coconut flour

1/2 cup coconut milk

3 eggs, separated

3/4 cup soaked dates in 3 tbsp hot water

1/2 tsp vanilla

1/2 tsp baking soda

1/4 tsp low sodium salt

1 tsp lemon rind

Frosting

2/3 cup coconut cream (from the top of a can of coconut milk)

2 tbsp almond milk

1 tbsp Stevia

3 tsp lemon juice

¼ cup coconut oil, room temperature

Instructions

Put dates in a heat safe bowl or container and pour 3 tbsp boiling water over them and let soak for about 15 minutes. You can chop the dates before soaking to speed up the process, but it's not necessary.

Separate the eggs with yolks in one bowl and whites in one large stainless steel, glass or ceramic bowl. When you go to whip the egg whites, it helps if they are at room temperature.

Once dates have soaked put them in a food processor along with remaining water and mix until you have a paste-like consistency. Add coconut flour, milk, egg yolks, vanilla, baking soda, salt and lemon rind and mix.

Whip the egg whites until foamy and stiff peaks form. This is much easier if you have a stand mixer with the whisk attachment or a hand mixer. It is possible to do it by hand, but takes time.

Gently fold egg whites into the batter. Grease a standard sized loaf pan. Put batter in pan and even out the top with a spatula or spoon.

Bake in a 350° oven for 20-30 minutes or when a toothpick inserted comes out clean.

For the frosting

Coconut cream can be purchased in cans or you can skim the cream of the top of cans of coconut milk, however you may have to use multiple cans of coconut milk. Put coconut cream in a bowl and whisk for a few minutes to make it lighter and creamier.

Add coconut oil, milk, stevia and lemon juice and whisk until fully incorporated.

Allow the cake to cool completely before frosting. Once the cake has cooled, cut small squares or circles out of the cake and skim some cake off of the top with a knife to make it even. There will be leftover scraps, but they make a great snack!

Cut the squares in half and frost the middle. You can use the prepared frosting, but it will be very thin.

Drizzle the prepared frosting over the small cake squares and use a spatula or knife to frost the sides evenly. Once you've frosted each petit fours, refrigerate to allow the frosting to harden. Top with a bit of lemon rind.

444. Blushing Blueberry Cupcakes

Ingredients:

1/2 cup almond flour

1/2 cup coconut flour

1/2 cup hazelnut flour

1 tbsp coconut sugar

1 tsp baking soda

¼ tsp low sodium salt

3 eggs

3 tbsp unsweetened almond milk

5 drops stevia liquid (May need a few more – please taste test)

1 tsp vanilla extract

½ cup blueberries

Instructions

Preheat oven to 350°.

Combine dry ingredients (both flours, sugar, baking soda, and salt) into a bowl and mix.

In a separate bowl, whisk eggs together; add milk, stevia and vanilla and stir.

Fold wet ingredients into dry ingredients.

Stir in the blueberries by hand.

Line muffin tin with muffin liners and spray each one with a bit of nonstick spray (optional but recommended).

Pour batter evenly to your cupcake tray

Bake for 10-15 minutes or until batter is no longer in liquid form.

Drizzle with extra stevia if desired.

Enjoy!

445. Delicious Morning Cupcakes

Ingredients

1/3 cup mashed sweet potato

3 eggs

¼ 5 drops stevia liquid (May need a few more – please taste test)

1 teaspoon pure vanilla extract

1 cup grated carrot (1 large)

1 cup grated apple (½ large Fugi)

2 teaspoons fresh ginger, peeled and grated, optional

2 cups blanched almond flour

1 cup unsweetened shredded coconut (or flaked coconut)

2/3 cup raisins

2/3 cup raw walnuts, chopped

2 teaspoons ground cinnamon

1 teaspoon baking powder

¼ teaspoon baking soda

½ teaspoon low sodium salt

Instructions

Preheat the oven to 350 degrees F and line a 12-cupcake tray with baking cups.

Whisk together the mashed sweet potato, eggs, stevia, grated carrot, apple, and ginger until well-combined (wet ingredients).

In a seperate mixing bowl, stir together the almond flour, raisins, walnuts, cinnamon, baking powder, baking soda, and salt (dry ingredients).

685

Pour the dry mixture into the bowl with the wet mixture and stir well until a thick batter forms.

using an ice cream scoop or small measuring cup, scoop batter into the lined muffin tray, filling the cups 3/4 of the way up.

Place cupcake tray on the center rack in the preheated oven and bake for 30 to 35 minutes, until cupcake test clean when poked with a toothpick.

Allow cupcakes to cool at least 20 minutes before mowing them down < - if you try to eat the cupcakes before letting them cool, they will stick to the cupcake cups like whoa.

446. Cheerful Coffee Cupcake

Ingredients:

6 eggs

1/4 cup ghee

1/4 cup coconut flour

1/4 cup water chestnut flour 2 Tbsp grade B stevia 2 Tbsp vanilla

5 drops stevia liquid (May need a few more – please taste test)

1/4 tsp low sodium salt

1/2 tsp cinnamon

Topping Ingredients:

1/2 cup pecans (chopped)

5 drops stevia liquid (May need a few more – please taste test)

4 Tbsp ghee

2 Tbsp almond flour

1 tsp cinnamon

1/8 tsp low sodium salt

Instructions

Preheat oven to 350 degrees.

Put eggs in a large mixing bowl and mix thoroughly with an immersion blender until frothy.

Add remaining ingredients and mix well.

Fill muffin pan evenly (should make 1 dozen).

Place in oven and set timer for 20 minutes.

Now combine ingredients for the topping in a separate bowl.

At the 20 minute mark take out the muffins and add the topping evenly between all the muffins.

Put them back in the oven for another 10 minutes.

Broil for an additional 2 minutes and remove quickly.

Let cool.

Enjoy with a hot cup of coffee! Ok, I guess I'll let you do tea if you insist

447. Luscious Lemon Poppy Seed Cupcake

Ingredients

1 1/4 cup almond flour

2 tbs coconut flour

1 tbs poppy seeds

1 tsp baking soda

1 tsp baking powder

1/4 tsp low sodium salt

5 drops stevia liquid (May need a few more – please taste test)

1/4 cup fresh lemon juice, plus the zest of 1 lemon

3 eggs whisked

3 tbs coconut oil

1 tsp vanilla extract

Instructions

Preheat oven to 350-degrees F

In a small bowl, mix all the wet ingredients together

In a medium bowl, combine all the dry ingredients

Now pour the wet ingredients into the dry ingredients bowl, and stir into a batter

Let batter set for a few minutes, then stir it again

Grease a muffin tin or use muffin liners and fill each well or cup about two-thirds full

Bake about 15-20 minutes, or until a toothpick inserted into a muffin comes out clean

Serve and enjoy!

448. Strawberry chia Cupcake

Ingredients

½ c + 2 tbsp (56g) coconut flour

1 tsp xanthan gum

¾ tsp baking powder

¾ tsp baking soda

¼ tsp low sodium salt

1 tbsp (13g) chia seeds

1 tbsp (5g) lemon zest (about one medium)

1 tbsp (14g) coconut oil or unsalted butter, melted

1 large egg, room temperature

1 tsp vanilla extract

¼ c (60g) plain nonfat Greek yogurt

¼ c (60mL) agave

3 tbsp (45mL) freshly squeezed lemon juice (about one medium-large)

½ c (120mL) unsweetened vanilla almond milk

2 scoops (84g) vanilla protein powder

1 c (140g) frozen unsweetened strawberries, thawed slightly and diced

Instructions

Preheat the oven to 350°F, and lightly coat 9 standard-sized muffin cups with nonstick cooking spray.

Whisk together the coconut flour, xanthan gum, baking powder, baking soda, salt, chia seeds, and lemon zest in a medium bowl. In a separate bowl, whisk together the coconut oil or butter, egg, and vanilla. Stir in the Greek yogurt until no large lumps remain. Stir in the agave, lemon juice, and almond milk. Mix in the protein powder. Add in the coconut flour mixture, stirring until fully incorporated. Let the batter rest for 10 minutes. Gently fold in the diced strawberries

Divide the batter between the prepared muffin cups. Bake at 350°F for 25-28 minutes, or until a toothpick inserted into the center comes out clean. Cool in the pan for 10 minutes before carefully turning out onto a wire rack.

Notes: Any milk (cow, soy, cashew, etc.) may be used in place of the almond milk.

449. Triple Coconut Cupcakes

Ingredients

1 cup almond flour

3 tbsp coconut flour

1 cup shredded coconut

1½ tsp baking powder

¼ tsp low sodium salt

5 drops stevia liquid (May need a few more – please taste test)

4 eggs, separated

¼ cup coconut oil

1 tbsp vanilla extract

Instructions

Preheat the oven to 350F. Grease a muffin tin or line with muffin cups.

Combine almond flour, coconut flour, shredded coconut, salt and baking powder in a medium mixing bowl.

Mix the egg yolks, stevia, coconut oil and vanilla extract in a small mixing bowl. Add to the almond flour mixture and combine thoroughly.

Using a hand mixer, whip the egg whites until they form stiff peaks.

Stir the egg whites into the rest of the ingredients, spoon the batter into the muffin tin.

Bake for 25 minutes (or until the tops are nicely browned and a tester comes out clean.

450. Lemon-Coconut Muffins

Ingredients

1 1/4 cup almond flour

1 cup shredded unsweetened coconut

2 tbs coconut flour

1/2 tsp baking soda

1/2 tsp baking powder

1/4 tsp low sodium salt

5 drops stevia liquid (May need a few more – please taste test)

1/3 cup fresh lemon juice, plus the zest of 1 lemon

1/4 cup full-fat coconut milk

3 eggs, whisked

3 tbs coconut oil

1 tsp vanilla extract

Instructions

Preheat oven to 350º F

In a small bowl, mix all the wet ingredients together

In a medium bowl, combine all the dry ingredients

Now pour the wet ingredients into the dry ingredients bowl, and stir into a batter

Let batter set for a few minutes, then stir it again

Grease a muffin tin or use silicone muffin liners (paper liners not recommended) and fill each well or cup about two-thirds full

Bake about 18-23 minutes. Test for doneness > insert toothpick into muffin center; if it comes out clean they're done

Serve and enjoy!

451. Chocolate Banana Muffins

Ingredients

2 medium super ripe bananas (each banana was 185 grams with the peel and 143 grams without)

5 drops stevia liquid (May need a few more – please taste test)

2 teaspoon vanilla extract

2 eggs

1/4 cup (56 grams) refined coconut oil, melted

200 grams (~2 cups but please weigh!) blanched almond flour

3 tablespoons (27 grams) coconut flour

1/3 cup (42 grams) Dutch process cocoa powder

1 teaspoon baking soda

1/4 teaspoon low sodium salt

1 cup (180 grams) semi-sweet chocolate chips ,additional mini chocolate chips for sprinkling, if desired

Directions

Preheat the oven to 350°F (175°C) and line a muffin tin with 12 muffin liners.

In a large bowl, mash the bananas with the bottom of a glass. They should almost be like a puree.

Add the stevia and vanilla and stir.

Add in the eggs and oil and stir until well combined.

In a medium bowl, mix together the almond flour, coconut flour, cocoa powder, baking soda and salt.

Stir just until combined and then stir in the chocolate chips.

Spoon the batter into the muffin liners and sprinkle on additional chocolate chips, if desired.

Bake for 18 minutes or until a toothpick inserted in the center comes out clean. Be careful not to confuse a melted chocolate chip with the batter.

Let the muffins cool for 5 minutes in the pan and then turn out onto a wire rack to cool completely.

Place in an airtight container and store in the refrigerator for up to 5 days.

Notes: Use can use unrefined coconut oil if you don't mind a slight coconut taste.

452. Delicious English Cupcakes

Ingredients

For the regular option

¼ cup almond or cashew flour

1 tablespoon coconut flour

¼ teaspoon baking soda

⅛ teaspoon low sodium salt

1 egg

½ tablespoon coconut oil

2 tablespoons water

For the cinnamon raisin option add the following to the regular option above

¼ teaspoon cinnamon

½ 5 drops stevia liquid (May need a few more – please taste test)

1½ tablespoons golden raisins

Instructions

Whisk together the dry ingredients in a small bowl.

Add the remaining wet ingredients and whisk again until fully incorporated.

Transfer the mixture into a greased microwave safe ramekin

Microwave for 2 minutes.

Remove from the ramekin, slice the muffin in half and toast for 2-3 minutes in a toaster oven.

Serve with softened butter.

453. Amazing Almond Flour Cupcakes

Ingredients:

2-1/2 cups almond flour or almond meal

¾ tsp baking soda

½ tsp low sodium salt

3 large eggs

⅓ cup unsweetened pumpkin puree, thawed winter squash puree, butternut squash puree, unsweetened apple sauce, or mashed very ripe banana

2 drops stevia, agave nectar or stevia

2 tablespoons coconut oil (melted) or vegetable oil

1 teaspoon vinegar (white or cider)

Optional Flavorings: 1 teaspoon extract (e.g., vanilla, almond), citrus zest, dried herbs (e.g., basil, dill), or spice (e.g., cinnamon, cumin)

Optional Stir-Ins: 1 cup fresh fruit (e.g., blueberries, diced apple) or ½ cup dried fruit/cacao nibs/chopped nuts/seeds or

Instructions:

Preheat oven to 350F. Line 10 cups in a standard 12-cup muffin tin with paper or foil liners.

In a large bowl whisk the almond flour, baking soda and salt (whisk in any dried spices or herbs at this point, if using).

In a small bowl, whisk the eggs, pumpkin, stevia, oil and vinegar (add any extracts or zest at this point, if using).

Add the wet ingredients to the dry ingredients, stirring until blended. Fold in any optional stir-ins, if using.

Divide batter evenly among prepared cups.

Bake in preheated oven for 14 to 18 minutes until set at the centers and golden brown at the edges. Move the tin to a cooling rack and let muffins cool in the tin 30 minutes. Remove muffins from tin.

454. Delightful Cinnamon Apple Muffins

Ingredients:

1 cup unsweetened applesauce

4 eggs

1/4 cup coconut oil, melted

1 tsp vanilla

Stevia to taste

1/2 cup coconut flour

2 tsp cinnamon

1 tsp baking powder

1 tsp baking soda

1/4 tsp low sodium salt

Instructions:

Preheat oven to 350 degrees F. Line a muffin tin with liners. In a large bowl, add applesauce, eggs, coconut oil, stevia, and vanilla. Stir to combine.

Stir in the coconut flour, cinnamon, baking powder, baking soda, and low sodium salt. Distribute the batter evenly into the lined muffin tins, filling each about two-thirds of the way full.

Bake for 15-20 minutes, until a toothpick inserted into the center comes out clean. Serve warm or store in the refrigerator in a resealable bag.

455. Delish Banana Nut Muffins

Ingredients:

4 bananas, mashed with a fork (the more ripe, the better)

4 eggs

1/2 cup almond butter

2 tbsp coconut oil, melted

1 tsp vanilla

1/2 cup coconut flour

2 tsp cinnamon

1/2 tsp nutmeg

1 tsp baking powder

1 tsp baking soda

1/4 tsp low sodium salt

Instructions:

Preheat oven to 350 degrees F. Line a muffin tin with cups. In a large bowl, add bananas, eggs, almond butter, coconut oil, and vanilla. Using a hand blender, blend to combine.

Add in the coconut flour, cinnamon, nutmeg, baking powder, baking soda, and low sodium salt. Blend into the wet mixture, scraping down the sides with a spatula. Distribute the batter evenly into the lined muffin tins, filling each about two-thirds of the way full.

Bake for 20-25 minutes, until a toothpick comes out clean. Serve warm or store in the refrigerator in a resealable bag.

456. Paleo Vanilla Cupcakes

Serves: 6 cupcakes

Ingredients

¼ cup coconut flour

⅛ teaspoon celtic sea salt

⅛ teaspoon baking soda

3 large eggs

¼ cup room temperature coconut oil

5 drops stevia liquid (May need a few more – please taste test)

1 tablespoon vanilla extract

Instructions

In a food processor, combine coconut flour, salt and baking soda

Pulse in eggs, shortening, honey and vanilla

Line a cupcake pan with 6 paper liners and scoop ¼ cup into each

Bake at 350° for 20-24 minutes

Cool for 1 hour

Frost with Paleo Chocolate Frosting

Serve

457. Apple Cinnamon Muffins

Ingredients

5 eggs

1 cup homemade applesauce (store bought should work too)

½ cup coconut flour

2-3 TBSP cinnamon

1 tsp baking soda

1 tsp vanilla (optional)

¼ cup coconut oil

5 drops stevia liquid (May need a few more – please taste test)

Instructions

Preheat the oven to 400 degrees F.

Grease a muffin pan with coconut oil.

Put all ingredients into a medium sized bowl and mix with immersion blender or whisk until well mixed.

Let sit 5 minutes.

Use ⅓ cup measure to spoon into muffin tins.

Bake 12-15 minutes until starting to brown and not soft when lightly touched on the top.

Let cool 2 minutes, drizzle with honey (if desired) and serve.

458. Apple Cardamom Cupcakes

Ingredients

½ cup applesauce

⅓ cup honey

4 large eggs

¼ cup coconut flour

½ teaspoon baking soda

¼ teaspoon salt

1 teaspoon cinnamon

¼ teaspoon nutmeg

¼ teaspoon cloves

½ teaspoon cardamom

For frosting:

1 cup coconut milk

1 cup honey

pinch of salt

1 teaspoon vanilla

2 tablespoons arrowroot powder

1 tablespoon water

1 cup coconut oil, melted

Instructions

Preheat oven to 350 degrees. Prepare muffin/cupcake pan with liners.

Using an electric mixer or by hand, combine applesauce, honey, and eggs until smooth.

Sift together all dry ingredients, making sure to get out any lumps in the coconut flour.

Combine dry and wet ingredients, mixing thoroughly.

Divide batter amongst 10-12 cupcake liners, filling each one about ⅔ of the way up.

Place in oven and bake for 35-45 minutes, or until top is lightly browned and toothpick comes out clean.

Meanwhile, begin making frosting. In a medium saucepan, heat coconut milk, honey, salt, and vanilla and allow to simmer for 10 minutes.

In a small bowl or ramekin, combine arrowroot powder and water to form a thick paste.

Add arrowroot mixture to pan, whisk vigorously, and bring to a boil.

Remove pan from heat and very slowly add melted coconut oil while mixing with an electric hand blender.

Allow pan to cool slightly, then place whole thing in refrigerator for at least an hour or until it is cool and has turned white.

Remove from refrigerator and use electric hand blender to whip until fluffy.

Spread a dollop on each cupcakes (this frosting is quite sweet, so you don't need a lot but let your tastes be the guide!).

Sprinkle with cinnamon for garnish.

459. Chocolate Olive Oil Cupcakes

Ingredients

2 tablespoons cocoa powder

2 tablespoons coconut flour

1 teaspoon baking powder

1/4 teaspoon ground cinnamon

2 eggs

3 tablespoons honey

1/2 teaspoon vanilla extract

2 tablespoons olive oil

Icing

1 tablespoon coconut oil (melted)

1 tablespoon cocoa powder

1 tablespoon honey

Instructions :

Preheat oven to 160 C.

Combine the cocoa, coconut flour, baking powder and cinnamon.

Add the eggs, honey, vanilla and olive oil.

Mix until smooth and well combined.

Spoon 4 lined cup cake tins.

Bake cupcakes for about 20 – 25 minutes.

Remove from the oven and allow to cool.

Instructions for Icing

Melt the coconut oil.

Mix in the cocoa powder.

Mix in the honey until all well combined.

Allow to harder then spread over muffins.

(Note: I didn't wait long enough for the icing to harder and the cupcake drank it up but it still tasted great!)

460. Pretty Vanilla Cup Cake

Ingredients

For the cupcakes:

¾ cup coconut flour

6 large eggs

¾ cup raw honey

½ cup melted coconut oil

1 tablespoon pure vanilla extract

¾ tsp baking powder

¼ tsp salt

For the icing:

1 can coconut milk (full fat) refrigerated overnight, scoop out coconut cream

1 tsp pure vanilla extract

2 heaping tablespoons pure coconut palm sugar or cane sugar

Instructions

Preheat the oven to 350 degrees.

Using a muffin pan, line each cup with a cupcake liner and spray generously with olive oil cooking spray or if not using cupcake liners grease very well with melted coconut oil.

In a bowl add the dry cupcake ingredients and mix to combine. In another small bowl whisk together the wet cupcake ingredients and add to the dry. Mix until completely smooth.

Pour the batter equally among the greased cups and bake in the oven for 16-18 minutes.

Allow the cupcakes to cook completely before removing from tin or removing from liners.

While the cupcakes are baking add the coconut cream to a large bowl with the vanilla and sugar. Use an electric beater and whip until frothy. Place in the fridge to chill.

Wait until the cupcakes are completely cooled and then pipe the coconut cream on each cupcake.

Place cupcakes back in the fridge for 3-4 hours to chill and the icing will firm up.

Top each cupcake with a halved fig slice, sprinkles, or other garnish of choice.

461. One-Bowl Coconut Flour Cupcakes

Ingredients

½ cup coconut flour

½ teaspoon baking powder

¼ teaspoon fine sea salt

4 large eggs (preferably brought to room temperature)

½ cup maple syrup, honey or agave nectar

⅓ cup coconut oil, warmed until melted (or vegetable oil of choice)

2 tablespoons dairy or nondairy milk of choice milk

2 teaspoons vanilla extract vanilla extract

Instructions

Preheat oven to 350°F.

IMPORTANT: Line 8 muffin cups with paper or silicone liners; spray insides of cups with nonstick cooking spray or oil/grease (to prevent sticking).

In a large bowl, whisk the flour, baking powder, and salt until blended. Whisk in the eggs, syrup, oil, milk, and vanilla until completely blended and smooth.

Divide the batter equally among the prepared muffin cups.

Bake in preheated oven for 18 to 22 minutes or until golden and a toothpick inserted in the center comes out clean.

Transfer baking tin to wire rack and cool 10 minutes.

Carefully remove the cupcakes from the tin and place on wire rack; cool completely.

Notes

Sore in an airtight container at room temperature for up to 2 days, in an airtight container in the refrigerator for up to 1 week, or freeze (unfrosted) for up to 2 months.

462. Meatloaf Cupcakes

Ingredients

1.5-2 pounds of ground beef (grass-fed if possible)

3 eggs

¼ cup almond flour (or enough to thicken- this will depend partially on the fat content of the meat and the texture of the almond flour)

1 teaspoon dried basil

1 teaspoon garlic powder

1 medium onion

2 tablespoons Worcestershire sauce

Salt and pepper to taste

5-6 sweet potatoes

¼ cup butter or coconut oil

1 teaspoon sea salt or Himalayan Salt

Instructions

Preheat the oven to 375 degrees

Finely dice the onion or puree in a blender or food processor.

In a large bowl, combine the meat, eggs, flour, basil, garlic powder, pureed onion, Worcestershire sauce, and salt and pepper and mix by hand until incorporated.

Grease a muffin tin with coconut oil or butter and evenly divide the mixture into the muffin tins to make 2-3 meat "muffins" per person. If you don't have a muffin tin, you can just press the mixture into the bottom of an 8x8 or 9x13 baking dish.

Put into oven on middle rack, and put a baking sheet with a rim under it, in case the oil from the meat happens to spill over (should only happen with fattier meats if at all)

For sweet potatoes: if they are small enough, you can put them into the oven at the same time, if not you can peel, cube and boil them until soft.

When meat is almost done, make sure sweet potatoes are cooked by whichever method you prefer, and drain the water if you boiled them.

Mix with butter and salt or pepper if desired and mash by hand or with an immersion blender.

Remove meat "muffins" from the oven when they are cooked through and remove from tin. Top each with a dollop of the mashed sweet potatoes to make it look like a cupcake.

463. Paleo Chocolate Cupcake with "Peanut Butter" Frosting

Ingredients

Cake Ingredients

1/4 cup coconut flour

3 large eggs

1/4 cup cup unsweetened cacao powder

1/3 cup raw honey

1/4 cup coconut oil

1/2 tsp baking soda

1 tsp vanilla

Pinch of salt

Frosting Ingredients

3/4 cup sunflower butter

3/4 cup Tropical Traditions Palm Shortening –or– 3/4 cup organic butter

1/3 cup raw honey

2 tsp vanilla

pinch salt

Instructions

Make your frosting first

Frosting Instructions

Using a stand mixer or hand mixer, combine sunflower butter and shortening on medium-high speed until fluffy. Takes about 3 minutes.

Add honey, vanilla and pinch of salt. Whip on high for another couple of minutes.

It should look like frosting, thick enough to spread on a cupcake.

Place in fridge while you bake your cupcakes

Cake Instructions

Combine dry ingredients together in a bowl: coconut flour, cacao powder, baking soda, salt

Whisk eggs in another small bowl and add melted coconut oil, honey and vanilla

Combine with dry ingredients and mix

Pour into muffin cups of your choice

Bake at 350º F for 15-18 min.

Makes about 6-8 cupcakes

Once cooled, frost those yummy cakes!

We sprinkled on a few mini dark chocolate chips just for fun :)

Frosting holds up well, but refrigerate if you don't eat them all right away.

464. Paleo Apple Pie Cupcakes with Cinnamon Frosting

Ingredients:
WET INGREDIENTS

- 5 Eggs, room temperature

- 1/2 cup applesauce (you can make your own or use a sugar-free pre-made brand)

- 1/2 cup raw honey, melted

- 1/3 cupcoconut oil, melted

DRY INGREDIENTS

- 1 1/4 cup finely ground blanch almond flour

- 1/2 cup coconut flour

- 1/2 tsp. sea salt

- 1/2 tsp. baking powder

FROSTING INGREDIENTS:

- 1 cupcoconut oil

- 3 Tbsp. raw honey

- 2 tsp. cinnamon

- Dash sea salt

Equipment:

- Muffin tin

- 12 baking cups

- 2 medium mixing bowls

Hand mixe

- For

Directions:

1. Preheat oven to 350F. Line muffin pan with baking cups.

2. Combine all wet ingredients in a medium sized mixing bowl. Beat on medium with a hand mixer for about 30 seconds.

3. Combine all dry ingredients in another medium sized bowl. Mix together with a fork to break apart any clumps.

4. Add the dry ingredients to the wet ingredients and beat for about 20 seconds. Make sure all ingredients are combined.

5. Fill each lined muffin tin about 3/4 of the way full. Bake for 25-30 minutes or until a toothpick comes out clean in the center.

6. Take the cupcakes out of the oven and set aside to cool completely. All the way cooled! But feel free to sneak one to nibble on while the rest cool off.

7. Once the cupcakes have cooled, make the frosting! Combine all of the ingredients into a medium mixing bowl and beat on medium speed for about 30 seconds until well combines. Ice those cupcakes and get to eating!

465. Black Forest cupcakes

Ingredients

125g/4½oz butter, softened

175g/6oz caster sugar

2 free-range eggs

200g/7oz self-raising flour

2 tbsp cocoa powder

125ml/4fl oz milk

100g/3½oz dark chocolate (minimum 70% cocoa solids), melted, plus extra to serve

1 x 360g/12½oz jar black cherries in kirsch

½ tsp arrowroot or cornflour mixed with a little water to make a smooth paste

300ml/10fl oz double cream, lightly whipped

Instructions

Preheat the oven to 170C/325F/Gas 3. Line a 12-hole muffin tray with paper cases.

Beat the butter and sugar together in a bowl until light and creamy. Gradually add the eggs, one at a time, until well combined. Sift in the flour and cocoa powder and mix until well combined. Fold in the milk and melted chocolate.

Spoon or pipe the mixture into the muffin cases and bake for 18-20 minutes, or until well risen and springy to the touch.

Remove the cakes from the tin and set aside to cool on a cooling rack.

Drain the cherries in a sieve collecting the kirsch in the bowl below. Pierce the cakes with a skewer and carefully pour about a teaspoon of the kirsch over each cake.

Heat the kirsch and arrowroot paste in a small saucepan until just boiling. Remove the pan from the heat and beat until thickened.

Using a small knife make a well in the top of each cake by removing a disk of cake

Pipe or spoon a swirl of cream onto the cakes, top with a few cherries and drizzle with the thickened kirsch. Just before serving, grate over some chocolate.

466. Perfect Pizza Muffins

Makes 12 large muffins.

Ingredients:

4 cups almond flour

4 tablespoons ground flaxseed + 12 tablespoons water (or 4 eggs)

¼ cup arrowroot flour (or coconut flour)

½ cup melted ghee (or coconut oil)

1 tablespoon garlic powder

1 tablespoon parsley

1 tablespoon oregano

4 links of italian sausage, finely chopped or ground in a food processor

8 slices of cooked bacon, finely chopped or ground in a food processor

½ cup spinach, finely chopped or ground in a food processor

Instructions

Preheat the oven to 375 degrees.

Mix together the flaxseed and water and let it sit for a minute.

Mix all of the ingredients together, then scoop into the muffin tin. I used silicone muffin cups as liners. Fill each tin all the way to the top.

Bake for about 30-45 minutes, or until firm.

If you would like to use cheese, you can mix in about 1 cup with your batter before baking or melt some on top of the cooked muffins. Dip them in your favorite sauce and enjoy.

467. Honey Cream Hottie

Ingredients:

Stevia to taste, plus more for topping

Steamed almond milk (or any milk you love) and foam

2 shots (or more) of espresso

Instructions:

At the bottom of a mug, add honey.

Pour a little steamed/warm milk into the mug and stir to mix in honey.

Add the shots of espresso then pour the rest of the steamed milk in along with the foam. Drizzle honey over the top.

468. Cheeky CHURROS

Ingredients

1/2 C Water

7 Tbsp softened Ghee

1/2 tsp fine Sea Salt

½ C Cassava Flour

1/4 cup Arrowroot

3 Eggs

Stevia to taste

1 tsp Cinnamon

1 C frying Oil

Instructions

Combine the Cassava Flour, Arrowroot powder and Salt in a small bowl.

Over low heat melt the Ghee in the Water. Once it is brought to a low boil quickly add in the flour mixture

Stir quickly until a ball is formed (30 seconds)

Remove from heat and let cool about 5 minutes.

Add one egg at a time, stirring vigorously after each addition.

The dough will look stringy an oily, that is normal. Just keep stirring and making a ball.

Once all the eggs have been incorporated and the dough is well blended, spoon the dough into a piping bag.

Heat your oil of preference in a deep pot or a deep fryer. I used Coconut Oil.

Once the oil is hot enough, carefully pipe the dough into the hot oil.

Fry until golden brown on each side, about 1 min on each side

Remove the Churros from the oil and place on a plate prepared with paper towel to absorb the extra oil.

469. Beautiful Banana Bread

Ingredients

1 cup almond flour

2 medium soft bananas

3 eggs

1 tablespoon solid coconut oil

1 teaspoon baking powder

1 teaspoon vanilla

1/8 teaspoon stevia (optional)

1/4 teaspoon salt

Method

Preheat the oven to 350 degrees and line a small baking pan with parchment paper.

Combine all of the ingredients in a high powered blender or food processor (this combine all the ingredients into the smoothest texture and makes a big difference in the consistency and texture, so it is highly suggested to use a blender or food processor in combining).

Once the batter is smooth, pour it into the bread loaf pan and cook on 350 degrees for 1 hour and 10 minutes.

470. Eggie Egg Muffin Cups

INGREDIENTS

1 tablespoon olive oil

4 whole eggs

4 egg whites

2 cups baby spinach - roughly chopped (measured/packed before chopping)

1 cup red pepper (measured after chopping)

1 cup green pepper (measured after chopping)

1 cup yellow onion (measured after chopping)

1 cup mushrooms (measured before chopping)

2 cloves garlic, minced

Salt, to taste

Hot sauce, optional for drizzling on top!

INSTRUCTIONS

Start by chopping some veggies: red pepper, green pepper, yellow onion, mushrooms, and baby spinach! I like chopping everything pretty small, because I'm not a fan of big chunks, but the size of veggie is up to you! Now mince some garlic and crack some eggs! I used 4 whole eggs and 4 egg whites. Whisk the eggs together in a large four cup measuring cup and set aside. I like whisking the eggs in the measuring cup, because it makes pouring the mixture into the muffin tin easier later on!

Now, heat a non stick pan over medium heat. Once hot, add in olive oil. Then add in the red pepper, green pepper, yellow onion, and a pinch of salt. Saute for about 5-7 minutes, or until the peppers are tender. Add in spinach and mushrooms and cook for another 2 minutes. In the last 30 seconds, add in minced garlic.

Taste and re-season with salt if necessary!

Pour the cooked veggies into the whisked eggs. Stir to combine. If you like, you could even add in a little hot sauce.

Preheat the oven to 350 degrees F and grease a muffin pan with cooking spray.

Pour the egg/veggie mixture evenly into the muffin pan. You'll have enough for all 12 muffin slots!

Bake for about 15 minutes, or until the tops are firm to the touch or if an inserted toothpick comes out clean.

Let cool in the pan for a few minutes, before removing! Serve immediately or let finish cooling on a cooling rack. Store in an airtight container in the fridge for no longer than 4 days. You can, however, store these individually in the freezer! To thaw, remove from the freezer the night before and store in the refrigerator. Then just pop it in the microwave in the morning until warm.

NOTES

Calories are for one muffin, so eat up and serve this with a side of toast, your morning coffee, yogurt, etc!

471. Totally Tropical Granola

Ingredients

6 ounces Macadamia Nuts, coarsely chopped

6 ounces Slivered Almonds

6 ounces Cashews, coarsely chopped

6 ounces Dried Mango(unsweetened), coarsely chopped

½ cup Flaked Coconut(unsweetened)

¼ cup Coconut Oil, melted

Stevia to taste

1 Small Egg White

¼ teaspoon Cinnamon

⅛ teaspoon Chili Powder

½ teaspoon Coarse Salt

1 teaspoon Vanilla

Instructions

Preheat the oven to 250 degrees.

In a large mixing bowl, toss together the macadamia nuts, almonds, cashews, mango, and coconut.

Place half of the mixture in a food processor and pulse several times until about ½ of the mixture is broken down into smaller pieces.

Add the mixture back into the mixing bowl and toss again.

In another small bowl, whisk together the coconut oil, honey, egg white, cinnamon, chili powder, salt and vanilla.

Pour over the nut mixture and stir until well coated.

Spread the mixture in a single layer on top of a parchment or non-stick mat lined baking sheet.

Bake in the preheated oven for 1½ hours.

Watch closely in the last 15 minutes of baking to make sure they do not darken too much.

Remove when the granola is golden brown.

Let granola sit on the baking sheet until fully cooled.

Break up into pieces and store in an airtight container.

472. Apple cinnamon delight Recipe

INGREDIENTS

1 cup riced cauliflower, packed

1/3 cup full fat coconut milk

2/3 cup sweet apple cider

1 tsp ground cinnamon

1/4 tsp freshly grated nutmeg

pinch Himalayan salt

2 tbsp raisins

2 tbsp pecans, chopped

2 large eggs, beaten

2 tbsp flaxseed meal

INSTRUCTIONS

By far, my favorite way to rice cauliflower is in the food processor. Simply cut the cauliflower into very small florets, throw them in the bowl of the food processor without overcrowding it and pulse a few times until the cauliflower has the desired coarseness. 10 to 15 short pulses usually do the trick.

A Ninja Prep Master works wonders for small quantities such as this, but you could also use a box grater if you wanted to.

Once your cauliflower has been riced, add a cup of it to a medium saucepan, along with raisins and pecans.

In a measuring cup, mix the the coconut milk, sweet apple cider, salt and spices and add that to the saucepan. Bring to low boil over medium heat and cook until cauliflower is tender and cooking liquid is almost completely absorbed, about 10 minutes or so.

Remove from heat and pour the eggs in a steady stream while whisking constantly so they don't cook and curdle on you. Add flax seed and resume whisking until completely incorporated.

Serve right away, garnished with more coconut milk and a few pieces of nuts.

473. Fabulous Brownie Treats

Ingredients:

1 1/2 cups walnuts

Pinch of low sodium salt

1 tsp vanilla

1/3 cup unsweetened cocoa powder

Instructions:

Add walnuts and low sodium salt to a blender or food processor. Mix until the walnuts are finely ground.

Add the vanilla, and cocoa powder to the blender. Mix well until everything is combined.

With the blender still running, add a couple drops of water at a time to make the mixture stick together.

Using a spatula, transfer the mixture into a bowl. Using your hands, form small round balls, rolling in your palm.

474. Rose Banana Delicious Brownies

Ingredients:

2 red beets, cooked

2 bananas

2 eggs

1/2 cup unsweetened cacao powder

1/3 cup almond flour

1 tsp baking powder

3 tablespoons crushes mixed nuts

Stevia to taste

Instructions:

Combine all ingredients in a food processor, and blend until smooth.

Stir in the nut bits

Pour into a well-greased pan about 8x8 inches

Bake at 325 for about 40 minutes.

475. Pristine Pumpkin Divine

Ingredients:

2 cups blanched almond flour

½ cup flaxseed meal

2 teaspoons ground cinnamon (optional)

Stevia to taste

½ teaspoon low sodium salt

1 egg

1 cup pumpkin puree

1 tablespoon vanilla extract

Instructions:

Mix together the almond flour, flaxseed meal, cinnamon, and low sodium salt

In a separate bowl, whisk the egg, pumpkin and vanilla extract using a rubber spatula.

Gently mix dry and wet ingredients to form a batter being careful not to over mix or the batter will get oily and dense.

Spoon the batter onto a 9-inch pan lined with parchment paper or grease the pan

bake at 350°F until a toothpick inserted into the center comes out clean, approximately 25 minutes.

476. Secret Brownies

Ingredients:

1 c. raw almonds

1/2 c. raw cashews

4-5 Tbs. cocoa powder

1 Tbs. cashew butter

Stevia to taste

Instructions:

Combine all ingredients in the food processor.

Whir until somewhat smooth.

Press into 8×8" glass baking dish.

Chill until ready to serve.

477. Spectacular Spinach Brownies

Ingredients:

1 ¼ cups frozen chopped spinach

6 oz sugar free chocolate

½ cup extra virgin coconut oil

½ cup coconut oil

6 eggs

Stevia to taste

½ cup cocoa powder

1 Tspn vanilla pod

¼ tsp baking soda

½ tsp low sodium salt

½ tsp cream of tartar

pinch cinnamon

Instructions:

Preheat oven to 325F. Line a 9"x13" baking pan with wax paper or use a silicone baking pan.

Melt coconut oil and chocolate together over low heat on the stove top or medium power in the microwave. Add vanilla and stir to incorporate. Let cool.

Mix cocoa powder, baking soda, cream of tartar, low sodium salt and cinnamon.

Blend spinach, egg, together in a food processor or blender, until completely smooth (2-4 minutes).

Add coconut oil to food processor and process until full incorporated.

Add melted chocolate mixture and 3 or 4 drops stevia liquid to egg mixture slowly and processing/blending constantly.

Mix in dry ingredients and process/stir to fully incorporate.

Pour batter into prepared baking pan and spread out with a spatula.

Bake for 40 minutes. Cool completely in pan. Cut into squares. Enjoy!

478. Choco-coco Brownies

Ingredients:

6 Tablespoons of coconut oil

6 ounces of Sugar free Chocolate

4 Tablespoons of Packed Coconut Flour (20g)

¼ cup of Unsweetened Cocoa Powder (30g)

2 Eggs

½ teaspoon of Baking Soda

¼ teaspoon of low sodium salt

Extra coconut oil for pan greasing

Stevia to taste

Instructions:

Preheat the oven to 350F. Grease an 8x8 baking pan and line with parchment paper.

Ensure eggs are at room temperature. You may run them under warm water for about 10 seconds while shelled.

Gently melt the semisweet chocolate and oil in a double boiler. You may use the microwave at 50% heat at 30 second intervals with intermittent stirring.

Stir in unsweetened cocoa powder.

Sift together the superfine coconut flour, baking soda, stevia and low sodium salt.

Beat the eggs and add the dry ingredients. Beat until combined

Add the rest of the wet ingredients and beat until incorporated.

Pour the batter into the lined 8x8 pan.

Bake for 25-30 minutes at 350F until a toothpick inserted into the center of the batter comes out clean.

When done, remove from the oven and let cool in the pan for at least 15 minutes.

479. Coco – Walnut Brownie Bites

Ingredients:

2/3 cup raw walnut halves and pieces

1/3 cup unsweetened cocoa powder

1 tablespoon vanilla extract

1 to 2 tablespoons coconut milk

2/3 cups shredded unsweetened coconut

Instructions:

Pulse coconut in food processor for 30 seconds to a minute to form coconut crumbs. Remove from food processor and set aside.

Add unsweetened cocoa powder and walnuts to food processor, blend until walnuts become fine crumbs, but do not over process or you will get some kind of chocolate walnut butter.

Place in the food processor the cocoa walnut crumbs. Add vanilla. Process until mixture starts to combine.

Add coconut milk. You will know the consistency is right when the dough combines into a ball in the middle of the food processor.

If dough is too runny add a tablespoon or more cocoa powder to bring it back to a dough like state.

Transfer dough to a bowl and cover with plastic wrap. Refrigerate for at least 2 hours. Cold dough is much easier to work with. I left my dough in the fridge over night. You could put it in the freezer if you need to speed the process up.

Roll the dough balls in coconut crumbs, pressing the crumbs gently into the ball. Continue until all dough is gone.

480. Best Ever Banana Surprise Cake

Ingredients:

Bottom Fruit Layer:

2 tbsps coconut oil, melted

1 small banana, sliced, or ¼ cup blueberries for low carb version

2 tbsps walnut pieces * optional, can omit for nut free.

Stevia to taste

1 tsp ground cinnamon.

Top Cake Layer:

2 eggs, beaten.

Stevia to taste

¼ cup unsweetened coconut milk, or unsweetened almond milk.

1 tsp organic GF vanilla extract, or 1 tsp ground vanilla bean

½ tsp baking soda.

1 tsp apple cider vinegar.

1 small banana, mashed, or ¼ cup blueberries for lower carb version.

⅓ cup coconut flour

Instructions:

Preheat oven to 350 F, and lightly grease a 9 inch cake pan.

Place 2 tbsps coconut oil into cake pan, and put pan into preheating oven for a couple minutes to melt butter or oil. Once melted, make sure butter or oil is evenly distributed all over the bottom of the pan.

Sprinkle 2-4 drops stevia sweetener all over the melted oil.

Sprinkle 1 tsp cinnamon on top of sweetener layer.

Layer banana slices or blueberries on top of butter- sweetener layer, as seen in photo above. Add optional walnut pieces to fruit layer. Set aside.

In a large mixing bowl combine all the "top cake layer" ingredients except for the coconut flour. Mix thoroughly, then add the coconut flour and mix well, scraping sides of bowl, and braking up any coconut flour clumps.

Spoon cake batter on top of fruit layer in cake pan

Spread cake batter evenly across entire pan.

Bake for 25 minutes or until top of cake is browned and center is set.

Remove from oven and let cool completely.

Use a butter knife between cake and edge of pan and slide around to loosen cake from pan. Turn cake pan upside down onto a large plate or serving platter.

Slice and serve.

Should be stored in fridge, if serving later.

481. Choco Cookie Delight

Ingredients:

1/2 cup dark chocolate sugar free chips

1/2 cup coconut milk (thick fat from top of can)

2 eggs

1 cup almond flour

pinch of low sodium salt

1/2 teaspoon vanilla extract

1/4 teaspoon baking powder

Vanilla glaze:

1/2 cup coconut butter, liquid

Stevia to taste

1 /2 teaspoon vanilla extract

Chocolate Glaze:

1/2 cup chocolate chips

Stevia powder for decoration

Instructions:

Place a small sauce pan over low heat and melt your chocolate and coconut milk together (only keep the heat on long enough to melt them together)

While melting, place your 2 eggs in a stand mixer with the whisk, or use a hand mixer with the whisk and beat your eggs until they are fluffy, about 1 minute

Add your coconut milk and chocolate to your eggs and mix well

Stir in your almond flour, low sodium salt, vanilla extract and baking powder

Mix well ensuring everything is combined

Pipe your batter into the cookie wells ensuring you fill higher than the halfway point

Remove from the cookie maker, gently insert the sticks and place everything in the freezer for 30-45 minutes

Vanilla Glaze:

Combine your coconut butter, stevia, and vanilla extract in a small glass to make it easy to dip

You can keep this glass in hot water to keep the glaze more liquidy to make the dipping easier

Chocolate Glaze:

Melt your chocolate chips over a double boiler and keep the heat low and them liquid – then spread over cooled cookies!

482. Choco Triple Delight

Ingredients:

Cake:

1 cup almond flour (or 3 oz ground raw pumpkin seeds for nut-free version)

3 tbsp Raw Cacao Powder

1 tbsp coconut flour

1 tsp baking powder

1/2 tsp baking soda

1/8th tsp Stevia

3 tbsp melted Raw Cacao Butter or coconut oil)

Pinch of low sodium salt

1 large pastured egg

2 tbsp coconut milk (or dairy of choice)

1 tsp pure vanilla extract

2 oz 80% cocoa bar, chopped

Top with 2 tbsp chopped nut of choice,

Optional: 1/8th tsp low sodium salt sprinkled on top of cake before baking

Chocolate Drizzle:

2 tbsp coconut cream concentrate, warmed

3 tbsp water (or coconut milk)

3 tbsp Cacao powder

1/2 tbsp pure vanilla extract

Stevia to taste

Instructions:

Preheat oven to 350 degrees F.

Oil the sides and bottom of 8 inch cake pan.

Line the bottom of the pan with parchment paper and set aside.

In a medium bowl, add dry ingredients. Use a sifter to insure that all ingredients are blended well and that there are no lumps.

Add remaining ingredients (except nuts and optional salt) to dry ingredients and mix. Taste for sweetness and adjust if necessary.

Press (or spread with angled spatula) into a 8 inch cake pan. Sprinkle with nuts. Bake for 11-14 minutes.

DO NOT OVER BAKE! Remove from oven and serve warm or allow to cool and top with Chocolate Drizzle.

Chocolate Drizzle:

In a small bowl, blend coconut cream concentrate and water until smooth.

Add cacao powder, vanilla and stevia. Whisk until creamy.

Taste for sweetness and adjust if necessary. Drizzle over the cake.

483. Peach and Almond Cake

Ingredients:

2 whole peaches

300g almond meal

6 eggs

Stevia to taste

1 tsp baking soda

Instructions:

Cover the peaches in water in a saucepan and boil for about 2 hours.

Preheat the oven to 180 degrees Celsius and line the bottom of a 24cm pan with baking paper.

Lightly beat the eggs.

Blend the eggs and peaches (quarter them first) thoroughly in a food processor.

Add the rest of the ingredients to the food processor, again blending thoroughly.

Pour mixture into the lined tin and bake for roughly an hour.

484. Apple Cinnamon Walnut Bonanza

Ingredients:

For the cake:

1 cup almond flour

2 tablespoons coconut flour

Stevia to taste

1 tablespoon cinnamon

1 teaspoon baking soda

1/4 teaspoon low sodium salt

1 tablespoon coconut butter, plus more for greasing the pan

2 eggs

1/2 cup cream from a can of refrigerated coconut milk

1 teaspoon vanilla

1 cup grated apple (about 1 large apple)

For the topping:

1 1/2 cups walnuts (or pecans, if you prefer)

1/2 cup almond flour

4 tablespoons melted coconut butter

Stevia to taste

1 tablespoon cinnamon

pinch low sodium salt

Instructions:

Preheat your oven to 350° and grease a 8 x 8 baking dish.

Make the topping: pulse the walnuts in a food processor 10-12 times or until they are course crumbs. Add the remaining ingredients and pulse 2-3 more times until combined. Set aside.

Wipe out and dry the bowl of your food processor and add your dry cake ingredients. (almond flour through low sodium salt) Pulse a few times to mix.

Cut the tablespoon of butter into smaller chunks and add it to the dry ingredients. Pulse 8-10 times or until it's cut in to the dry ingredients, similar to if you were making a pie crust.

In a small bowl, mix your wet cake ingredients (eggs through vanilla) and whisk until well combined. Stir in grated apple.

Add to the food processor and mix until combined. Scrape down the sides once or twice to make sure it's well mixed.

Pour into the prepared baking dish and sprinkle the topping over, as evenly as you can.

Bake for 30-35 minutes, or until a toothpick inserted into the center comes out clean.

Allow to cool, and enjoy!

485. Chestnut- Cacao Cake

Ingredients:

100g (1 cup + 1 heaping tablespoon) chestnut flour

50g (1/2 cup) ground almonds (almond flour)

3 eggs, separate

1/2 teaspoon cream of tartar

35g (1/2 cup) raw cacao powder

Stevia to taste

3/4 cup coconut milk

1/2 teaspoon baking soda

Crushed chestnuts

Instructions:

Preheat oven to 180C fan (350F).

Grease a pie/tart pan.

In a clean mixing bowl, beat the egg whites and cream of tartar until stiff peaks form. Set aside.

In another mixing bowl, cream the egg yolks, chestnut flour, ground almonds, stevia, raw cacao, baking soda and coconut milk.

Fold in the egg whites and blend until the white is no longer showing.

Pour into the pie/tart mold.

Sprinkle with crushed chestnuts, if desired.

Bake for 35-40 minutes on the middle rack.

486. Extra Dark Choco Delight

Ingredients:

1 egg

½ very ripe avocado

¼ cup full fat canned coconut milk

2 tbsp cacao powder

1 tbsp carob powder

pinch low sodium salt

pinch cinnamon

1 scoop vanilla flavored hemp protein powder

10g raw hazelnuts

2 tbsp unsweetened shredded coconut

Instructions:

Add the egg, avocado and coconut milk to a small food processor and process until very smooth and process until very smooth and creamy.

Add cacao powder, carob powder, low sodium salt, cinnamon and protein powder and process again until well combined and creamy.

Add hazelnuts and shredded coconut and give a few extra spins until the hazelnuts are reduced to tiny little pieces.

Serve immediately or refrigerate until ready to serve.

Garnish with a little dollop of coconut cream and cacao nibs or shredded coconut and crushed hazelnuts.

This will keep in the refrigerator for a few days in an airtight container.

487. Nut Butter Truffles

Ingredients:

5 tablespoons sunflower seed butter

1 tablespoon coconut oil

2 teaspoons vanilla extract

¾ cup almond flour

1 tablespoon flaxseed meal

pinch of low sodium salt

¼ cup sugar free dark chocolate chips

1 tablespoon cacao butter

chopped almonds (optional)

Instructions:

Add sunflower seed butter, coconut oil, vanilla, almond flour, flaxseed meal and low sodium salt to a large bowl. Please note that you may find a thin layer of oil in the sunflower seed butter jar that separates from the butter and rises to the top. Be sure to mix oil and butter together before scooping into bowl.

Using your hands mix until all ingredients are incorporated (I like using gloves when mixing so the oils from my skin do not get into the mixture)

Roll the dough into 1-inch balls and place them on a sheet of parchment paper and refrigerate for 30 minutes (using 2 teaspoons for each truffle will yield about 14 truffles)

Melt the chocolate chips in a double boiler along with the cacao butter

Dip each truffle in the melted chocolate, one at the time, and place them back on the pan with parchment paper

Top with chopped almonds and refrigerate until the chocolate is firm

488. Fetching Fudge

Ingredients:

1 cup coconut butter

1/4 cup coconut oil

1/4 cup cocoa

1/4 cup cocoa powder + 1 Tbsp

Stevia to taste

1 tsp vanilla

Instructions:

In the pot, gently melt the cocoa butter on low (number 2)

When it is half melted add the butter, the coconut oil and the coconut spread and gently mix with the whisk as it melts

Add vanilla, and stevia and whisk in well

Add the cocoa powder and whisk in well

Be sure to take the pot off the heat when the fat is melted and keep whisking until it is smooth and all the lumps are out — you don't want to overheat this

Pour into the 8 x 8 pan that is lined with parchment paper

Refrigerate for 1 – 2 hours

When solid, pull the parchment paper out of the pan, put the block of fudge on a flat surface and cut into small squares

Enjoy! This will melt rather quickly — but it won't last long!

489. Choco – Almond Delights

Ingredients:

1 c. toasted hazelnuts

1 c. raw almonds

2/3 c. raw almond butter

5 Tbs. raw cacao powder (or unsweetened cocoa powder)

1/2 tsp. vanilla extract

1/4 c. unsweetened, shredded coconut

Instructions:

Combine all the ingredients, except for the coconut, in the food processor. Whir until smooth. This will take a few minutes and may require scraping down the sides of the bowl one or more times.

Line a mini muffin tin with plastic wrap. Spoon dollops of the sweet mixture into the lined tin cups and form into "mounds." Freeze until well formed. Remove mounds from plastic and tin and flip for presentation. Sprinkle with shredded coconut.

490. Chococups

Ingredients:

4 eggs

Stevia to taste

1/3 cup coconut flour

1/4 cup cacao powder

1/2 teaspoon baking soda

1/4 cup coconut oil (melted in microwave)

1/4 cup cacao butter (melted in microwave)

For topping:

1 can coconut cream (chilled in fridge overnight)

Cacao nibs to decorate.

Instructions:

Heat oven to 170 degrees Celsius (338F)

Grease 10 muffin pans with coconut oil.

Beat eggs with electric beaters.

Add coconut flour, baking soda and cacao powder.

Beat well and add stevia

Add melted coconut oil, cacao butter and mix.

Spoon mixture into 10 greased muffin pans.

Bake for 12-15 minutes until risen and top springs back.

Cool in pans.

Beat the solid coconut cream with electric beaters until creamy. Add honey to taste if you wish.

Pipe coconut cream onto top of cakes.

491. Choco Coco Cookies

Ingredients:

Stevia powder – 1 teaspoon

1 cup coconut flour

½ cup coconut oil

½ cup coconut milk, (from the can)

2 Teaspoons vanilla extract

¼ Teaspoon low sodium salt

2½ cups finely shredded coconut

1 cup big flake coconut

⅔ cup dark sugar free chocolate chunks or chocolate chips (I used 80% dark chocolate)

Optional: ½ cup almond or cashew butter

Instructions:

In a large saucepan, combine the, coconut oil, and coconut milk. Bring the mixture to a boil, and boil for 2-3 minutes.

Remove from the heat and add the vanilla, low sodium salt, and coconut flour and coconut. Stir to combine. If you're using the almond or cashew butter, mix it in thoroughly. Finally, add the chocolate chunks and combine, stirring as little as possible to keep the chunks intact.

Portion the cookie on a parchment lined baking sheet and let cool. This version of no-bakes takes a full 3-4 hours to fully set up, but you don't have to wait that long because they're really good warm and gooey.

492. Apple Spice Spectacular

Ingredients:

1 cup unsweetened almond butter

Stevia to taste

1 egg

1 tsp baking soda

1/2 tsp low sodium salt

half an apple, diced 1 tsp cinnamon

1/4 tsp ground cloves

1/8 tsp nutmeg

1 tsp fresh ginger, grated on a microplane

Instructions:

Pre-heat oven to 350 degress F.

In a large bowl, combine almond butter, stevia, egg, baking soda, and low sodium salt until well incorporated. Add apple, spices, and ginger and stir to combine.

Spoon batter onto a baking sheet (you may have to spread the batter a little to get it into a round shape) about 1-2 inches apart from each other--they'll spread a bit.

Bake about 10 minutes, or until slightly set.

Remove cookies and allow to cool on pan for about 5-10 minutes. Then finish cooling on a cooling rack.

493. Absolute Almond Bites

Ingredients:

1 1/2 cups almond flour

1/4 teaspoon low sodium salt

1/4 teaspoon baking soda (gluten-free, if necessary)

1/8 teaspoon cinnamon

2 tablespoons melted coconut oil

Stevia to taste

1 1/4 teaspoon vanilla extract

1/4 teaspoon almond extract or almond flavoring

12 to 15 whole almonds; sprouted or soaked and dehydrated

Instructions:

Preheat oven to 325°F. Line a baking sheet with parchment paper.

In a medium bowl combine almond flour, low sodium salt, baking soda, and cinnamon. Mix well, breaking up any lumps.

In a small bowl, place coconut oil, vanilla, almond extract or flavoring. Whisk until well combined.

Add wet ingredients to dry ingredients and stir until combined...add stevia

Roll level-tablespoon-sized (using a measuring spoon) portions of dough into balls and place on baking sheet. Flatten slightly with the heel of your hand and press one almond into the center of each cookie.

Bake 15 to 17 minutes or until light golden brown. Allow to cool on baking sheet for a few minutes before transferring to cooling rack.

Store in an airtight container. Can be frozen.

494. Eastern Spice Delights

Ingredients:

1 3/4 cups + 4 tbsp almond meal

1/8 tsp low sodium salt

3/4 tsp ground ginger

3/4 tsp cinnamon

1/4 tsp ground cloves

1/4 tsp cardamom

1/8 tsp nutmeg

1/2 cup coconut oil (in solid form)

Stevia to taste

1 tsp vanilla extract

Instructions:

Preheat oven to 350F.

Combine all the dry ingredients in a large bowl. In a small bowl, mix together the oil, maple syrup, and vanilla until completely blended. Pour the wet ingredients over the dry ingredients and mix well.

Drop the cookie dough on a cookie sheet. It will spread a bit as it cooks (and thus flatten), but not an awful lot.

Bake for 10-12 minutes. These cookies will not look golden when they're done. Makes two dozens.

495. Berry Ice Cream and Almond Delight

Ingredients:

For the Ice Cream:

1 can full fat coconut milk

Stevia to taste

2 tbsp vanilla

1 cup fresh strawberries cut into fourths

For the crisp:

1/3 cup almond flour

3 tbsp sunflower seed butter (or almond butter)

1/2 tsp vanilla

1 tbsp honey

low sodium salt to taste

Instructions:

For the ice cream:

Combine coconut milk and vanilla together in a small saucepan over medium heat and stir until ingredients are well combined (just a few minutes).

Transfer milk mixture to a small bowl and place in the freezer for two hours.

Next, add strawberries to a small saucepan and bring to a low boil.

Turn heat to medium-low and allow to cook until they start breaking down into a sauce-like mixture, leaving small chunks.

Place strawberries in refrigerator while the ice cream hardens.

For the crisp:

Combine all ingredients and mix until you get a "crumble' consistency.

Place crisp in refrigerator until ready to use.

After two hours, place milk mixture into your ice cream maker along with the strawberries and use as directed.

When ice cream is ready, scoop and serve with crisp sprinkled on top.

496. Creamy Caramely Ice Cream

Ingredients:

Delicious Instant Caramel Topping:

2 heaped tablespoons of hulled tahini

Stevia to taste

2 tablespoons of coconut milk

1/2 teaspoon of vanilla

Delicious Instant Ice Cream:

4 frozen bananas, chopped

4 tablespoons coconut milk

1 teaspoon of vanilla

Instructions:

Spoon the tahini and stevia into a cup and stir with a fork to combine. Mix in the coconut milk and vanilla. Refrain from eating it while you make your ice cream.

Place the ingredients into food processor or blender, blend until the mixture is an ice cream consistency.

Spoon the ice cream into bowls, drizzle generously with the caramel topping, sprinkle with low sodium salt if you desire. Enjoy!

497. Cheeky Cherry Ice

Ingredients:

14oz. cans 365 Coconut Milk (Full Fat)

Stevia to taste

1 ½ tsp. vanilla extract

2 cups fresh cherries, pitted and diced

Instructions:

In a large bowl, combine coconut milk, stevia and vanilla and stir well.

Chill for 1-2 hours.

Transfer to ice-cream maker and process according to manufacturer directions.

Add diced cherries to the mixture during the last 5-10 minutes of processing.

498. Creamy Berrie Pie

Ingredients:

Crust:

3 cups almonds

½ Teaspoon cinnamon

½ cup honey

2 Tablespoons coconut oil

1 Tablespoon lemon zest

1 Teaspoon almond extract

A pinch of low sodium salt

Filling:

2 Teaspoons plant-based gelatin, dissolved in 2 Tablespoons hot water

⅓ cup freshly squeezed lemon juice

Stevia to taste

1 can coconut milk, chilled

4 cups blueberries for serving

Instructions:

Place the almonds and cinnamon in a food processor and pulse until your desired texture is reached. I like to leave some bigger pieces for texture. Add the rest of the crust ingredients and pulse until a sticky dough forms. Pat the crust into a pie plate, (use water to keep your hands from sticking to the crust).

For the filling, mix the gelatin and water together. Stir to dissolve and immediately add the lemon juice. If the gelatin gets clumpy, place the mixture over hot water until it melts again. Pour the coconut milk into an electric mixer, add the stevia and whip on high until peaks form, about 15 minutes. Add the gelatin mixture to the whipped cream. Pour the filling into the crust. The filling will seem thin, but don't worry it will set up in the refrigerator.

Chill for at least 4 hours until set, and serve with lots of berries!

499. Peachy Creamy Peaches

Ingredients:

3 medium ripe peaches cut in half with pit removed

1 tsp vanilla

1 can coconut milk, refrigerated

1/4 cup chopped walnuts

Cinnamon (to taste)

Instructions:

Place peaches on the grill with the cut side down first. Grill on medium-low heat until soft, about 3-5 minutes on each side.

Scoop cream off the top of the can of chilled coconut milk. Whip together coconut cream and vanilla with handheld mixer. Drizzle over each peach. Top with cinnamon and chopped walnuts to garnish.

500. Spiced Apple Bake

Ingredients:

2 apples of your choice

1/4 cup walnuts

1/4 tablespoon nutmeg

1/4 tablespoon cinnamon

1/4 tablespoon ground cloves

Instructions:

Preheat oven to 350 degrees Fahrenheit.

Slice the very top and very bottom off of each apple. (The top allows for more room to stuff with goodies, the bottom allows the apples to soak up all the nice sauce).

Core both apples to the bottom, but not all the way through.

Mix spices, walnuts, and raisins in a small bowl.

Pour half of the spice mixture into each apple.

Place on baking sheet and bake 20-25 minutes, or until apples are soft. I like to pour any remaining sauce mixture into the bottom of the pan so the apples can soak up the flavors.

500 Paleo Anti Inflammatory Instant Pot, Bone Broth and Dessert Recipes By Mercedes Del Rey

About the Author

If you're a sufferer from any kind of immune deficiency disorder, I especially want to extend a warm welcome to you. Welcome, my friend, to my wonderful world of completely safe and natural healing. My name is Mercedes del Rey but my friends and patients call me Merche and I am truly fortunate to live in one of the most beautiful places in the world. My home is in sunny Andalusia in the south of Spain, the place where I was born and where I grew up before travelling to the US to complete my higher education. My life has been blessed in so many ways but, like so many people, I've also had to contend with plenty of problems along the way.

Despite growing up in such a wonderful place, my health has not always been very strong. For example, my immune system was a constant source of worry and I suffered from a series of acute and often debilitating allergies throughout my childhood, sometimes reacting to certain foods and then to the chemicals in ordinary household articles like hand soap and shampoo. I seemed to pick every bug and infection that was going round. A deficient immune system can do that. Eventually, the conditions became severe and I began my long exposure to the medical profession and a cocktail of drugs that were supposed to balance my immune system and calm my allergies but, in the end, they only succeeded in making my life more miserable because of all the unpleasant side effects. Doctors rarely mention the negative consequences of the drugs they prescribe but I could see that my condition was becoming worse rather than getting better.

There were times when I suffered from bouts of depression and a complete lack of confidence, always conscious of the rashes and the embarrassing marks on my skin, the unexplained outbreaks of eczema and the fear of being disfigured by the horrible patches that appeared on my face and body. Sometimes it seemed that my immune system was attacking me rather than protecting me. In some ways, growing up was a nightmare. Like so many other unhappy people, I turned to food as a source of comfort and then I started to gain weight, which made me feel even worse! I was highly strung, super-sensitive, borderline depressed and often miserable. The drugs were no help whatsoever. The fact is that my immune system had been further compromised by the constant stream of allergies and by the medication that had been prescribed for my various conditions. And then, as if out of the blue, I met someone who turned my life around completely.

A friend was very concerned about me. She knew I wasn't sleeping well, that my allergies were a constant source of discomfort and embarrassment, that I was depressed and that I'd hit a low spot in my life where I no longer knew where to turn for help. She recommended someone to me, a very special person, a lady who understood exactly what was wrong with me and who showed me how to change my life forever using the most natural remedies imaginable. Her name is Beran Parry and her knowledge of herbalism opened my life to an extraordinary world of natural healing. Beran has a very wide knowledge and experience of health, nutrition and all the factors that can contribute to complete wellbeing. The results of her advice and guidance were simply astonishing. My allergies and have disappeared and my immune system is functioning perfectly. I don't even get colds or 'flu anymore, and that in itself is quite remarkable! My mood swings have vanished. I sleep wonderfully and my confidence has soared. I was so impressed by her knowledge and passion for natural healing that I became her pupil and studied with her for several years. She has inspired me to travel the world on my quest to research and investigate herbal medicine and all that it entails.

I visited China, India, Germany, the USA and Canada and met with so many wonderful Naturopathic Doctors and Herbalists along my learning path.

I now practice as a Holistic Nutritionist and I advise my own clients on the use and application of herbal remedies. It was Beran, of course, who encouraged me to write this book and she assisted me with my research and studies. My dearest hope is that it proves to be as useful and helpful to you as her teaching has been to me.

This is not a medical advice book so please always check any remedy with your medical and naturopathic doctor at all times!

May the force of Nature be with you!

FREE FROM THE PUBLISHER

DOWNLOAD YOUR FREE PALEO EPIGENETIC DIET EBOOK

AND START LOSING WEIGHT TODAY

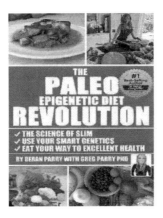

Please search this page over the internet

www.skinnydeliciouslife.com/free-epigenetic-diet-ebook

500 Paleo Anti Inflammatory Instant Pot, Bone Broth and Dessert Recipes By Mercedes Del Rey

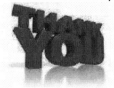

I am so delighted that you have chosen this book and it's been a pleasure writing it for you. My mission is to help as many readers as possible to benefit from the content you have just been reading. So many of us are able to take new information and apply it to our lives with really positive and long lasting consequences and it is my wish that you have been able to take value from the information I have presented.

Thank you for staying with me during this book and for reading it through to the end. I really hope that you have enjoyed the contents and that's why I appreciate your feedback so much. If you could take a couple of minutes to review the book, your views will help me to create more material that you find beneficial.

I am always delighted to hear from my readers and you can email me via the publisher at beranparry@gmail.com if you have any questions about this book or future books. Let us know how we can help you by sending a message to the same email address.

Thanks again for your support and encouragement. I really look forward to reading your review.

Stay Healthy!

Please go to the product page to write your review

365 Days of Paleo Keto Diet Recipes

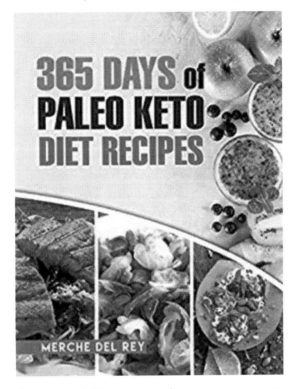

Please search this page over the www.amazon.com

amzn.to/2sXsvSz

365 Days of Anti-Inflammatory Recipes

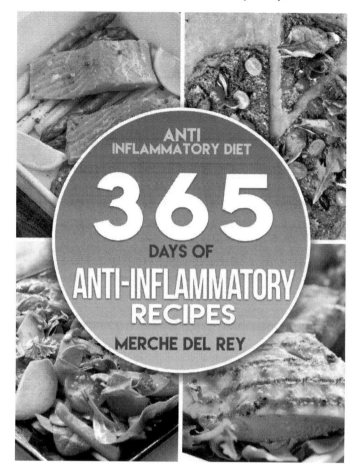

Please search this page over the www.amazon.com

amzn.to/2tgANEF

365 Days of Perfect Paleo Air Fryer Recipes

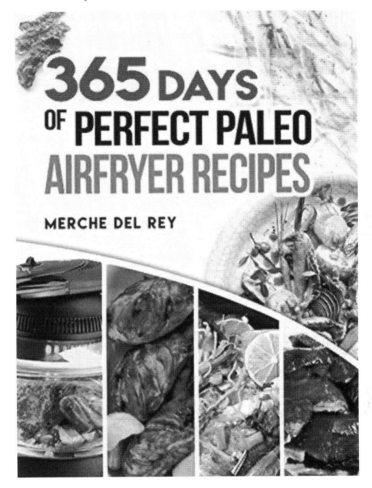

Please search this page over the www.amazon.com

amzn.to/2sv7Dm2

74205005R00423

Made in the USA
Columbia, SC
26 July 2017